The PowerRev Way
DEVELOPING THE TOTAL ATHLETE

International Performance Sciences

ISBN: 979-8-9865860-2-1 (Paperback)

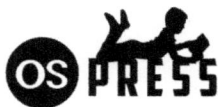

OS PRESS

Published By OS Press, Fuquay-Varina, NC

TABLE OF CONTENTS

Section 1: Coaching Essentials

Section 2: Activities, Training, Tools

Section 3: Create Your Program

Section 4: Recovery & Nutrition

Section 5: Program Evaluation & Testing

Section 6: Auxiliary Training Methods

FOREWORD BY CHIP MORTON

To coach someone means you are taking on much responsibility – because it's not just about coaching the sport – it's about coaching an individual who is unique and wonderful in their own way. I believe that an effective coach is the person who can come alongside an athlete and build a relationship. Through relationships, a coach can come to "see" into the hearts and minds of the people under their care and can help draw out the best in those individuals, not only on the field or court, but in life. By knowing their heart, you learn their deepest goals and desires. Good coaching entails hard work and individualization for each athlete. The character, care, knowledge and experience of the coach are qualities that are continually being developed and refined.

The PowerRev Way is a thorough resource for the coach who wants to work at their craft, but also see the opportunity to develop themselves to live better in all areas of life. PowerRev Way doesn't stop with the development of the coach; the information regarding development for their athletes is comprehensive, detailing the physiology behind performance, principles to guide the coach in the application of all the movements and athletic drills. The PowerRev Way may truly be considered a coaching reference manual, presented with an informative, easy to understand delivery that a coach will go to again and again when designing effective daily workouts and long-term one-of-a-kind progressions.

The content of PowerRev Way is powerful because it captures years of experience of the educators and coaches who put their thoughts and ideas into words for the benefit of the reader! They are professors, mentors, instructors and coaches who have read all the research or have contributed to the current body of knowledge. These authors have dedicated their careers to learning and then sharing insights and experiences gleaned in the pursuit of the development of human performance. Time on task - in many cases, years - dedicated to drawing out the BEST in the people they have mentored, trained, coached and cared for, is now passed on to YOU, all within the pages of this book.

Section One of the book will draw you in as you learn the truth about HOW to move people to live fulfilled, purposeful lives and how to train the physical body. It speaks to the importance of the coach's role and the value and necessity of coming alongside the athletes you train through service and care. The importance of building relationships is followed by the physiological principles that will help you understand the body's response to training and the rationale that underlies effective program design.

Section Two covers all aspects of training in-depth with exercise and drill descriptions for the development of Strength & Power, Speed & Agility, and Jump training. Section Three outlines how to combine these exercises and drills when writing programs and progressions to develop all those essential athletic qualities.

Section Four, in true "reference manual" form, presents methodologies and specific techniques to augment recovery from training, with an in-depth chapter sharing sound nutrition and hydration practices to support improved performance. It includes a summary of how to "Press RESET" with movements that honor our design and will therefore restore health and vitality—a must-read for all coaches. Section Five speaks to measuring the effectiveness of your program with testing protocols to keep the athletes progressing. In keeping with the completeness of PowerRev Way, the final section addresses future directions in training within an interesting presentation of a new and effective training modality.

PowerRev Way is a very complete and practical book full of sound training advice. In my opinion, it should be required reading for coaches, educators and athletes interested in a detailed source of information for developing athletic performance qualities and the athlete as a whole person. The authors are all experts in their fields of study and having all their expertise in one book will be sure to help you reach your full potential as a coach (and/or athlete).

ABOUT THE CONTRIBUTORS

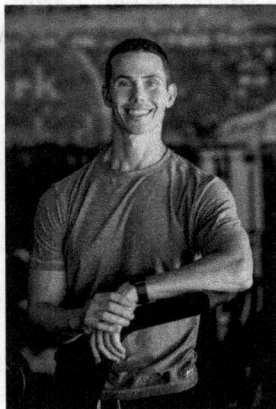

Tim Anderson is an author, speaker, teacher, and trainer in the area of movement education. His motto is "It feels good to feel good," and he loves helping people learn how to feel amazing in their own bodies. Tim is also the creator of the Orginal Strength System, a system for restoring a person's movement patterns.

He is passionate about Health Wholeness, focusing on the whole person (body, mind, and spirit). He teaches this wholeness through movement, humor, and an invitation to experience the wonder of your own body.

Tim has authored several books, including Original Strength, Becoming Bulletproof, Pressing RESET, Habitual Strength, and Discovering You. He has also been featured in many news broadcasts and publications, and he has presented his Original Strength System all over the world.

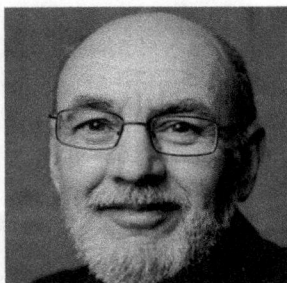

Phil Bishop, EdD is Emeritus Professor of Exercise Science of the University of Alabama (1984 - 2016). He has over 200 refereed science publications and 350 professional presentations. He has been a visiting scientist at NASA's Johnson Space Center, a visiting researcher at the Swedish National Winter-Sport Center, and a Fulbright Fellow at the University of Botswana. He served with Dr. Dornemann working with the Philippine Olympic Coaches in 2011.

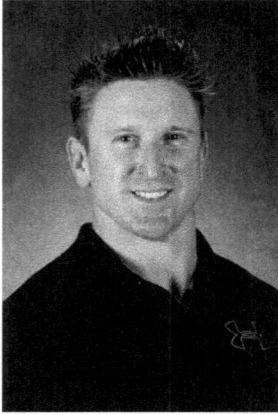

Paul Cater has worked as a Strength and Conditioning Professional for 20 years. After playing football at UC Davis and in Barcelona, he has gone on to work at a high level both internationally and in the US, primarily with rugby and baseball including London Wasps (2005-2010) and Baltimore Orioles (2012-2018). During this time, he has concurrently earned his Master's degree at Middlesex University, London and is now working towards his PhD through University Pablo de Olavide surrounding the topic of rotary inertia flywheel resistance. Through Cater's early affiliation with Athletes In Action he met Craig Schink, which set the course to cross cultural barriers to contribute innovative methodology across the major international sports. Meeting Tim Dornemann has helped further cast a vision to administer advanced methods in feasible ways where time and resources may be limited in more austere scenarios. Cater is currently working for the Los Angeles Angels and helping to develop high performance training centers on the West Coast of California with his wife and two daughters.

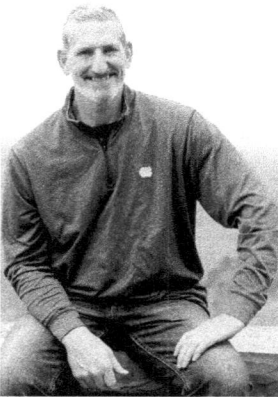

Ben Cook has worked as a Strength and Conditioning Professional for 35 years. He earned a Bachelor's degree in Exercise and Sports Science from Pfeiffer University and a Master's degree in Exercise Science from the University of North Carolina at Chapel Hill. He is the author of *52-Week Football Training*, *Total Basketball Fitness: A 52-Week, Year-Round Training Program* and co-authored of *Jumpmetrics*.

Cook has trained athletes from every sport, with his career highlights being the Strength and Conditioning Coach for the University of North Carolina Tar Heels men's basketball (1993-2001). In the early 2000s he began working with Evernham Motorsports (2003-2006), Red Bull Racing (2006-2009), Michael Waltrip Racing (2009-2011) and Richard Petty Racing (2015) as one of NASCAR's first full-time strength coaches. Ben and Tim Dornemann were classmates in graduate school at UNC-Chapel Hill, where Tim served as the instrument of God that led Ben to the Tar Heel Men's basketball team.

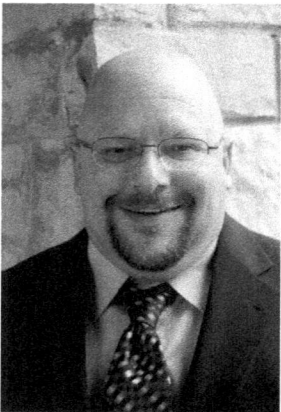

Tim Dornemann is an associate professor in and director of the exercise science program at Barton College. Dornemann oversees both the undergraduate in exercise science and the master of science in kinesiology programs at Barton College. In addition to his academic responsibilities, Dornemann previously served as the director of sports performance at Barton, where he oversaw the strength and conditioning programs for all athletic teams. Dornemann volunteers as the director of educational programs for Sports Performance Sciences (SPS), an organization that conducts performance-enhancement education programs internationally and develops conditioning programs combined with character development programming domestically. Two of the projects Dornemann developed for SPS have been published by Linus Publishing— *PowerRev "Four Laws of Victory" Character Development Program: Build*

Successful Teams and Athletes by Teaching Lessons That Transcend Sports and *PowerRev Youth Athletic Development Program: Building Champions in Sports and in Life*. He completed his doctorate of education in sports management with an emphasis in sports fitness and health and a specialization in leadership from the United States Sports Academy.

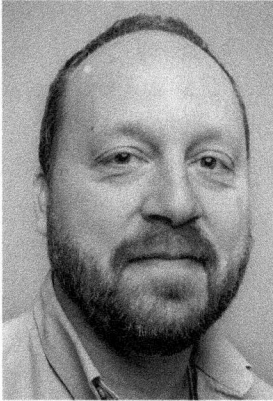

Brian Edlbeck is a Clinical Assistant Professor of Exercise Science along with human performance at Carroll University in Waukesha, Wisconsin. He earned his Bachelor of Science degree in dietetics in 1999 from the University of Wisconsin-Stevens Point and his Master's degree in kinesiology from UW-Milwaukee in 2004. Brian is currently pursuing his Ph.D. in the field of Human Performance at Concordia University-Chicago. Prior to joining the Carroll University faculty, Brian interned as the assistant strength and conditioning coach at UW-Milwaukee. Prior experiences include interning with the Colorado Rockies as a minor league strength and conditioning coach and being a personal trainer for twenty years. He is a NSCA certified strength and conditioning specialist and certified personal trainer.

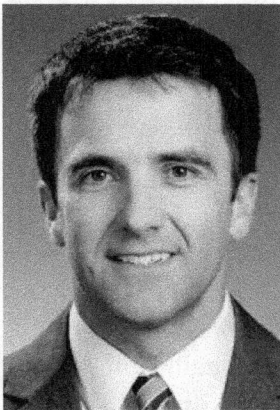

Dave Kemble earned both his BS and MA degrees from East Carolina University ('03 & '06). He is currently an instructor in the Department of Kinesiology and serves as the Program Coordinator for the Health Fitness Specialist undergraduate degree and the Assistant Director of the Activity Promotion Laboratory. At ECU, Dave teaches courses in Strength and Conditioning, Personal Fitness Training, and Fitness Education. Dave is the owner of East Carolina Weightlifting & Sports Performance, LLC. in Greenville, North Carolina. The gym caters to youth and junior athletes from a variety of sports including Olympic-style weightlifting. Prior to joining the faculty at East Carolina University, Dave worked in the health club industry for three years. He is Certified Strength and Conditioning Specialist through the National Strength and Conditioning Association and a National Coach through USA Weightlifting and Lead Instructor of Coaching Courses offered by USA Weightlifting. He is the 2010 recipient of the Health and Human Performance Ray Martinez Teaching Excellence Award.

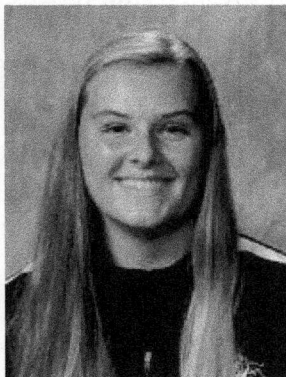

Carson Molaro graduated with honors from Barton College. Carson double majored in Sports Management and Exercise Science and completed her honors research comparing loaded and non-loads neural resets. Carson completed her master's degree in exercise science with a concentration in strength and conditioning from the University of Louisville. Her thesis research was on the force relationship between seated and non-seated cycling positions, and she has had an academic research article published. Carson works for the University of Louisville as a sports performance coach for women's soccer, women's tennis and golf.

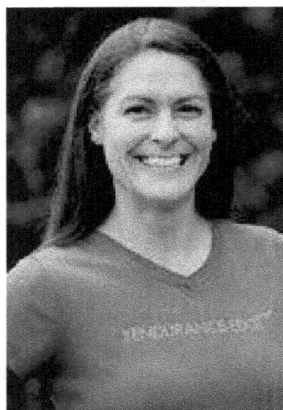

Chris Newport, MS, RDN, LDN, CISSN, EP-C is the Founder, Head Coach and Performance Dietitian at The Endurance Edge, a company that provides endurance coaching, sports and wellness nutrition, and sweat and metabolic testing. She started her fitness career in 1999 as a Certified Personal Trainer, then pursued her dietetics license and Master of Science in Nutrition from Meredith College focusing on the nutritional management of a type 1 diabetic athlete during a 12-hour mountain biking trial. She is a Certified Exercise Physiologist and Certified Specialist in Sports Nutrition. With that skill set, she's able to help translate the science of nutrition and exercise into practical solutions for athletes and fitness enthusiasts for healthy living and optimal performance. She enjoys running, off-road triathlon, hiking, camping, skiing, baking, gardening and spending time with her family.

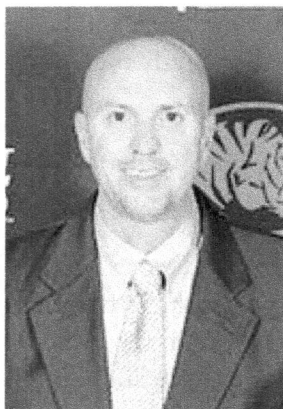

Scott O'Dell, Master Strength and Conditioning Coach from the CSCCa, CSCS, USAW Level-I, USATF Level I, FMS, practitioner in Jeet Kune Do with a current ranking of Brown Sash (Instructor). He is currently a director of Sports Performance at East Central University of Oklahoma, but has also had many roles coaching collegiate level football and leading sports performance and strength and conditioning programs around the United States. He is the author of the book *The Power Revolution* and a Speaker for the NSCA, Nike Coach of the Year Clinics, and Frank Glazier Football Clinics.

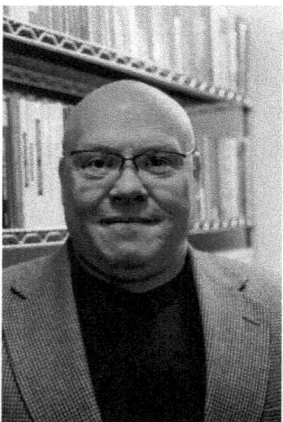

Jeff Valodine is the director of Every Thought Captive, Inc. He studied mechanical engineering at the Milwaukee School of Engineering before becoming an analyst for the Naval department. He received degrees in theology and church history from Lincoln Christian University. While serving as campus minister at the University of Illinois he enrolled in his doctoral studies, working simultaneously as a missionary in Prague for several years. He has since served as adjunct professor at Florida Christian College, Marquette University, and Mid-Atlantic University. Due largely to Covid-related shut downs, Jeff is back in the classroom, dissertating on the topic of mystical theology at Columbia International University. He is affiliate staff with Athletes in Action and Sports Performance Science. He enjoys powerlifting, skiing, wrestling, rugby, water skiing, baseball and bicycling.

INTRODUCTION

1
THE POWERREV WAY

By: Tim Dornemann, Ed. D., CES, PES, CSCS, OS Pro
Exercise Science Program & Kinesiology Director, Barton College
Associate Professor of Exercise Science, Barton College

Developing the Total Athlete

THE POWERREV WAY is **to develop the total athlete** – meaning their body, mind and heart – through sports performance training. This book is designed to encourage, equip and enable individuals and coaches with the tools to design safe and effective training programs for any sport.

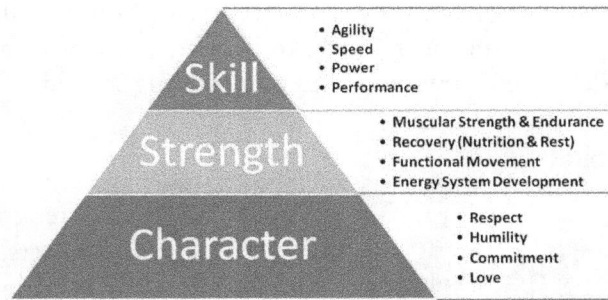

- Agility
- Speed
- Power
- Performance

- Muscular Strength & Endurance
- Recovery (Nutrition & Rest)
- Functional Movement
- Energy System Development

- Respect
- Humility
- Commitment
- Love

PowerRev Performance Pyramid

The pyramid pictured above is like your map. Now, let's get going.

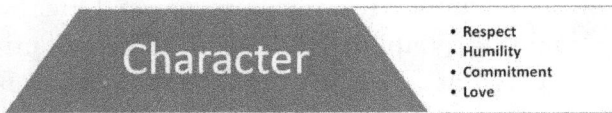

- Respect
- Humility
- Commitment
- Love

PowerRev's Four Laws of Victory provide a way to teach character through the themes of respect, humility, commitment and love. Once the foundation of good character is in place, then a sports person or team can begin to reach their full potential.

You could design the perfect program for an athlete, but if there is no commitment from them, that program will fail. To optimize performance, one has to be committed physically and also one needs to be committed in all other aspects of their lives. This means being committed mentally and emotionally and includes things like following the program designed for them, showing up on time and maintaining the right attitude. Being *fully* committed means to be fully committed to the whole process. Physical training only takes a fraction of the day, but what someone does the rest of the day can either enhance or ruin the effects of their training. For example, the proper amount of sleep and proper diet are key to optimizing the impact of a training session. A program can be designed perfectly to develop muscle, however, without the proper protein intake the athlete will not be able to increase the size of the muscle. To optimize training one needs to be committed in all aspects of their lives, picking and choosing areas to be committed to will not result in an athlete who can maximize their abilities.

To get this level of full commitment a coach must coach beyond the sport. The coach needs to coach the whole individual: body, mind and heart. Coaches must be coaches of influence to truly get the best out of their players.

Strength

Strength

- Muscular Strength & Endurance
- Recovery (Nutrition & Rest)
- Functional Movement
- Energy System Development

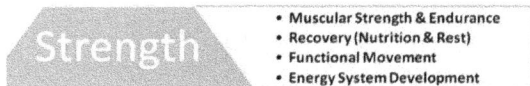

Character and commitment provide the basis for strength. Building strength is foundational to almost every sports skill. Training the muscles to move properly and work together through functional exercises and to be able to produce maximal strength (e.g., muscular strength) and have stamina (e.g., muscle endurance) is key to optimal performance.

Developing the energy system or systems utilized in a sport is vital to success. Fatigue can inhibit success, which is why the better conditioned team often wins at the end of close competitions.

Coaches often overemphasize physical training and underestimate the value of nutrition and recovery. It is easy to obsess on skill practice and physical training programs, but if proper nutrition and recovery are not implemented the benefit of training can be lost. While the time spent in activity is important, the time spent recovering is just as important, if not more important. If you are going to practice and/or train two to four hours a day, what you do the other 20 to 22 hours in a day is what will determine how successful that training session is.

Skill

Skill

- Agility
- Speed
- Power
- Performance

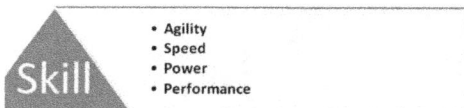

Strength, power, speed and agility are key elements for most players, regardless of sport. Developing these skills in sport prepares one for the development of the physical skills that are required for that sport.

Power & Performance

Power is defined as force times distance over the time it takes to create that force.

Strength - also known as the ability to produce force - is the basis for producing power. Often in sport, the best players are powerful. Throwing, hitting, sprinting, jumping, striking and kicking all utilize power. Training with fast movement velocities through activities, like plyometrics, that utilize one's body weight or explosive lifting movements that utilize triple extension (extension of the ankles, knees and hips) are essential tools for building power.

Speed

Whether utilized directly in track and field or indirectly in field and court sports, speed is a key factor in success of a sport. Speed combined with skill makes a great athlete. The ability to triple extend and push off the ground with maximal ground reaction force will determine how fast someone runs. Speed is a combination of stride length and stride frequency. The more ground reaction force one can produce pushing into the ground, the more distance will be covered in each stride as the body is propelled forward.

Direction

Change of direction is a key feature of agility that is important in many sports. To efficiently and effectively change direction you have to decelerate, stop and aggressively change direction. Decelerating from top speed and stopping puts a great deal of stress on the body. Strength not only protects the body from potential injury, it also provides the ability to quickly change the body's momentum from one direction to another. Once the body is stopped, strength and power are required to move quickly in a new direction.

All of these work together. Speed is a display of the power that can be produced, but strength is what develops the body's capacity to produce that power and agility.

How to Use this Book

This book will help you develop your players in all aspects of the performance pyramid, which will allow you to develop the total athlete: body, mind and heart.

Section 1: Coaching Essentials

Chapters 2-3 cover how to become a coach of influence and the basics of exercise science to catch you up if you have not had previous exposure to the science of exercise.

Section 2: Activities, Trainings and Tools

Then, chapters 3-10 provide guides to the practical activities that you will use in your programs. Consider these the tools that are in your toolbox. This section covers dynamic warm-up and cooldown, core conditioning, strength development, power development, agility training, speed training and plyometric training.

Section 3: Create Your Program

Chapters 11-14 will teach you how to utilize all the tools in the toolbox from the previous chapters and create your program. These chapters are about resistance training programming, athletic development programming, energy system development and periodization. The resistance training chapter covers how to develop resistance training for a sport starting with the needs analysis, and guides you through how to set up a resistance training workout. Athletic development training teaches how to design speed, agility and plyometric programs to optimally develop your players. The energy system development chapter will show you how to design programs to develop the stamina needed for your sport. The periodization chapter provides strategies to help vary training to promote continued improvement over time and create an annual plan.

Section 4: Recovery & Nutrition

Chapters 15-17 cover recovery and nutrition. This section includes chapters that cover general recovery strategies, sports nutrition and neural resets. Neural resets help enhance mobility and performance. These chapters provide the information to help optimize the effectiveness of your programming.

Section 5: Performance Testing & Evaluation

Chapters 18-19 go into detail about performance testing and program evaluation. The programming process is a cycle that begins and ends with testing. Chapter 19 teaches how to properly test the target areas of your program. For example, if a basketball team is being trained to be more explosive and to jump higher, a vertical jump can be used to measure improvement in producing vertical power. Program evaluation is the ability to interpret your testing results. A good programmer knows what aspects of a sport the training program emphasizes and tests at the beginning to establish a starting point, then tests periodically to monitor improvement. If the desired progress does not occur, then changes need to be made.

Section 6: Auxiliary Training Methods

The last chapter, chapter 20, is a bonus chapter on auxiliary training methods. This chapter focuses on eccentric training and use of flywheel technology. The benefits of eccentric training and how to apply eccentric training in almost any situation are explained. Additionally, the use of flywheel technology to train eccentrically is covered in the instance when one has access to flywheel equipment or can acquire flywheel equipment in the future.

Basic Exercise Principles

Before you begin the rest of the book, here are some basic exercise principles that are foundational to successful training.

SAID Principle: Specific Adaptations to Imposed Demands

The SAID principle applies to all training regardless of the targeted outcome. Training places stress or imposed demands on the body to cause a specific adaptation to occur. For example, lifting weights that push the muscle past its normal limits makes that muscle adapt and get stronger to be able to meet that demand. To produce power, plyometrics are done quickly and explosively to challenge the neuromuscular system to produce force quicker and more powerfully. Manipulating the heart rate during aerobic training is done to produce improvements in the cardiorespiratory system. Everything goes back to the SAID principle. Programming is about designing activities to stress the body in ways to produce the desired improvements.

Basic Training Principles

- **Overload:** In order for a muscle to become stronger, it must be worked beyond its normal limits.
- **Progressive Resistance:** Once a muscle adapts to an exercise stimulus, a progressively harder stimulus needs to be used in order for improvements to be made.
- **Specificity of Training:** In order to make the gains one is striving for, one has to implement a program to specifically meet those needs.
- **Use/Disuse:** When an exercise stimulus pushes the muscle past its normal limits then gains will be made, but when that stimulus is absent the gains will be lost.
- **Individuality:** No exercise stimulus affects everyone in exactly the same way. Everyone's response to exercise is different.

Now that you have a map of the journey that this book will take you through and you know the principles that guide the process, let's get started.

SECTION 1

COACHING ESSENTIALS

2
INFLUENCE OF A COACH

By: Jeffery Valodine, PhD
Director of Every Thought Captive*

EVERY FEBRUARY IN the United States the eyes of American football fans turn to Indianapolis, Indiana and the hundreds of college football players invited to participate in a series of physical and skill evaluations where their talent and athleticism can translate into value and subsequent placement in the upcoming draft. Welcome to the NFL Scouting Combine. These elite athletes are subjected to a series of physical and mental tests that include the 40-yard dash, 225 pound bench press repetition, the vertical and broad jumps and a series of cone drills, including position-specific drills and standardized aptitude tests. NFL executives and coaches from all 32 professional franchises scrutinize and evaluate each player and every move they make. An athlete's performance during the Scouting Combine can affect their draft status, salary and ultimately their career as a professional athlete.

After scoring a mind-boggling 122 touchdowns in his last two years of high school football, this receiver-turned-quarterback would go on to win the Heisman Trophy, awarded to the best football player in the nation, as a college freshman. With victories over four top-ranked teams, including the number one ranked Alabama, this dynamic playmaker accounted for 5,116 yards of offense and 47 touchdowns. The entire nation celebrated the arrival of "Johnny Football." He would forgo his college career at Texas A&M after a strong sophomore season to be selected by the Cleveland Browns in the first round of the 2014 National Football League (NFL) Draft. Mr. Texas Football would go on to play less than 2 years in the NFL, throwing for only 1,675 yards, seven touchdowns and seven interceptions. Cleveland released Johnny Manziel in March, 2016.

Success and failure are part of sports. Even if one never reaches the pinnacle of their sport and hoists the championship trophy overhead, all coaches and athletes cannot escape the two certainties of winning and losing. We have taken up mantras to highlight the varieties of both "the thrill of victory and the agony of defeat" that highlight the ups and downs, highs and lows of athletic competition.[1] The world of sports has the ability to tell the background stories of our culture, as the game of baseball

---

[1]   See Jim McKay's introduction to ABC's Wide World of Sports, 1961.

did in 20th century America, and as World Cup Soccer has done in Europe and South America. However, many of the most remembered events in sports history highlight its negative side. The Black Sox Scandal in 1919 in baseball, the murder of Columbian footballer Andrés Escobar in 1994, the use of performance-enhancing drugs (PEDs) in sports–especially in track and field and the Tour de France–all reveal the ugly side of competition. "Do whatever it takes to win," has become modern sports mantra.[2] People will take extreme measures for a win.

The Larger Scope of Sport

Athletic competition is integrated into the human psyche and into our souls. Since sport is an external event, separate from the individual athlete themself, it functions as a standard-bearer for all who participate. The nature of competition sets these standards in which we then evaluate our own progress, success or failure. Athletes are not just competing against each other in the moment, but against the benchmarks that have been established over time; they compete against history. When they take their position on the starting line and gaze left and right, they see not only their immediate competition, but also all those who have run the same race thousands of times throughout history. They not only want to beat the runner next to them, they want to beat the 9.58 posted in Germany in 2009 as well. And everyone *knows* this mark. What will an athlete do for the whole world to recognize them as the fastest or strongest or most talented person on earth? Apparently, anything.[3] In many cases, the list of competitors chasing immortality doubles as a PED's "Most Wanted" poster.

The history of mankind could be told by the stories of athletic competition. Many popular sports around the world started out as physical challenges brought on by statements like, "I bet you can't do this," or "my pals could beat you and your pals any day of the week." Others have a competitive nature as an extension of real life, developing everyday tasks like chores, school or work into contests of who can do it better and faster. Since the rebirth of the ancient Greek games into the modern Olympic Games in 1896, sports and athletics have become separated, not only from the life events that gave them their start, but also, in many cases, from the everyday rhythm of social life. The modern world now has professional sports, an entity we've endowed with a special place in modern culture, simultaneously creating modern heroes and wealthy millionaires. However, Superman does not share his superpowers and the wealthy do not fill the offering plate at church.

Elitism in sports has created an us-versus-them dichotomy in the world of coaching, developing and nurturing elementary youth into active adulthood. This dichotomy was clearly evidenced during the reign of the USSR when the State would separate out youth with genetic or aggressive potential and raise them up as elite athletes. The modern athlete must somehow be brought into relation with the rhythm of life that not only gave them birth but that continues to give them life, not some artificial environment created out of test tubes with genetic modification nor with dehumanizing training methods and mere functionalism. An emphasis must be placed on the holistic development of the athlete, not limited to hitting occasional peak performances a few times in their lives, but in creating a system of lifelong fitness inside athletic competition that transcends sport itself. Our focus should be to create an ethos in athletic development that provides wise, healthy and active people who operate in all areas of

---

[2] See Henry Russell ("Red") Sanders, "Winning isn't everything; It's the only thing" (1950, 1953, 1956); Vince Lombardi's address to the Packers before training camp 1959, "Winning isn't everything. The will to win is the only thing" (Michener, James A – Sports in America. Fawcett Crest, 1987).

[3] See the history of the 100 meter world record progression at Wikipedia, 2021. "100 Meters." Last modified 19 April 2021.

their lives with a grounded moral compass and who place highest value on something outside the quest of winning or losing.

Those of us who are fortunate to have both our occupation and vocation centered around sports, coaching and athletic development must take time to see our profession from 30,000 feet: above the specificity of any one area of focus to a wider scope that includes the greatest potential for overall sustained success. We should focus on the tens of millions of children who almost naturally begin participating in one kind of sport or another early in life. We should also pay attention to the hundreds of millions of adults who remained engaged in some sort of athletic endeavor throughout their entire lifespan. We need to ask ourselves how, as coaches, we can make systemic impact in those we are working with that will result in lifelong physical, spiritual, intellectual and emotional well-being. In addition to training athletes physically, we need to ask how we can coach future coaches, pastor future pastors or instruct future intellectuals.

- How can I model what it means to be a responsible human being?
- How can I best represent what it means to be a faithful loving husband or wife and a caring, nurturing father or mother?
- Do my athletes see me as someone who can speak into the complexities of their emotional ups and downs?
- How can I come alongside the precious people I am blessed to influence in order to mold them and shape them into the very best person they can be?

These ontological questions are arguably more important to resolve in the overall development of the entire life of a person than bodily performance and skill development. However, many would argue that it's not the responsibility of a coach to deal with anything except an athlete's physical attributes.

What You Win Them WITH is What You Win Them TO

It is often said, "Success comes on the practice field before it shows up in the game." This principle has its counterpart in coaching. If you want to see your athlete shine as brightly as the sun, you must be a star yourself. We see the moon not because it has illuminated itself, but because sunlight reflects off of it. Only stars shed light. However, coaches and trainers are not the source of light themselves, but we function as a prism—diamonds if you will. The source or sources of light we allow into us thus illuminate the world around us. A wise man once said, "The eye is the lamp of the body. If your eyes are healthy, your whole body will be full of light. But if your eyes are unhealthy, your whole body will be full of darkness. If then the light within you is darkness, how great is that darkness!"[4] All coaches understand the importance of a healthy diet, proper hydration, adequate sleep, dynamic warmup and the value of hard work. We want to see these things in our athletes—in fact we demand them. You cannot out-exercise a bad diet. Don't borrow time from tomorrow by staying up too late today. Hydrate or die. We know these things. There is a right way and a wrong way towards athletic progress. A good coach will insist that development be accomplished in a proper manner, on and off the field. This is to the benefit of everyone involved, not only for the athlete and coach, but also for the team, for the university, for the country…

---

[4] See the New International Version Bible, 2011, Matthew 6:22-23. This wisdom comes directly after instructions against chasing after temporal things in lieu of eternal things and is preceded by the brilliant conclusion: "Do not run after these physical things. but seek first his kingdom and his righteousness, and all these things will be given to you as well."

for everyone. To even suggest that some sort of propriety exists in the realm of coaching seems to violate the cultural climate of the 2020s. Postmodernity, with its incredulity towards metanarratives, the death of dialectics brought on by the escalating cancel culture, and the reimagining of the historicity of the world, has exacerbated the entire scope of sports to the point where athletes are increasingly looked at as mere commodities—objects that entertain us and as products with which we can make money. Rather than being viewed as role models, contributing citizens or even decent human beings.

If you are a coach you are a person of influence. And as a person of influence, you must decide not only who you will affect, but also how you will impact them and what you emphasize (or deemphasize) in your role as coach. A person's influence is directly tied to their character.

I like to think of a person's character as who they are when no one is watching them. This speaks about the inner, authentic self of a person, and not the outer, projected self.[5] Character is about one's ontological being and is not about one's disposition. Coaching athletic character, in my opinion, has a much higher systemic value than coaching the physical attributes. Young people are counting on you to move from being convinced to being convicted. "If you are convinced character is important in sports, then start living with conviction! Make it the priority of your program and mission as a coach. Become intentional by investing your time, money and resources into making it a reality."[6] A combination of development, both of the inner person and the outer physical representation of that person, yields an athlete who will shine brightly on and off the field of competition. We refer to this as holistic coaching and this type of holistic method is what this book is about. We know of the extremes: champion athletes who live ugly, destructive lives or the nice guys who always finish last. It is our intent to teach and impress, first within you as a coach, then through you into your students, a coaching perspective that produces champions both 'on the court' and more importantly, 'off the court' and throughout their lives. However, there is a catch. It is impossible to help someone financially if you yourself are bankrupt; it is impossible to provide academic wisdom if you are ignorant; it is also impossible to coach holistically if you are unaware of the depth and breadth of the scope, and increasingly impossible to give something you don't already have. If I was to draft a tentative plan of action for a coach that could produce highly-productive athletes that are men and women of character and integrity, the list may look like (in order of importance):

1. Get your internal self right
2. Get your external self right
3. Get another person's internal self right
4. Get their external self right
5. Produce champions.

I wrestled with categorizing these steps in such a large scope and ambiguous way but this was done on purpose. This allows for rigidity in *structure* but allows for freedom in *details*. Foundational development is crucial (structural); how we function from our base of operation is specific (details). Commitment to

---

[5] John Wooden, coach of the UCLA men's basketball team: "Be more concerned with your character than your reputation, because your character is what you really are, while your reputation is merely what others think you are." Abraham Lincoln, America's sixteenth President: "Character is like a tree and reputation its shadow. The shadow is what we think it is and the tree is the real thing."

[6] J.P. Nerbun, as quoted on the website https://thriveonchallenge.com/4-ways-to-coach-character/

God and His Kingdom and *strength and conditioning* are two excellent examples of building core structure without being outcome-based or sport-specific.

The first structural key is to build your life on a strong foundation. If you are interviewing a candidate for a head coaching position ask them to explain who they ARE rather than what they've DONE. As general manager or athletic director it is easy to see their win-loss record. However, it's not easy to identify their character traits, their moral and ethical integrity, their coaching philosophy nor their philosophical worldview. How then, should the interior of a person be built? On a "liquid foundation" where the issues of right/wrong, morals/ethics and pride/power are relative and ambiguous? Or on a strong, solid foundation that meets the highest demands of both the physical and metaphysical world? It is wise to build on a solid foundation. Early in His ministry, Jesus of Nazareth went up onto a Judean hillside and taught the crowd a series of timeless truths, concluding that wise people build their lives not on the shifting sands of life but on a solid foundation, the truth of His Word.[7] In a similar fashion, I submit to you that, just as Christianity forms the proper metaphysical attributes of an athlete/coach, strength and conditioning form the proper physical attributes of an athlete/coach. This combination gives us the best opportunity to not only BE a better athlete/coach, but also to create better athletes/coaches. Christianity must be looked at as more than merely a religion or a philosophy–Christianity is *the* Way of Life. Strength and conditioning must be looked at as more than general health or fitness. Rather, it must be the physical foundation on which all athletics and sports are founded. Strength and conditioning is focused on sports performance and, when combined with athletic coaching and sports-specific instruction, creates a unique way of life.

The "way of life" of a complete athlete/coach has both a solid spiritual foundation and a strong physical foundation. On top of these two pedestals we can add two more fundamental elements: proper diet and proper instruction. Perhaps you've heard of the statements, "You are what you eat," or "Garbage in, garbage out." Proper diet plays a key role in the performance of your athlete. A standardized healthy diet for athletes is nothing new, but proper nutrition is much more scientific in the modern world. Without proper diet and hydration it is impossible to reach your maximum potential in sport. When working part-time as a strength and conditioning coach in Prague, Czechia the world champion decathlete Roman Šebrle once heard me describe my favorite hot dog, to which he responded, "Jeff, I haven't had 'junk food' for so long I cannot remember what a hot dog tastes like." It takes discipline to go a long time following any type of regimen. The key word is discipline. If you want to become a better athlete you must be disciplined in the proper structures that build a strong foundation. You must have a dedicated Way in Life. This not only is important in your days as an athlete but also in your latter years as an active adult and during your time as a coach. Long ago, I discovered that my time in competitive sports had a short window, so I made the best of it. I wasn't very big nor was I a particularly gifted athlete so I trained hard, played hard, and I enjoyed 20+ seasons competing at the collegiate level in several sports. Then one day I woke up and realized that my body wasn't able to respond to the demands I was placing upon it. But because I learned how to compete with men much bigger than me, men with more natural skills, I became a student of the game(s). Moreover, I became known as a gym rat, patterned after the legendary Wisconsin Badger Iron Mike Webster.[8] I am confident that my dedication to proper strength and conditioning kept me competitive through my playing days and has continued to serve me well as

---

[7]   See the New International Version Bible, 2011, Matthew 7:24-27

[8]   Mike Webster was an undersized center at the University of Wisconsin who went on to become a Hall of Fame player in the NFL. At only 6-1 and 255 pounds he was able to bench press 455 for six sets of eight reps. See the article by Colin Webster at https://startingstrength.com/article/reflections_in_iron_mike_websters_training_methods

I transitioned into coaching and into other sporting avenues. But as much as physical training has paid dividends thus far, the most important, most crucial thing I did was to make my peace with God. Why do I make such a claim? Because I know myself. Now, after 30 years in examining the human condition as well as investigating the claims presented by Christian theism, I can say that what was true for me is also true for everyone, whether they know it or not.

It's Not the Title but the Towel that is Important

We are all born into a world that is both vast and majestic, but yet small and domestic. The small and domestic nature of *our* world helps us remain sane when thinking about the vastness of the universe. But the grand expanse of the universe, its harshness and distant coldness, is tempered by proximity and care. These are most often experienced in a home that provides both parents and a place to dwell. If the universe is uncreated and undirected, we would expect it to be random and chaotic. However, we experience just the opposite. The world seems particularly designed for us. Evidence from science, philosophy and experience tend to parallel the historical narrative found in the Judeo-Christian Scriptures. This then summarizes the idea of the physicality of the universe and the meta-physicality of humanity, consciousness and being together in one grand narrative. Both the universe and everything in it was created by God and for God, it was meant for us and we for it. Likewise, when we consider the physicality of sport and the meta-physicality of our athletes, God created everything in our discipline; coaches exist for athletes and athletes for coaches. I learned of this truth by a paradigmatic shift shortly after my conversion to Christianity. As a student-athlete I had been striving to succeed in both the classroom and in athletic competition. Thinking with merely a physical brain and lacking compassion from a merely physical heart, I developed severe anger issues, was willing to win at any cost, avoided or ignored inferior teammates and basically lived as though I was my own god. The passion and humility of Christ changed me by softening my heart. God did this in many ways. First, He was God and didn't need my help, although I needed His. Second, He got my internal self corrected with a spiritual house-cleaning. Third, He ordered my external self, the person that engages with the world I inhabit, through His Word and through active obedience. Then fourth, He called me to do the same with the people I interact with throughout my life. My life was transformed. I stopped living for myself and started living for God and for others. I stopped striving for personal victories and started living to advance God's Kingdom and the lives of those around me. God changed the way I thought about the world and everything within it. One of my colleagues says of himself, "God first entered my life with a brain transplant," after he had a similar experience to mine. If space would allow, I would offer up a six-fold plan that speaks to this transformation and development that covers (1) spiritual development, (2) intellectual development, (3) character development, (4) physical development, (5) social development and (6) practical development.[9]

In the spring of 2011, a group of spiritually aligned ragamuffins descended upon the Philippines to tangibly do the very things I'm suggesting. On this trip, the physical and metaphysical worlds collided in a majestic and yet humbling fashion. Men representing several American universities and a few different Christian ministries spent six weeks coaching, teaching and pastoring hundreds of Filipino professors, coaches and athletes on a program designed to build up holistic athletes and coaches for a lifetime. This book represents that vision. I vividly remember being swept off to venue after venue for training

---

[9] See appendix A for a short diagram I use with athletes as a series of devotions entitled "Embracing the D." "Embracing the D" is © Every Thought Captive, Inc. 2005.

among the national and olympic coaches and their staff. Then it was on to the University of Makati, then Benguet State University north of Baguio, then also to Tacloban at the University of the Philippines Visayas Tacloban College. After eight to nine hours of dynamic coaching and team building, Tim Dornemann and I would spend each evening building out the seven modules program, the dynamics of coaching modules and preparing to engage our audiences on the necessity of having a spiritual foundation. This book represents this initial work. We received tremendous blessings throughout our many trips to Southeast Asia over the years but one event stands out among them all. After an exhausting four days of training with the Philippine Olympic teams, coaches and staff, the national director of Athletes in Action Totie Andes and I shared the truth of how God has wed the physical and spiritual worlds together and how they coalesce in Jesus, the Son of God. You could have heard a pin drop. Afterward we prayed for everyone and offered a copy of the Bible to anyone who was interested. Four large cases of the Scriptures were gone in less than a minute. At first I thought the rapid distribution of the Text might simply be because it was free. However, I doubt this was the case because of the conversations that followed. Instead of getting questions concerning lifting technique, periodization or dynamic stretching, the conversations were about the nature of God, the church and how to grow in the Christian faith. I remember retiring that evening with a deeply satisfied spirit. It has been encouraging to me to see God's faithfulness at work over the years as I witness coaches grow in their faith and succeed with their athletes, their families and in themselves. Coach Andes always reminds his audience that we coach three things, "the Head, the Heart, and the Hands," referring to the intellect, the being and the production of an individual.

The most difficult thing for me about graduating from Seminary wasn't the classes, the tens of thousands of pages I read, the papers or the exams, nor even the thesis. No, it was meeting the list of 15 graduation requirements - many of which I was unaware of. One requirement stands out among the rest. It reads something to the effect of, "The Seminary reserves the right to withhold degree or diploma, or even dismiss a student at any time during their academic journey for failures in moral or spiritual conduct, even if all other requirements of sought degree have been satisfied." During my exit interview with university leadership I inquired as to the intent of such a seemingly harsh requirement. The answer was brilliant. In essence, they explained that the university was preparing students, not merely to have cognitive awareness of principles nor merely to provide certain skill sets to be used when they work 'in the real world.' No, their purpose was to graduate disciples of the Lord Jesus Christ into the worldwide mission field to advance His Kingdom, without regard to location, vocation or occupation and a student's character and integrity could disqualify them for such a task. This principle is also true when considering coaching and athletic development. The world of sports is littered with stories of individuals who crash-and-burn after their 15 minutes of fame. Stories of million dollar basketball players caught begging for money less than ten years after they leave the court. Cyclists who have their Tour de France championships stripped away for cheating. Athletes who may seem like superstars on the field but who have successive martial failures, paternity suits, and caustic egoism.

During the graduation ceremony after Seminary, the university has a tradition that puts your hard work into perspective. First, the registrar hands you your degree. Second, your academic advisor ceremoniously hoods you. And last, the university president congratulates you, places a towel over your arm and says, "Remember, it is not the *title* (i.e., degree) but the *towel* (e.g., humble service) that matters." Likewise, when we coach we must become a servant to those we serve.[10] Vince Lombardi, legendary coach of the Green Bay Packers, told his team, "Men, when you get across that goal line act like you've

---

[10]   See Philippians 2:1-11

been there before." Instill deeper internal qualities into your athletes; timeless traits, tradition and patterns that will pay out over time. Become a master of your game, wisest among your peers and yet coach those under you with the care of a dove with her chicks. Recognize the negative habits of the proud and arrogant among you and steer them in the other direction. Do not avoid the difficult person but see them as a challenge not only to you but to themself. Set your eyes on the prize but be satisfied in a job well done. These challenges bring us back to the importance of having good eyesight. C.S. Lewis said, "I believe in Christianity as I believe that the Sun has risen, not only because I see it but because by it, I see everything else."[11] Lewis uses this as both metaphor, the ability to see and as agent, the reality of the thing shown. As light illuminates both sides of the universe—the physical and the metaphysical—so too can we see the outcome of holistic athletic coaching, training and development. Ribbons and trophies may come and go but the compliment, "well done my faithful servant," is reserved for those who do it well and in the right way. The real legacy we leave as a coach is in the life of our athletes.

Sport is not ultimate. There isn't an exit exam for sport at the end of life. However, Jesus does offer us a life challenge in John 15 when he calls us to, "Remain in me and I in you so you can bear fruit." He furthers, "As the Father has loved me, so I have loved you. Love one another. Bear fruit that will last." Coach as if life itself depends upon it.

References: Chapter 2

1. *See Jim McKay's introduction to ABC's Wide World of Sports, 1961.*

2. *See Henry Russell ("Red") Sanders, "Winning isn't everything; It's the only thing" (1950, 1953, 1956); Vince Lombardi's address to the Packers before training camp 1959, "Winning isn't everything. The will to win is the only thing" (Michener, James A – Sports in America. Fawcett Crest, 1987).*

3. *See the history of the 100 meter world record progression at Wikipedia, 2021. "100 Meters." Last modified 19 April 2021.*

4. *See the New International Version Bible, 2011, Matthew 6:22-23. This wisdom comes directly after instructions against chasing after temporal things in lieu of eternal things and is preceded by the brilliant conclusion: "Do not run after these physical things. but seek first his kingdom and his righteousness, and all these things will be given to you as well."*

5. *John Wooden, coach of the UCLA men's basketball team: "Be more concerned with your character than your reputation, because your character is what you really are, while your reputation is merely what others think you are." Abraham Lincoln, America's sixteenth President: "Character is like a tree and reputation its shadow. The shadow is what we think it is and the tree is the real thing."*

6. *J.P. Nerbun, as quoted on the website https://thriveonchallenge.com/4-ways-to-coach-character/*

7. *See the New International Version Bible, 2011, Matthew 7:24-27*

8. *Mike Webster was an undersized center at the University of Wisconsin who went on to become a Hall of Fame player in the NFL. At only 6-1 and 255 pounds he was able to bench press 455 for six sets of eight reps. See the article by Colin Webster at https://startingstrength.com/article/reflections_in_iron_mike_websters_training_methods*

9. *See appendix A for a short diagram I use with athletes as a series of devotions entitled "Embracing the D." "Embracing the D" is © Every Thought Captive, Inc. 2005.*

10. *See Philippians 2:1-11*

11. *C.S. Lewis, in the essay entitled "Is Theology Poetry" found in The Weight of Glory.*

[11]   C.S. Lewis, in the essay entitled "Is Theology Poetry" found in *The Weight of Glory*.

3
PRINCIPLES OF EXERCISE PHYSIOLOGY

By: Phillip Bishop, Ed. D.

Professor Emeritus of Exercise Science, University of Alabama

THE HUMAN BODY is composed of many integrated systems. The excellent working of all these systems is essential to good health and great sports performance. Some of these systems play a key role in sports performance and will be introduced in this chapter. This is not comprehensive of any of these systems necessary to body function.

The Cardiovascular System

The cardiovascular system is composed of the heart and blood vessels. For us to remain alive, we need this system to deliver vital oxygen and nutrients throughout our entire body. The number-one cause of death in the USA in coaches, retired sportsmen and the general public is cardiovascular malfunction.

In sports, where prolonged muscle contractions are required, training the cardiovascular system is essential. For example, long distance runners, cyclists, skiers and swimmers must be able to pump large quantities of oxygen to provide energy for muscle contractions over the entire length of their event. In these athletes, the heart is doing two things - it is pumping large quantities of blood each beat and it is beating very fast for the duration of the event.

If you examine a healthy heart in any athlete - or even from a pig, large goat or cow - you will notice a few of the same details. The heart is actually a large left chamber wrapped around a smaller right chamber. You have to look closely to see the two small chambers (the atria) sitting on top of the left and right heart. There are thin valves that often function over 70 years without external maintenance. The right side of the heart is small, relative to the size of the left side of the heart because the right heart only needs to move blood a few inches to fill the lungs since the heart is located in the upper-middle of the left lung.

If the lungs are healthy and functioning well, the blood pumped there will be exposed to oxygen. The hemoglobin in the blood picks up a full supply of oxygen for future use to produce energy for the muscles. The oxygenated blood from the lungs is pumped back to the left heart and the left heart has the task of pumping blood to the muscles all over the body - from foot to brain. Moving large amounts of blood requires a large, healthy left-heart muscle. Training the heart requires gradually exposing it to high workloads in training.

All athletes need a good supply of hemoglobin to carry oxygen. Low hemoglobin, more common in women, can hurt the performance of any athlete. Utilize your team physician to evaluate the hemoglobin levels of your endurance athletes and recommend proper treatment for those who have low hemoglobin levels. Blood doping, a common phrase used in professional sports, is an illegal manipulation of the blood to supply it with extra hemoglobin thereby raising the oxygen-carrying capacity of the blood.

The pumping action of each side of the heart is accomplished by valves. The mitral valve in the left heart must close and remain sealed when the left-heart powerfully contracts, or squeezes. Consequently, in some athletes, often long-distance runners, the valve leaks. This creates a heart murmur which reduces the heart's maximal output to the muscles. Athletes with leaky valves or valves that are pushed down into the heart chamber will not be able to perform at their best. Again, your sports physician will be able to detect this and may be able to offer some treatment in severe cases.

The blood vessels are distributed throughout the body and blood flow amounts are controlled by making these vessels bigger or smaller. The radius. i.e., the length from the center of a vessel to its inside perimeter, impacts the volume of flow by the fourth power. This means the radius of a blood vessel doubles the flow four times. For example, if the radius increases by a factor of two, the flow increases 2x2x2x2 or 16 times as much flow.

The left heart responds to endurance training by increasing in size over time. The more endurance training an athlete does, the larger the size of the left heart, which allows it to pump more blood with each beat. The amount of blood pumped in each beat (or stroke) is called **stroke volume**. Not all the blood is emptied from the left heart when it contracts. The percentage of blood ejected is called the **ejection fraction**. A strong left ventricle is able to eject most of the blood delivered to it from the lungs and has a high ejection fraction. The heart of a well-trained endurance athlete has a maximal beating rate slightly lower than when untrained, probably due to the increase in muscle mass. But the slight reduction in rate is overcompensated by the very high stroke volume, resulting in a very high amount of total blood pumped per minute. This is called **cardiac output**. Each year of life the maximal heart rate in humans tends to drop by about one beat per minute. This results in the maximal cardiac output lowering by about 0.5% for a 20-year-old getting a year older and partly explains some of the decline in performance when athletes age, especially past the mid-30's.

Training the Cardiovascular System

The cardiovascular system, like most body systems, adapts to the stressors placed on it. If the heart is stressed time and time again to pump more blood, the left chamber muscle will enlarge and the heart muscle will get stronger. This increases oxygen delivery capacity by the blood which increases energy output capacity and improves endurance performance. To train the cardiovascular system for maximum endurance, athletes should gradually increase the length and intensity of their training.

The blood volume of the heart also increases to meet the body's demands. If the heart is stressed to supply blood to more muscles, the response is greater. So, for example, cross-country skiing uses both the legs and the arms over long durations which requires more blood. Over time, this results in larger adaptive increases than running or cycling alone, which only use your legs. Swimming strokes requiring vigorous leg muscle engagement (e.g., breaststroke, butterfly) would produce larger cardio improvements than strokes with less leg muscle engagement. When practical, coaches may want to experiment during the off-season with different types of training utilizing more muscle groups, which will reduce monotony and joint stress and may produce better cardiac performance over time.

In very short, intense forms of exercise such as competitive weightlifting, the need for oxygen is low and oxygen delivery is not a limitation to exercise. Even though these types of athletes may not need endurance training for their performance, some endurance training will be beneficial to their overall health since heart disease claims many lives.

The Respiratory System

The respiratory system is chiefly made up of the trachea and lungs. When we inhale, or take a breath, the lungs receive air from the atmosphere by creating a lower pressure. The trachea has cartilage in it, making it stiff, such that it remains open at all times. In the breathing cycle, the low pressure is created by increasing the volume of the chest cavity. This is achieved by flattening the diaphragm (which is curved upwards into the chest) or by lifting the ribs with the respiratory muscles to make them rounder. When heavy breathing is needed, both approaches maximize the pressure drop and increase the amount of air with each respiratory cycle.

Exhaling happens when the diaphragm is relaxed, or the respiratory muscles relax to reduce chest volume, thereby making the pressure in the lungs higher than outside in the atmosphere. Fortunately, our respiratory capacity exceeds our ability to pump blood, so desaturation due to respiratory insufficiency does not usually occur in healthy athletes at or near sea level.

The role of the respiratory system is to move oxygen from the atmosphere into the blood for ultimate use by muscles (mostly) and other organs. It also transports the gaseous products of metabolism, carbon dioxide, from the site of energy production to the blood then to the lungs. Gas exchange happens when the gas exists in different concentrations on two sides of a membrane that allows the gas to pass through. For example, our hard breathing whilst running, mechanically delivers air from the atmosphere with an oxygen concentration of ~21% to the little chambers of the lungs, where, in heavy exercise, oxygen concentration can be almost 0%. But the oxygen level doesn't ever get this low in our bodies because we have blood returning not only from muscles working very hard (e.g., the leg muscles of a runner or the arm muscles of a rower) but also blood from unused muscles of the body, which ideally are relaxed and using only a little of the oxygen supplied to them.

God designed the lung tissue and the walls of the blood vessels which surround the lung cells to easily allow passage of oxygen into the blood and carbon dioxide out of the blood. So exercise situations requiring lots of energy for lots of muscles, such as cross-country skiing will use up much of the oxygen in the blood and produce lots of carbon dioxide. The limitation to performance in an endurance sport is the heart's ability to pump blood to the muscles and lungs for energy production in the muscles and delivery of carbon dioxide and pickup of oxygen in the lungs. In healthy athletes, the lungs will meet their demands readily. It is the heart and muscles that need to be trained to increase their capacities.

Altitude Training

As a person ascends to a higher altitude, the pressure of the atmosphere on the lungs diminishes simply because there is less air above us pushing down. Consequently, the partial pressure of oxygen declines as we ascend. So, if we take an endurance runner, cyclist, swimmer or skier to high altitude, the stressors on their respiratory and cardiovascular systems will rise, due to less oxygen delivery to the blood. The effects of pressure change become more noticeable at above 2,100 meters. At altitudes higher than this, the body will make short-term and longer-term adaptations in an attempt to deliver more oxygen to itself. Historically, the problem with taking athletes who have been training at altitudes below 2,100 meters to higher altitudes to train is that few can sustain their training volume and intensity at the higher altitudes and gains in system adaptation are overwhelmed by the detraining they experience.

This has led to a training concept of "Live-high, train low." Whereas this approach is impractical for most people, attempts have been made to use altitude chambers, oxygen-reduction equipment (not the same as pressure, but it works the same in our respiratory system) and other approaches to induce performance adaptations without having to commute up and down tall mountains. If this is of interest to you, we recommend you investigate this training possibility, since it is beyond the scope of this introductory text.

Regardless of your interest in altitude training, keep in mind that competitions held at altitudes greater than 2,100 meters will be especially challenging for some endurance athletes. If a competition is to be held at an altitude higher than what the athlete is typically training in, expose the athlete to the competition altitude for as long as practical prior to the competition. Altitude not only reduces oxygen delivery, it can also impact nutrition and sleep, both of which are vital to good performance.

Muscle Training

Muscle training is essential to improving most sports performance. The muscles of the body all work by shortening, or contracting. With few exceptions for skeletal muscle, the shortening of the muscle causes a bone to move, which allows us to lift a weight, throw an object, move the body or manipulate a ball or other object.

Muscles are connected to bones by tendons and bones are connected to other bones by ligaments. Where the muscle attaches to the bone via the tendon, in relation to the bone's attachment to another bone via the ligament determines the relative leverage force, or speed, of limb movement. In humans most agree that our anatomy generally favors speed over force.

The muscles are composed of actin and myosin filaments which ratchet past each other in one direction during contraction to exert muscle force. It is logical and accurate that the more fibers that ratchet, the stronger the force. In general, the larger the cross-section of the muscle, the more force produced. For example, the quadriceps muscles on the front of the leg have larger cross-sections than the biceps in the arms and can exert more force. It is also obvious that for a muscle to become stronger after the initial nervous adaptation, the increase in strength will be marked by an increase in muscle cross-section. Therefore, very strong athletes tend to be very large-muscled.

Basics of Muscle Training

Although we can make muscle training very complex, the basics are simple. Muscle groups, like all of the body's systems, are trained by stressing them, then providing nutrients and allowing them to respond during a recovery period. The adaptation the muscles make is directly related to the type of stress they experience. That is, muscles exposed to very short bouts of high contraction respond by increasing size and force production capacity. Muscles exposed to repeated lighter contractions over longer time intervals develop increased energy processing capacity and endurance increases. We use training cycles to facilitate recovery and adaptation.

The muscles, like all the adaptable systems of the body, respond to stress by changing such to reduce that stressor. This is called The General Adaptation Syndrome. This Syndrome says that if a stressor is applied (e.g., a resistance training workout), and nutrients and recovery are available, the part that is stressed will adapt in such a way to reduce the stress. Specificity means that the adaptation is specific to the type of stressor applied. Frequency of training is determined by how long it takes an athlete to recover and adapt which varies by the stressor and individual characteristics of each person. Intensity refers to how hard someone has to work to create stress. Duration, the length of a workout, likewise, is dependent upon how much stress is required to produce more adaptation. Mode of training is determined by what adaptations are desired.

For there to be an optimal adaptive response (e.g., increased sport performance) the training stimulus must be at a greater level of intensity and frequency than the person is accustomed to, which is basically the principle of overload. However, the overload stimulus must be applied in a gradual progression to allow recovery and to avoid injury and over-training responses.

Perhaps the most important principle of training is specificity. The specificity principle states that an athlete will get specific outcomes based on the type of exercise they perform. Simply stated, specificity says that an athlete will, "reap what they sow," with long-term training. If exercise is solely lifting heavy weights, the athlete will increase her ability to lift heavy weights—that is, strength training results in strength. If a coach has an athlete spend all her time running or cycling long distances, she will become very good at running and cycling long distances. If the coach wants to improve both muscular and cardiovascular fitness, then a combination of training approaches is required.

In general, each sport requires a unique training program that is designed to develop optimal levels of sport fitness within all parameters: body composition, flexibility, cardiovascular fitness, muscular strength and muscular endurance. A wise coach will GRADUALLY increase training. Too much overload too quickly vastly increases the possibility of injury.

Recovery plays an important factor in the athlete's ability to adapt to stress. If no recovery is allowed, the body is likely to over-train and become injured. The amount of recovery that may be needed is different for everyone and is related to many factors such as a person's sleep quality, diet, physical fitness level and psychological stress. An optimal training program must be structured to allow for sufficient recovery, even though it requires exercise on most days of the week. Typically, the type of workouts are alternated to allow for recovery of a given body part or physiological system, while continuing to train. Our experience and research demonstrates that some people need a longer recovery than others and, as much as possible, recovery should be tailored to the individual more than to the team as a unit.

What goes up must come down. This quote certainly applies to sport training. Physical adaptations achieved through training will disappear when training is reduced. Most of us coaches, in our enthusiasm, do not allow sufficient recovery, and consequently our athletes' bodies are too tired to perform as well as they could.

So, in summary, on the most basic level, muscle training programs must stress the muscles in the same manner that we hope to produce increased muscle function. Strength increases occur in tandem with size and are obtained by exposure to very high loads. Endurance adaptation occurs when endurance loads are applied. Regardless of the stressor, recovery is vital to allow muscles to adapt and to avoid over-stress and muscle injury and whole-body illness. Chapter 15 is devoted to recovery; you can learn more in that chapter.

Muscle Genetics

There are four factors that must align for an elite athlete to reach their potential:

1. Genetics—Optimal genetics for a specific sport or activity are vital for us to excel.
2. Opportunity—There are many people who never discover their capabilities due to lack of opportunity.
3. Desire—Despite favorable genetics and opportunity there is still much work required; some people do not have a desire to do what is required for sport success.
4. Coaching—Optimal training is usually a complex process of development, practice and recovery with skilled supervision; it is vital to achieve optimal performance in sport.

Genetic gifting is manifest in the muscles. To over-simplify, the muscles can be thought of as existing in two extremes—fast muscle and slow muscle. Whereas fast muscle can be trained to act with slower characteristics, slow muscle cannot be trained to act in the way fast muscles do. While muscles display a continuum of capabilities, we are merely discussing the extremes.

Fast-twitch muscle fibers can contract very fast. These fibers tend to be innervated by large and myelinated nerves (see section on the nervous system on page 21) which allow for fast nervous transmission of the signal to contract. They are able to rapidly contract and their fibers are large in diameter. Energy capabilities of fast twitch muscles are based on non-oxidative means such as glycolysis. Because their metabolic capacity for processing oxygen is limited, and because their larger size slows the diffusion of oxygen, they have high power capacity but relatively low endurance.

At the other end of the spectrum is the **slow-twitch muscle fiber**. As the name suggests, these fibers contract more slowly than the fast-twitch fibers. Slow-twitch muscle fibers are smaller in diameter to facilitate the diffusion of oxygen so that their oxygen-based metabolism can produce a lot of energy sustained over a long time. The nerves supplying these muscle fibers tend to be smaller.

You have probably noticed athletes who are rich in fast-twitch fibers and those who are rich in slow-twitch fibers. Those with an abundant population of fast-twitch fibers are weightlifting and sprinting sport competitors, for example. They tend to be muscular, can add muscle mass relatively quickly and are fast-moving but do not have high endurance. In contrast, athletes rich in slow-twitch fibers tend to be smaller, with smaller muscles and less ability to add muscle mass. They do not have high speed movement capabilities but respond very readily to endurance training, such as long distance runners and cyclists.

Many sports, like soccer or basketball, need both speed and endurance. The better players in these types of sports are not extremely fast- or slow- twitch but have a good mixture of both. As people age, the fast-twitch fibers become more slow-twitch. The peak performance age for fast-twitch sports (e.g., sprinting, weightlifting) tends to be younger than for slow-twitch (e.g., endurance) sports.

The body's ability to utilize oxygen to produce energy for sport performance is measured as the oxygen uptake expressed as volume of oxygen (VO_2) per minute. The maximal capacity is the VO_2max. The single best predictor of endurance sport performance is the VO_2max. The VO_2max is primarily limited by the body's ability to pump blood to the working muscle. The higher the slow-twitch fiber percentages, the higher the VO_2max is in response to training. And vice versa, a high percentage of fast-twitch fibers will result in lower VO_2max.

The Nervous System

The nervous system is the body's communication system. It coordinates all the actions and sensory information throughout each part. The nervous system controls:

- Movement, balance and coordination
- Sensations such as touch or hearing
- Breathing and heartbeat
- Interpretations of sensory information (e.g., vision and sounds)
- Mental function including learning and memory
- Sleep, healing and recovery
- Stress and responses to stress
- Body temperature
- Hunger, thirst and digestion
- And others (this list is not all encompassing)

The nervous system, through the brain, spinal cord and nerves, provides the signal for muscles to contract. In fact, when a new athlete or young person is initially exposed to resistance training, it is the nervous system that adapts first and provides the initial increase in strength.

The nervous system is extremely complex. It functions by using charged chemicals (ions) and allowing ions to move inside and outside the nerve to report sensations such as hot or cold, or to send a signal to a muscle to contract. Contractions can be both voluntary and reflex (or involuntary). In a voluntary contraction, nerves in our brain decide to contract a muscle. For example, to move our biceps in the way we want, a signal from the brain travels down the spinal cord where other nerves are stimulated and passed from nerve cell to nerve cell until the signal reaches the biceps, causing the muscle to contract. An example of a reflex contraction, is when you make a movement based on a sensory input without telling your brain to signal your body to do it - like the reflex causing you to withdraw your hand from a hot stove. The sensory nerves in your fingers send a signal to the spinal cord. Since we have a God-given reflex, it doesn't have to travel to the brain. Instead, to save time, the spinal cord sends a signal back to the muscles causing you to quickly withdraw your hand before incurring a serious burn.

The speed at which a nerve can conduct a signal is dependent on two factors: 1) The diameter of the nerve—the larger the faster—and 2) whether the nerve is covered in a myelin sheath which acts to isolate the conducting part of the nerve to speed signal flow. A highly coordinated skill, like throwing a fast-breaking curveball, requires training the neuromuscular system to apply the proper forces to the baseball to generate high speed and the appropriate spin. Anytime we are coaching skills, essentially we are training the nervous system to work with the muscles in an effective fashion.

The nervous system is also one of three integrated systems that control our heart. Nervous stimulation is what causes the heart to contract in a coordinated fashion, and if part of the heart's nervous system is damaged, the coordination will be disrupted to some extent. As we train endurance athletes, the left chamber of their heart enlarges and becomes more powerful, the nervous system adapts to slow the heart more at rest because the body's resting need for blood is mostly unchanged and more blood is ejected with every heartbeat. So, slower resting heart rate can be a good indicator of the adaptation of the heart to endurance training.

It should be clear that we cannot train athletes without training the nervous system. To develop motor skills or muscular power, muscle excitation and relaxation must be trained. To some extent, all training requires nervous system training.

The Endocrine System

In addition to the messages and control the body gets from the nervous system, the endocrine system is another signaling system within the body. For example, in addition to nerves controlling our heart rate as we mentioned, our endocrine system also influences heart rate by changing the level of the hormones called adrenaline and noradrenaline.

Hormones are produced by glands. Each gland produces one or more hormones, which communicate messages to our body. Some of the key glands include:

Gland	Location	Hormone	Function in the Body
hypothalamus	two triangular bodies which sit on top of each kidney	corticosteroid	controls salt and water balance in the body, the body's response to stress, metabolism, the <u>immune system</u>, and sexual development and function
		epinephrine (i.e., adrenaline)	increases blood pressure and heart rate when the body is under stress, such as immediately before and during competition.
pituitary	base of brain		produces many hormones that control many other endocrine glands
		growth hormone	stimulates the growth of bone and other body tissues and plays a role in the body's handling of nutrients and minerals, thus is key to training adaptations
		thyrotropin (pronounced: thy-ruh-TRO-pin)	stimulates the thyroid gland to make thyroid hormones
		corticotropin (pronounced: kor-tih-ko-TRO-pin)	stimulates the adrenal gland to make certain hormones
		antidiuretic hormone	helps control body water balance through its effect on the kidneys
			the pituitary also secretes endorphins which reduce feelings of pain. It also controls ovulation and the menstrual cycle in women.
thyroid	in the front part of the lower neck	thyroxine and triiodothyronine	control the rate at which cells burn fuels from food to make energy. Higher thyroid hormone cause faster chemical reactions. Thyroid hormones play a role in the development of the bones, brain and nervous system.

Gland	Location	Hormone	Function in the Body
parathyroids	just behind the thyroid glands	parathyroid hormones	control blood calcium levels
adrenals	on top of each kidney	corticosteroids (e.g. aldosterone)	controls fluid levels and blood pressure
		glucocorticoids (e.g. cortisol)	regulate metabolism
		adrenal androgens (eg. testosterone)	impact muscle growth and sexual development
		catecholamines (e.g. adrenaline)	impact the "flight or fight" responses.
ovaries	side of women's uterus	estrogen	there are three types of estrogen (estradiol, estrone, and estriosuch) that control the menstrual cycle, influence reproduction, body weight, and learning and memory.
testes	male testicles	testosterone	testosterone is produced in the testes, and plays an important role in increasing muscle size and strength. It has been illegally supplied and administered to athletes in an artificial form.

Another important part of the endocrine system is the pancreas. It makes insulin and glucagon which control the level of glucose (blood sugar). Insulin moves glucose from the blood to the cells. This glucose, as we said in the energy section above, is essential in supplying energy. When insulin levels are insufficient, diabetes (Type I) occurs, and when it is ineffective, Type II diabetes.

Acclimatization

In this chapter we have learned about various body systems that are important for athletic performance. One aspect that must be considered in training athletes is acclimatization - acclimating their body systems to various environments. Earlier we discussed acclimatization to high altitudes. Acclimatization to heat is perhaps even more important because many athletes compete in hot environments. The good news is that our bodies will adapt to improve performance in hot environments.

Muscle contraction generates a great deal of heat. In cold situations, this is positive for our bodies. In hot situations, this heat generation will reduce physical performance and expose athletes to the possibility of deadly heat stroke. Because of the dangers of heat stroke, coaches must monitor their athletes when exercising in the heat, and work intensity and volume will need to be reduced, at least initially. Heat acclimation, at a minimum, takes five to seven days of exposure and may take 10-14 days for full acclimatization for some. Heat acclimatization must be done slowly and carefully to protect people's health. Even a single sudden day of unseasonably warm temperatures can precipitate heat injuries. As the season turns from cool to warm, coaches must monitor the environment to protect their athletes.

Humans cool themselves by evaporating sweat from the surface of the skin. This requires two things: 1) sweat on the skin, and 2) an environment of sufficiently low humidity to allow evaporation to occur. Clothing causes air to be trapped under it, which raises the humidity of that air, and may also raise the temperature. In hot environments, the less clothing covering the skin, the better the heat removal.

Hypohydration (taking in less water than is lost from the body) is an added risk for exercise when sweating. Hypohydration reduces the blood volume (blood provides fluid to the sweat glands) which reduces oxygen delivery and also reduces blood flow to the skin. This blood flow is a major source of delivery of heat to the skin (where evaporation occurs) and the delivery of cooling to the muscles and internal organs. Hypohydration also contributes to heat injury. Coaches must ensure athletes consume sufficient water and electrolytes to replace the water and electrolytes lost in sweat, urination and breathing.

Sweat rates can be as high as just under four liters (or one gallon) per hour, depending on the size of the person. Some fluids ingested will be lost to urine production, so to maintain fluid levels most people will need to consume at least one liter per hour. Weighing athletes prior, during and after exercise and recording those weights is a simple and useful way to ensure athletes do not lose too much fluid by providing an indication of how much fluid needs to be replaced. This is NOT an issue to take lightly. People die every year from hypohydration and heat stroke.

The good news is that cold exposure, to a degree, is much less of an issue for sports. In general, for athletes the key danger in cold weather is frostbite. Frostbite is when the cells freeze and are damaged. This typically occurs in areas with large surfaces relative to their mass, and lower supplies of warmth-giving blood. The ears, tips of noses, toes and fingers are most susceptible to frostbite. Good clothing has been developed which provides adequate protection against frostbite. Coaches, as in warm weather, must also monitor and educate athletes about frostbite, about monitoring their teammates for frostbite and about wearing protective clothing.

SECTION 2

ACTIVITIES, TRAINING, TOOLS

4
POWERREV DYNAMIC MOVEMENT & WARM-UP GUIDELINES

By: Tim Dornemann, Ed. D., CES, PES, CSCS, OS Pro

Exercise Science Program & Kinesiology Director, Barton College
Associate Professor of Exercise Science, Barton College
&
Scott O'Dell
Director of Strength & Conditioning, East Central University

Dynamic Warm-Up

RESEARCH HAS SHOWN that traditional warm-ups featuring static stretching actually acutely reduce force and power production. Static stretching lengthens muscle beyond the muscle's resting length. Since muscles produce their greatest force at close to their resting length, lengthening the muscle during static stretching reduces force output. Dynamic warm-ups are excellent opportunities to teach athletes the correct movement techniques that will help them during their competition. Through increasing the pace of the warm-up from start to finish, a dynamic warm-up prepares players for the speed of the activity.

While static stretching is not the most appropriate way to warm-up before activity or competition, static stretching has been shown to be an effective way to increase flexibility. Long-term (chronic) flexibility training has been shown to reduce injury and enhance performance. Static stretching is excellent to include in a post activity cool-down.

A standard warm-up should progress from slow to faster movements to prepare the athletes for the expected tempo of the workout, practice or competition. A warm-up should include general movement, consisting of just moving the body, as well as some general movement technique exercises, such as dynamic stretches. This improves range of motion (ROM), gets the blood flowing and the body temperature warmed up. Depending on the sport, general movement technique is followed by 2-3 multiple direction movements chosen from the lateral and backwards movement lists. The movements and directions picked depend on the movement used in the sport. The warm-up finishes at higher tempo by using sprint and acceleration technique movements to focus on speed and agility. The linear warm-up movements will stimulate the central nervous system (CNS) and should be included prior to plyometric training sessions.

General Movement/Mobility

Get the body moving with a slow walk or jog. Arm circles or arm swings can be done while walking or jogging to add an upper body component to the warm-up.

General Movement Techniques (hip mobility)

All will emphasize good posture for increased force production, 90 degree elbows, knees up, toes up and heels up (moving stretches).

1. Knee Hugs
2. Hip External/Internal Rotation
3. Walking Hamstring
4. Lunge Walk with Rotation

Multiple Direction Activities

Lateral Movements

1. Side Shuffle
2. Short Carioca
3. Long Carioca

Backward Movements

1. Backward Run
2. Backpedal

Speed & Power Activities

All will emphasize good posture for increased force production, 90 degree elbows, knees up, toes up and heels up.

1. High Knees
2. Heel Kicks/Butt Kicks

Plyometric Linear Warm-Up Movements

All movements will emphasize good posture for increased force production, knees up, toes up and heels up. Ankle hops and flips are added into dynamic warm-up prior to plyometric training.

1. Power Skip

Dynamic Warm-up Template

Dynamic Warm-Up Design Template

Warm-Up Design Question: What movements are commonly used?
Ramp Protocol: Raise (temp., HR, resp., viscosity), Activate and Mobilize (through full ROM),
Potentiate (sport specific, progress to needed tempo)
General Warm-up: 5-10 minute walk or jog

<u>Example</u>

Slow → Fast	Phase	Movement	Slow → Fast	Phase	
	General Mobility	Walk with arm circles / swings		General Mobility	
		Knee Hugs			
		Hip Internal Rotation			
		Hip Extenal Rotation			
		Walking Lunge			
		Walking Hamstrings			
	Lateral	Lateral Shuffle		Lateral	
		Long Carioca			
		Short Carioca			
	Backward	Backward Run		Backward	
		Back Pedal			
	Speed & Power	High Knees		Speed & Power	
		Butt Kicks			
		Power Skip			

Warm-up for Speed, Agility & Plyometrics

Static stretching should not be performed immediately prior to speed, agility and plyometric training, as research has shown that static stretching before training does not aid in preventing injury and it also decreases force production (Landin, et al, 2008). When thinking of your muscles, picture a rubber band; the looser and more stretched out a rubber band is, the less likely it will stretch and recoil with pop or power. The thick, not so stretched-out rubber band can be stretched out and will recoil with much more pop or power. Try lining the loose, flimsy rubber band up on your arm and pull it back as far as you can, then let go. Then try a stiff, tight rubber band on your arm and pull it back as far as you can, then let it go. The second rubber band is going to have more power and would sting your arm when snapped against it. This is because the thick, stiff rubber band has more power when it is stretched. Muscles are elastic just like rubber bands.

Muscles contract in response to stretch–this is the stretch reflex. The stretch reflex is the involuntary reaction of your muscles to the eccentric contraction (lengthening of the muscle). Since muscles are elastic, the stretch reflex will tell your muscles to go into a concentric contraction (shortening of the muscle). This will naturally give the muscle more power due to its resistance to the eccentric contraction. This will be covered further in later chapters.

We have seen greater results in the vertical jump test when it is performed after one repetition of a power clean at maximum effort. The athlete's vertical jump would be higher when they tested their power clean immediately before as compared to testing the vertical jump by itself on a separate day. The reason for this was that the power clean would stimulate (or wake-up) their CNS before going for a max effort jump. For the purpose of the warm-up, it is critical to stimulate the central nervous system before training or competition so you are at your maximum speed and jumping ability.

Dynamic full range of motion movement results in more flexibility than from static stretching. An example of how flexibility is promoted during dynamic movement is an overhead squat. This is an exercise that we use in the first phase of training to promote flexibility, balance and stability; we theorize that if someone can do a proper, full range of motion, Olympic overhead squat (bar above their ears, hamstrings to calves and heels down) then they are ready to perform anything in the weight room through that demonstration of flexibility, balance and stability. Consistently, athletes will start their season not able to perform the overhead squat movement without their heels coming off the floor or do not have the shoulder flexibility to keep the bar directly above their ears. They practice their form and movement, even with a stick or a bar with no weights. Typically, in week three or four of the season every athlete on the team is able to perform the overhead squat with full range of motion and good technique.

In contrast, I have also coached under a routine with a lot of static stretching, and after four years in the program there are athletes who still do not have the flexibility to perform an Olympic overhead squat, an Olympic back squat or touch their toes with their legs straight. Through practical experience, it's been beneficial to compare and contrast various theories of flexibility improvement. The majority of static stretching should be done post-workout. This is when the muscles are the warmest and the most elastic to truly make increases in flexibility and static stretching at this time will not diminish any power production during the workout. Static stretching is a good tool to use and athletes will need it but, like everything, it has a time when it's most beneficial.

How to Perform Warm-Up Drills with Proper Technique

Utilize this section for more details on proper technique and form for warm-up drills.

General Warm Up

<u>Walking Arm Swings</u>

Swing arms across the chest, alternating right arm above left and then left arm above right, while walking.

<u>Walking Arm Circles (Large)</u>

While walking, make large arm circles with both arms. Perform half forward circles and half backwards circles.

<u>Walking Arm Circles (Small)</u>

While walking, make small arm circles with both arms. Perform half forward circles and half backwards circles

Technical Speed Warm-up Drills

These can be incorporated with the general warm-up prior to speed training.

<u>A-Walk/A-Skip</u>

Head up, good posture, toes up, heels up and elbows locked at 90 degrees throughout all ranges of motion.

- Bring the knee up above the hips with all forward action and keep the toes up while achieving triple extension with the leg in contact with the ground by driving upward through the balls of the feet.
- This can be performed at a walking or skipping pace.

<u>Slide Kick</u>

- Head up, good posture, toes up, heels up and elbows locked at 90 degrees.
- With a fast arm and high knee action bring the knee forward and up practicing positive shin angles while slightly moving forward.
- Assign foot contacts rather than distance to ensure an emphasis on practicing the positive shin angles and not trying to cover ground.

<u>Heel Walk</u>

- Keep the knees straight, flex the toes up towards the head. Keep the balls of the feet off the ground and walk on the heels.
- Strengthening the anterior tibialis to aid in shin splint prevention.

Heel Up/Toe-Up Walk

- Knees relaxed, walk on the balls of the feet, keeping the toes flexed up, and the heel off of the ground.
- Strengthening the ability for the body to move off of the balls of the feet.
- Strengthening the foot muscles; the gripping muscles of the feet.

Quick Feet Warm-up Drills

These can be incorporated with the general warm-up prior to agility training.

Rope/Line Jumping Drills

When looking to use agility as part of the warm-up or as a continuation of the warm-up, an effective tool is the jump rope. Thousands of different jump rope routines are not necessary, rather a handful of exercises to get skilled and quick at would be best. This is an effective tool to get a lot of repetition with the focus being on keeping the toes and heels up working off the balls of the feet for foot quickness and muscle recruitment.

- Two Feet - Keep feet together and jump over the rope on each revolution.
- Alternating - For one foot, repeat jumping with just one foot at a time jumping over the rope with each revolution. If alternating, switch feet with each revolution of the jump rope.
- Scissor - Move feet like scissors switching from front to back with each revolution of the jump rope.
- 360 - With feet together, move the body in a 360 degree turn and back, jumping over the rope with each revolution.
- Side to Side - Pick out a line on the ground and with feet together, jump from one side on the first revolution and back with the next revolution and repeat.
- Forward and Back - Pick out a line on the ground and with feet together, jump forward over the line on the first revolution and back with the next revolution and repeat.

Plyometric Warm-up Drills

These can be incorporated with the general warm-up prior to plyometric training.

Ankle Joint Movements

- Pogos - Toes up, heels up, slight bend in the knees, good posture. Block up with the arms and repeat with minimal contact time with the ground. Blocking up with the arms refers to forcefully using the arms ahead of the body to increase the vertical posture for increased force production. To block up with the arms, start with elbows bent at 90 degrees and using the shoulder drive the hands up while keeping the elbows at 90 degrees.

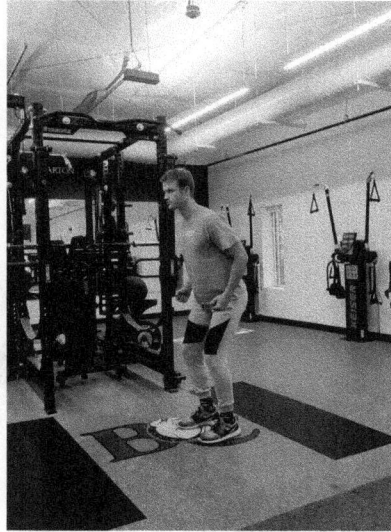

Block up starting position   Block up finishing position

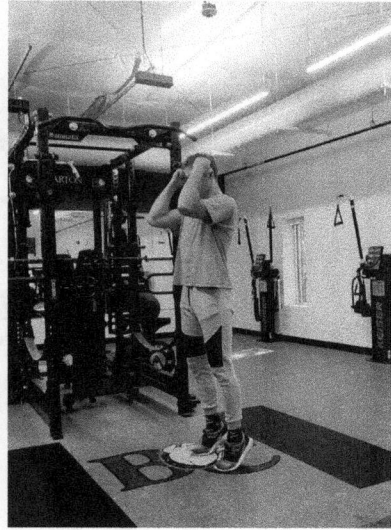

- Ankle Flips - Lean forward slightly from the ankles. Jump off the ground by extending the ankle joint with the forward lean propelling the body forward while keeping the knees straight but not locked.

Full Leg Movements

- Gallop - Place one leg forward and one back with the weight on the front leg and knee bent while the back leg stays straight. Drive forward off of the front leg, pick the same knee up and get ready to repeat upon the front foot landing. Leave the back leg motionless and extended back for balance.

Linear Dynamic Movements

Knee Hug

- Pull knee to chest and pause for a second
- Step and pull one knee to chest, while simultaneously raising up on toe of opposite leg (to work plantar flexion)

Walking Lunge

- Step out with front foot and lower down so both legs are at 90 degrees
  - Too long a stride if front knee is over heel
  - Too short a stride if front knee extends over or past toes
  - Correct stride if front knee is over arch to balls of feet
- Alternate into lunge on opposite leg
- An upper body twist can be added rotationally to one or both sides

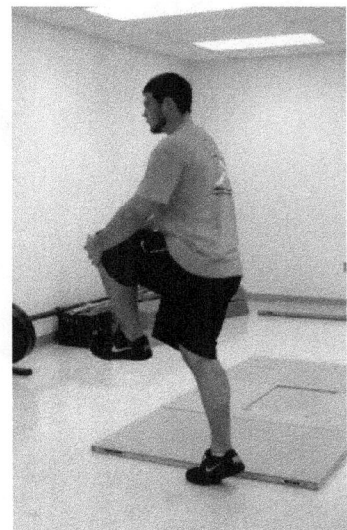

Knee Hug

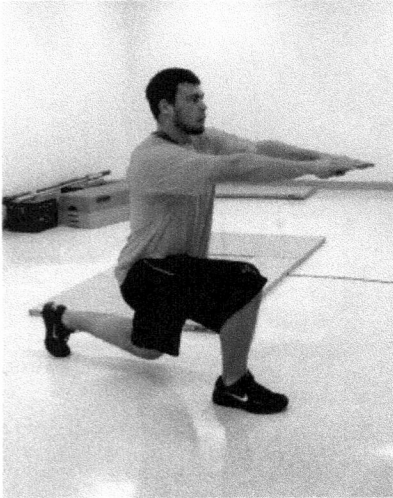

Basic Lunge

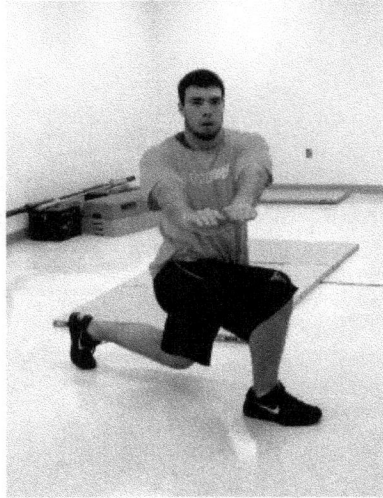

Lunge with right twist

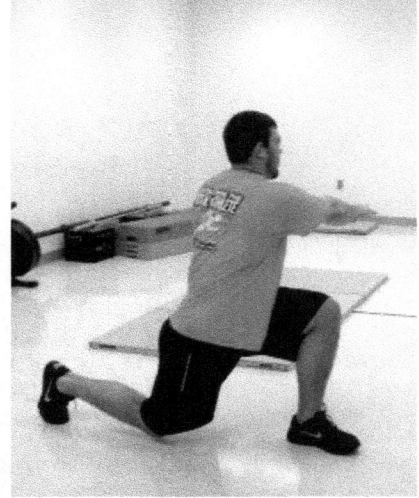

Lunge with left twist

Walking Hamstring

- Step out with one leg, reach down with hands for balance while raising up other leg behind
- The higher the one leg is raised behind while the other leg remains straight, the greater the hamstring stretch
- Alternate with other leg

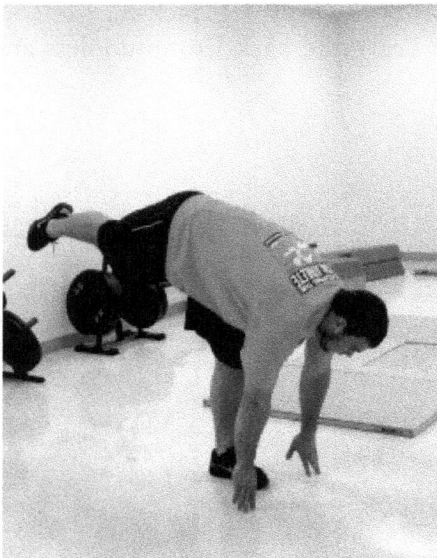

Basic Walking Hamstring

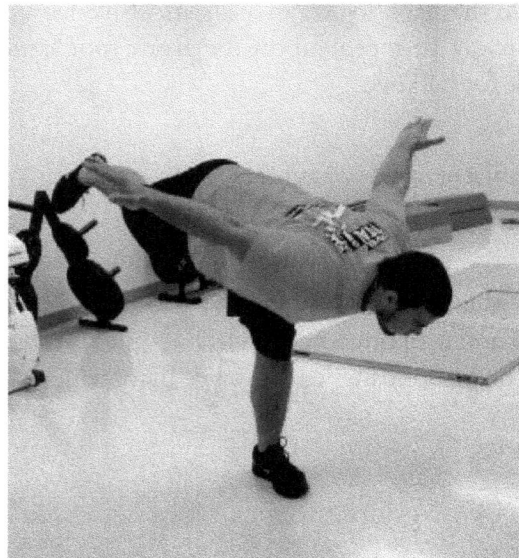

Walking Hamstring with balance

Internal Rotation

- Raise leg up to hip height with knee bent at 90 degree to the side and rotate leg to front of the body while stepping forward
- Alternate with other leg

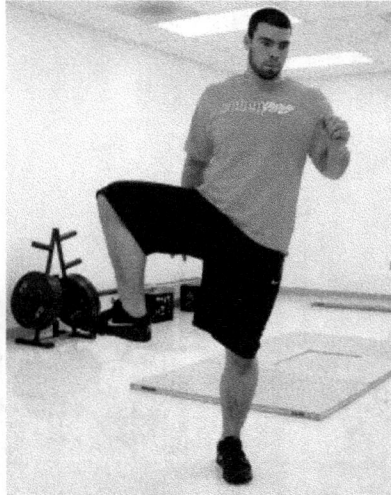

IR Starting position

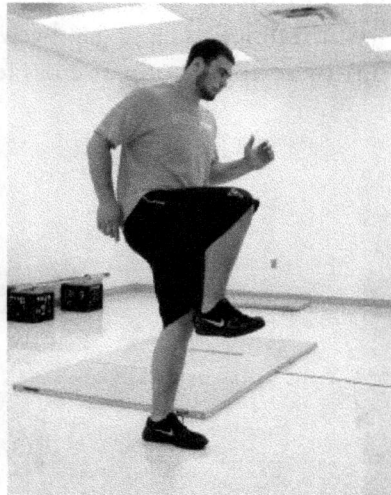

IR Finishing Position

External Rotation

- Raise leg up to hip height with knee bent at 90 degrees to the front and rotate leg to side of the body while taking a step backward
- Alternate with other leg

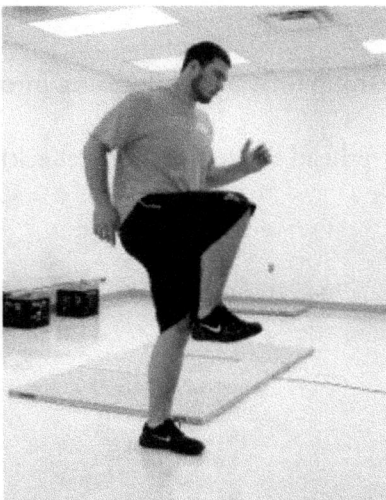

ER Starting position

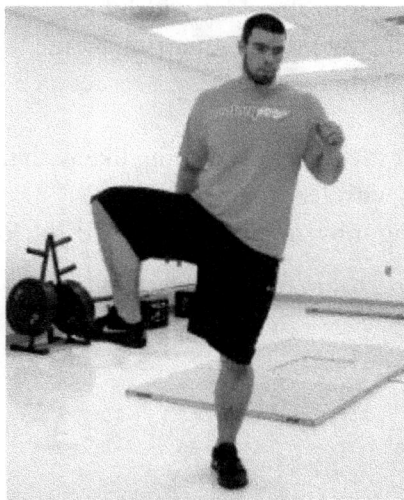

ER Rotate knee out

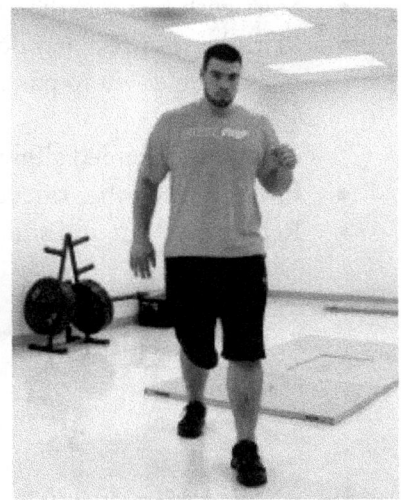

ER Step back

Lateral Movements

Side Shuffle

- Moving laterally keeping body low (maintaining athletic position)
- Step out laterally with front/lead leg, keep hips square
- Eyes look straight forward
- Push off of back/trail leg to close gap between feet
- Stay low, don't twist upper body or cross feet over

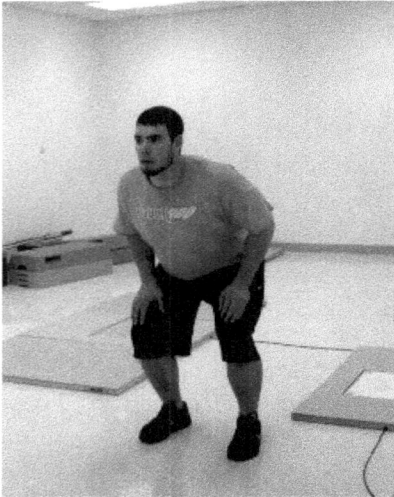

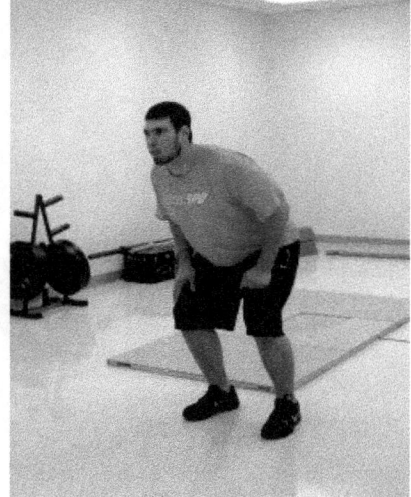

Side Shuffle Athletic Position   Side Shuffle Lateral step   Side Shuffle Closing step

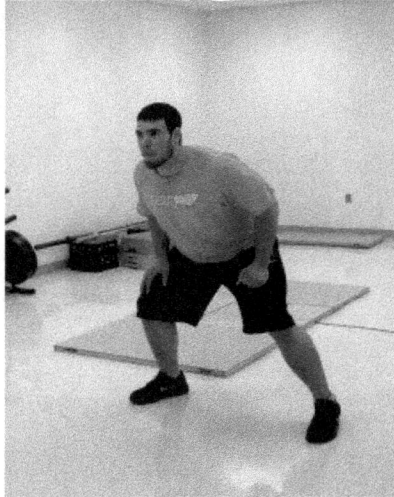

Lateral Walk

- Start with feet together, step out to shoulder-width base
- With hands up, squat down using proper squatting form
  - Going down to parallel, with knee tracking over feet, chest leaning forward while going into a squat
  - Arms extended allows for movement screening like with the overhead squat (flexibility check)
- Pivot to face other direction with feet together
- Repeat step out and squatting movement facing new direction

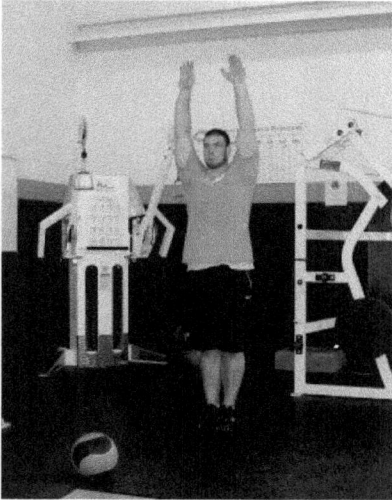

Lateral Walk Starting position

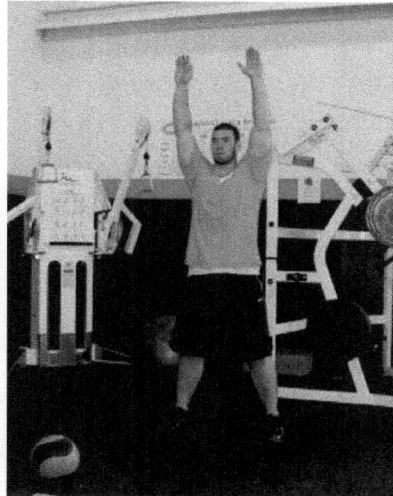

LW Step out

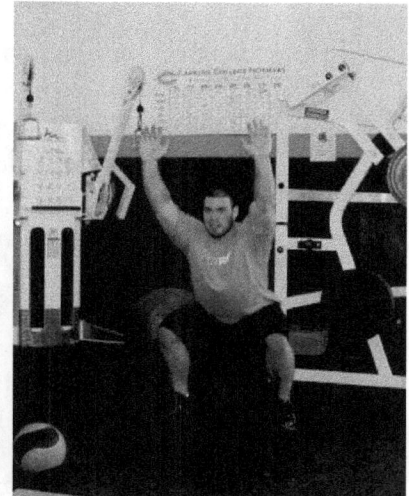

LW Squat

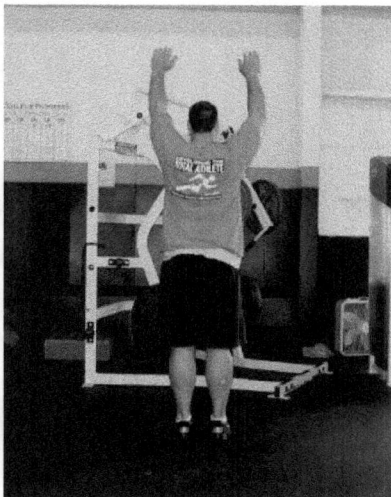

LW Pivot and turn

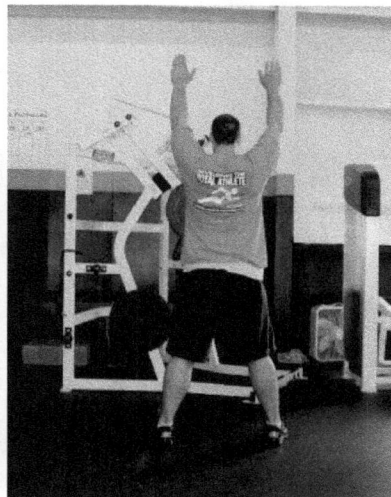

LW Pivot and turn Step out

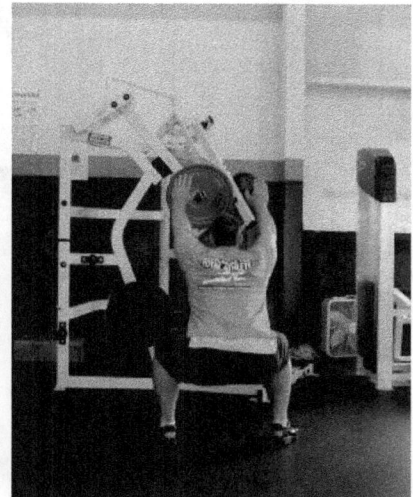

LW Pivot and Turn Squat

Carioca Movement

- Going Left
  - Start feet shoulder width apart (base position)
  - Moving left, cross right foot in front of left foot
  - Continuing left, step out to the side with left foot to base position
  - Moving left, cross right foot behind left foot
  - Continuing left, step out to the side with left foot to base position
  - Continue left repeating same foot pattern

- Going Right
  - Start feet shoulder width apart (base position)
  - Moving right, cross left foot in front of right foot
  - Continuing right, step out to the side with right foot to base position
  - Moving right, cross left foot behind right foot
  - Continuing right, step out to the side with right foot to base position
  - Continue right repeating same foot pattern

Long Carioca

- Working on developing explosive hip rotation
- Using Carioca movement
- When crossing leg in front drive (i.e., snap) the knee up high to waist height or higher
- Movement is done at a controlled pace
- Emphasize snapping the hip up every time the lead leg crosses in front

Short Carioca

- Using Carioca movement, concentrating on moving quickly and minimizing foot contact time
- Open up hip more
- Use short quick steps
- Stay on toes
- Perform in each direction as quickly as possible

Lateral Skip

- Moving laterally starting with feet together
- To the right
  - Step out to the right and drive the right knee up to hip height while skipping up using the left foot
  - Stay on toes
  - Repeat
- To the Left
  - Step out to the left and drive the left knee up to hip height as while skipping up using the right foot
  - Stay on toes
  - Repeat

Backward Movements

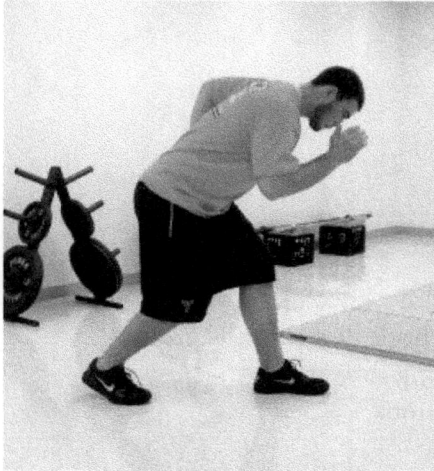

Backward - Correct body position   Backward - <u>Incorrect</u> body position

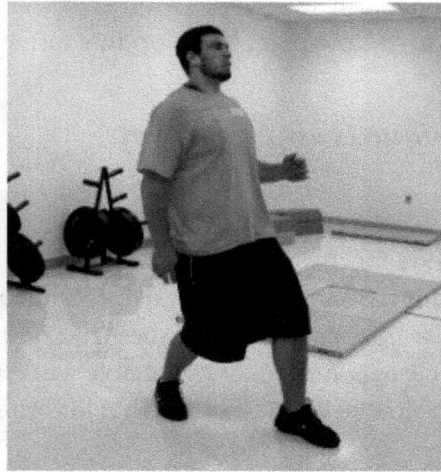

Backward Shuffle

- Similar to a five-cone shuffle without cones, but instead of moving forward move in backward direction, shuffling in a zigzag pattern while moving
- Use 45-degree drop steps to start the lateral shuffle and to change directions in the zigzag
- Use good shuffling technique, keeping the hips low
- Decelerate, drop and drive to change direction in the zigzags

Backward Run

- Lean forward keeping the chest over the feet to help maintain balance in all backwards movements
- Accentuate the backward kick of the back leg
- Drive that leg back while also reaching back with the back leg
- Push off the front foot and use proper arm swing
- Start with a slow pace, build up to a faster pace
- Do not sacrifice stride length (reaching back with leg/foot) for speed

Backpedal

- Lean forward, keeping the chest over the feet to help maintain balance in all backwards movements
- Use shorter, more natural stride than was used with the backward run
- Push off the front foot and use proper arm swing
- Start with a slow pace, build up to a faster pace

Backward Skip

- Lean forward keeping the chest over the feet to help maintain balance in all backwards movements
- Skip backwards off toes with ankles plantar flexed

- Drive front knee high and dorsiflex ankle
- Then drive foot down for next skip
- Use proper arm swing
- Start with a slow pace, build up to a faster pace

Speed Technique (Fast Movements)

<u>High Knees</u>

- Front side mechanics
  - o Front leg – ankle dorsiflexed, toes up and drive knee up to hip height
  - o Back leg – extend up on toes (run on toes, heels never hit the ground)
  - o Cycle legs as quickly as possible while moving forward
- Go at a slow pace, cycle through a lot of repetitions

<u>A Walk</u>

- The A walk combines features of the high knee and butt kick drill
  - o The front knee comes up high like with the high knee drill
  - o The heel of the front foot comes back as close to the butt as possible like in the butt kick drill
- The front foot stays dorsiflexed and is kicked out in front
- Back foot plantar flexes as while going up on toes
- Arms swing using proper running form

<u>A Skip</u>

- Same movement as the A walk, but a faster pace
- Add a skip with the back leg
- Front toe remains dorsiflexed
- Arms swing using proper running form

<u>Heel Kicks</u>

- Back side mechanics
  - o Front leg – extend up on toes (run on toes, heels never hit the ground)
  - o Back leg – ankle dorsiflexed, drive heel up to hamstrings, knee should come forward (leg should not be straight down from hip)
    - ▪ to reinforce good technique you should not be kicking yourself in the backside
    - ▪ instead the knee should come naturally forward and not back. Think about sliding the heel up a wall so that you stay compact and not creating backwards action (by staying compact you are cycling the foot back quickly to prepare for the foot to be driven back in the ground)
  - o Cycle legs as quickly as possible while moving forward
- Go at a slow pace, cycle through a lot of repetitions

Plyometric Linear Warm-Up Movement

<u>Ankle Hops</u>

- From the toes (plantarflexed position), gently hop up and down in place or over a set distance

<u>Ankle Flips</u>

- Balance on the heels, pulling up toes into a dorsiflexed position
- Take short steps, walk on heels

<u>Power Skip</u>

- Skipping powerfully
- Drive lead knee high
- Use arm swing to drive body upwards
- Powerfully triple extend with back leg skipping as high as you can

Cool-Down

- The cool-down period is 5-10 minutes of static stretching and core conditioning. The static stretching component, for enhancing flexibility, is individually prescribed by the coaches based on the specific flexibility needs of the athlete and the sport. Targeted muscle groups should be stretched for 1–3 repetitions with a 30-second static hold each time. Perform stretches for both sides of the body.

<u>Shoulder Stretch</u>

- Reach one arm across chest at shoulder height
- Give a gentle pull with other hand just past elbow
- Pull arm into and across chest to stretch the deltoids (shoulder)

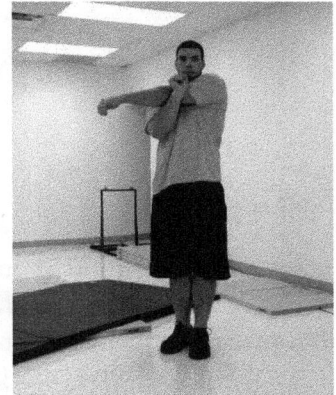

Shoulder Stretch

<u>Triceps Stretch</u>

- Reach one arm up and bend elbow dropping hand behind the neck so that elbow points up
- Reach the other hand up to place it on the top of the elbow
- Gently pull the elbow towards head to stretch the triceps
- An alternative is to place hand on the triceps and push arm up from underneath

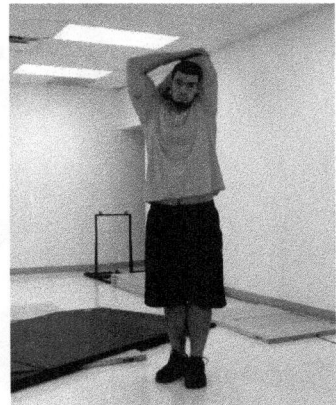

Triceps Stretch

Backward Lunge with a Twist Stretch

- Start with feet together, then step back into a lunge (knees at 90/90)
- Reach straight up with the arm on the side of back leg
- Reach out to the side with the arm on the front leg side
- Turn into the side of the front leg stretching the quads and hip flexors of the back leg

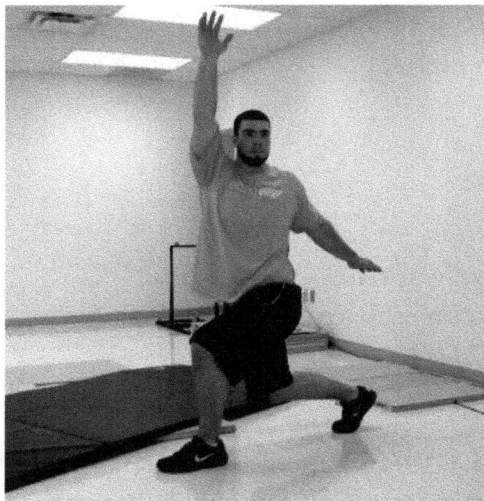

Back Lunge with a Twist Stretch

Side Lunge Stretch

- Start with feet shoulder width apart
- Step out to the right side, keep toes pointed straight ahead
- Squat down, sit into the right leg and keep left leg straight
- Squat as deeply as is comfortable to stretch inner thigh

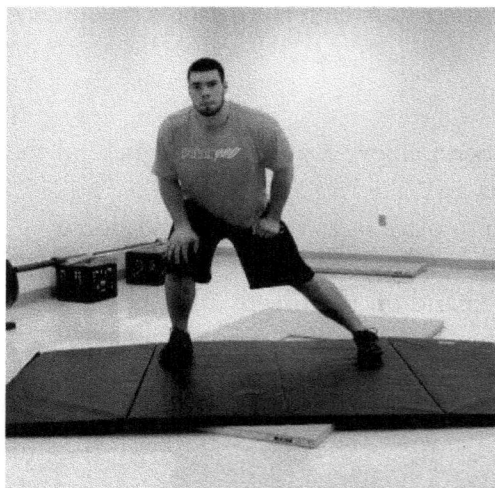

Side Lunge Stretch

Calf Stretch

- From a push-up position, cross one foot on top of the other heel
- With hips up high, pull toes towards the shin while pushing heel down towards the ground to stretch the ankle and calf
- Flexing the knee will shift emphasis of the stretch to the Achilles tendon
- This stretch can be performed by raising the heel up and then pushing the heel down for a couple seconds 2-3 times over a 30 second stretching duration

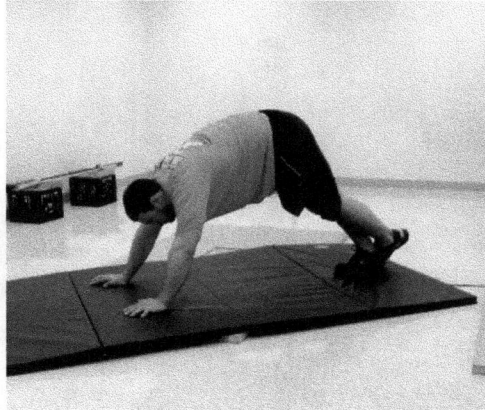

Calf Stretch

Modified Hurdlers Stretch

- Sit down with both legs extended out front, pull one foot back so that foot rests flat against other thigh
- Bend at the hip, shift the weight of upper body forward while bending towards the toes of the extended leg
- Reach forward until to feel a stretch in the hamstrings of the extended leg (you don't have to be able to touch your toes for the stretch to be effective)

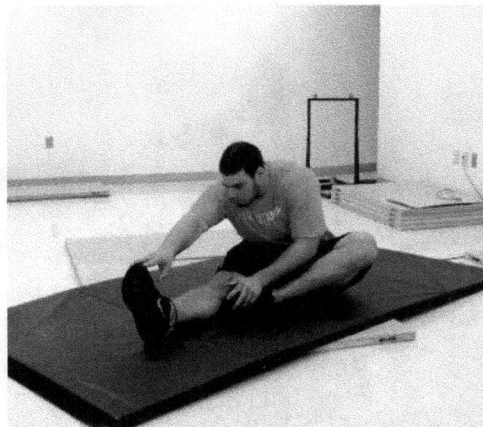

Modified Hurdlers Stretch

Butterfly Stretch

- Start with feet together and legs straight out in front
- Flex knees and pull bottom of the feet together and as close as comfortable to the trunk
- Keep back straight, place hands on the ankles and let knees drop towards the ground
- To accentuate the groin stretch, use forearms to gently push knees closer to the ground

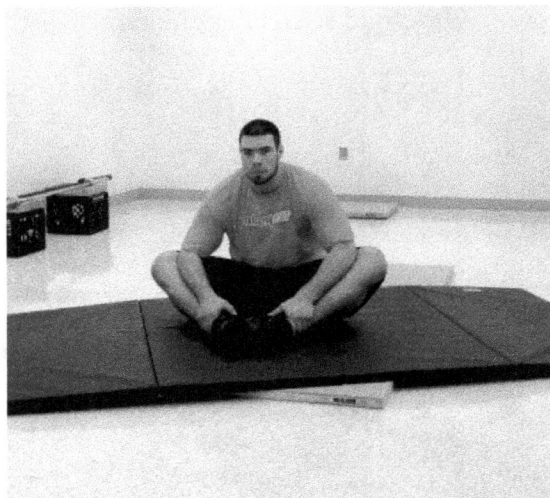

Butterfly Stretch

Lower Back Stretch

- Lie down facing up,
- Flex knee and bring it up towards chest
- Place hands on knee, gently pull leg to chest to stretch lower back
- This stretch can be done with both legs at the same time or with each leg individually

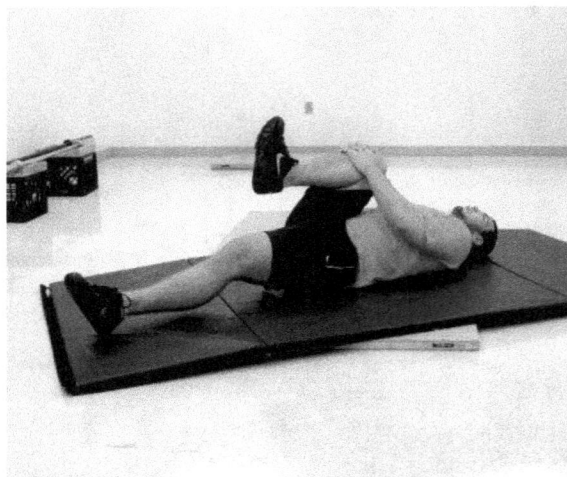

Lower Back Stretch

Hip (Piriformis) Stretch

- Lie on back with knees bent and feet flat on floor
- Cross one leg over, place ankle on top of the other knee
- Lift the leg (the leg that still has a foot on the ground) up and pull knee back to stretch the hip/piriformis
- Accentuate the stretch by either using hands to pull back gently on the thigh of the back leg or placing one hand on the ankle and the other hand on the knee of the cross leg and gently push on knee

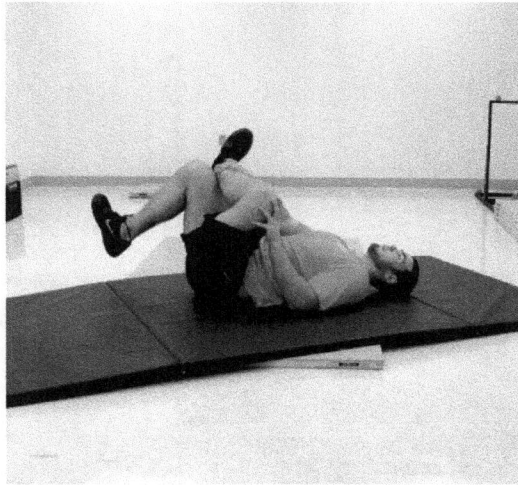

Hip (Piriformis) Stretch

Crossover Stretch

- Lie on back, face up and stretch out arms to the side
- Lift one leg straight up and lower leg across body towards the ground to stretch outer hip

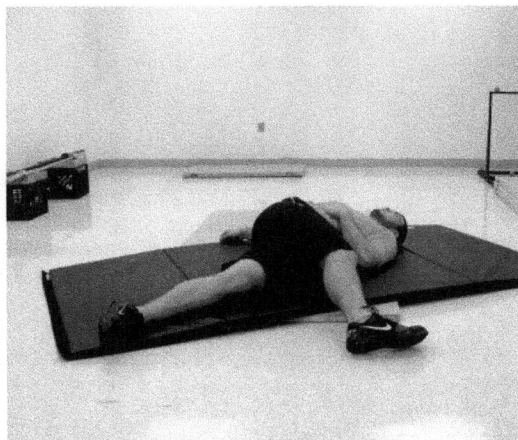

Crossover Stretch

References: Chapter 4

Sections in this chapter are adapted from previously published books by Dornemann and O'Dell:

1. Dornemann, T. M. *POWERREV Youth Athletic Development Program: Building Champions in Sports and in Life.* Ronkonkoma, NY: Linus, 2016.

2. O'Dell, S. *The Power Revolution: A Sports Performance Guide to Achieving Maximum Power.* Monterey, CA: Coaches Choice, 2015.

5
CORE TRAINING

By: Tim Dornemann, Ed. D., CES, PES, CSCS, OS Pro

Exercise Science Program & Kinesiology Director, Barton College
Associate Professor of Exercise Science, Barton College

CORE CONDITIONING STRENGTHS the abdominal and lower back muscles by enhancing muscular endurance. Strengthening these areas helps to prevent injury and enhances athletic performance. Specifically, core training that targets the lower back helps prevent lower back injuries that commonly occur in youth sports. Core strength helps tie the upper- and lower-body together; a strong core allows forces generated by the lower-body to be effectively transferred to the upper-body and vice versa. A weak core causes force to be lost between the upper- and lower-body, which negatively affects performance.

PowerRev core training includes four primary isometric exercises that can be modified by altering one's base width and changing arm and leg positions to make the exercise easier or harder:

Core Exercise	Muscle Group that is Activated and Strengthened	How to Modify
Floor Bridge	Glute Muscles	Raise and lower legs
Front Plank	Abdominal Muscles	More difficult when the base is narrowed (move arms closer together to decrease the stability) or when raising an arm and the opposite leg
Side Plank	Oblique Abdominal Muscles	More difficult by balancing on one leg, lift top leg or remove bottom leg from the base
Quad Exercise	Lower Back	More difficult when the base is narrowed (move feet and legs closer together to decrease the stability)

Core training should be done for 5-10 minutes at the end of each training session. PowerRev recommends using multiple sets of shorter holds initially with each exercise. A basic progression of the front plank entails holding a wide base plank for 5 seconds six times and progressing up to holding the plank position for a full 30 seconds. Once longer holds are established, the intensity can be increased by narrowing the base. After the exercise is mastered using a narrow base, manipulating the exercise can be done by raising the arms or legs to make the exercise more difficult. The final progression involves being able to perform an extended hold of a front plank with a narrow base and one arm and the opposite leg raised. The floor bridge, quad and side plank exercises can be progressed in a similar manner.

Altering the Base of the Primary Core Exercises

The front plank and quad can be modified by altering base width to make the exercises easier or harder.

Front Plank Bases

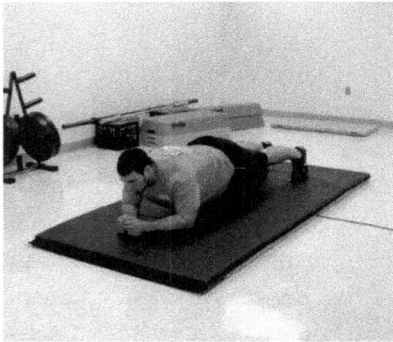

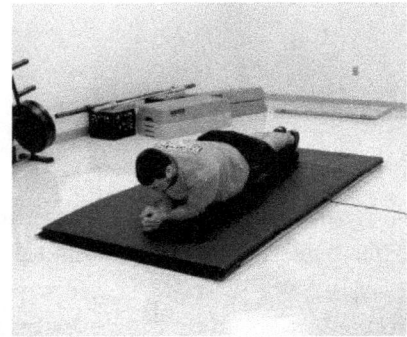

Wide Base Front Plank   Medium Base Front Plank   Narrow Base Front Plank

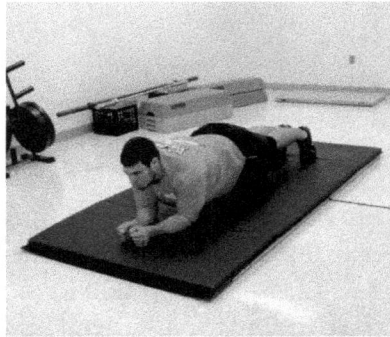

- *Wide Base Starting Position*
  Four points of contact, toes and elbows/forearms (both shoulder width apart)

- *Medium Base Starting Position*
  Four points of contact, toes and elbows/forearms (both elbows and toes 3-6 inches or 10 cm apart)

- *Narrow Base Starting Position*
  Four points of contact, toes and elbows/forearms (elbows as narrow as possible and toes together)

Quad Bases

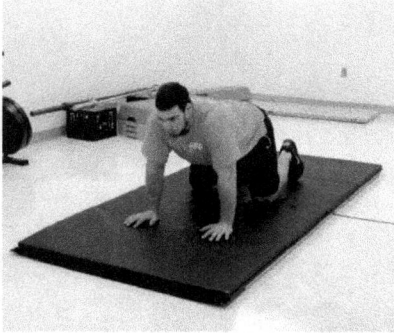

Wide Base Quad   Medium Base Quad   Narrow Base Quad

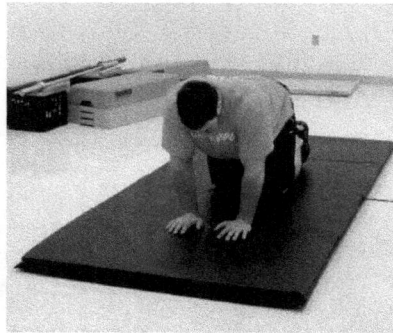

- ***Wide Base Starting Position***
  On hands and knees with back flat
  Place hands and knees shoulder width apart

- ***Medium Base Starting Position***
  On hands and knees with back flat
  Place hands and knees 3 - 6 inches (10 cm) apart

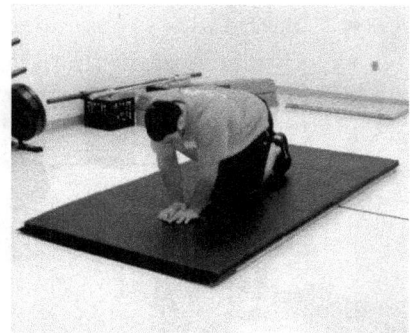

- ***Narrow Base Starting Position***
  On hands and knees with back flat
  Place hands together and knees together

Core Exercise Technique

Floor Bridge Series

<u>Floor Bridge</u>

- Starting Position - laying on back, knees bent shoulder width apart and toes pointed up
- Elevate hips so that knees, hips and shoulders are in a straight line
- Think of contracting glutes and pulling belly button to the spine
- Can be performed as repetitions (with a short hold) or as a prolonged hold

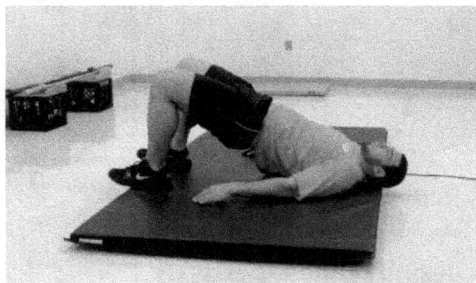

Floor Bridge (March)

- Starting Position - laying on back, knees bent shoulder width apart
- Elevate hips so that knees, hips and shoulders are in a straight line
- Think of contracting glutes and pulling belly button to the spine
- Lift one leg up with a 90-degree knee bend
- Can be performed as repetitions (with a short hold) or as a prolonged hold

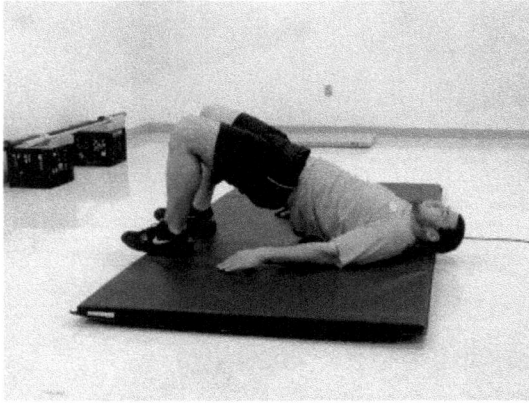

Floor Bridge March Bottom Position

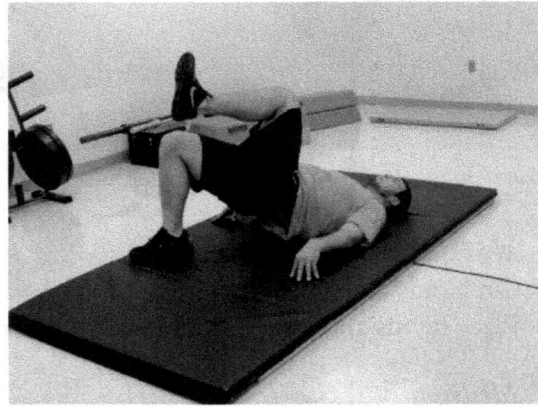

Floor Bridge March Top Position

Floor Bridge (90 degree hold)

- Starting Position - laying on back, knees bent shoulder width apart
- Elevate hips so that knees, hips and shoulders are in a straight line
- Think of contracting glutes and pulling belly button to the spine
- Lift one leg with 90 degree bent up, hold for 15 to 30 seconds and then alternate legs, hold other leg for 15 to 30 seconds
- Drop hips down to rest then repeat 5 to 10 times

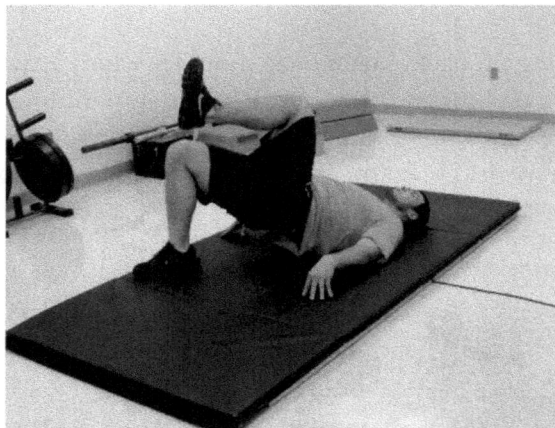

<u>Floor Bridge (Straight leg hold)</u>

- Starting Position - laying on back, knees bent shoulder width apart
- Elevate hips so that knees, hips and shoulders are in a straight line
- Think of contracting glutes and pulling belly button to the spine
- Lift one leg up in a straight position, hold for 15 to 30 seconds and then alternate legs, hold other leg for 15 to 30 seconds
- Drop hips down to rest then repeat 5 to 10 times

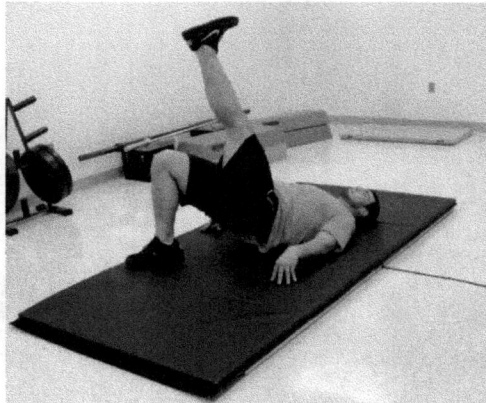

Quad Series

<u>Wide Base Quad</u>

- Starting Position – on hands and knees with back flat
- Place hands and knees shoulder width apart
- Elevate one arm and opposite leg so that a straight line can be drawn from toes to fingertips
- Do not raise arms and legs too high causing back to arch
- Can be performed as repetitions (with a short hold) or as a prolonged hold
- Alternate combination of arms and legs raised each repetition

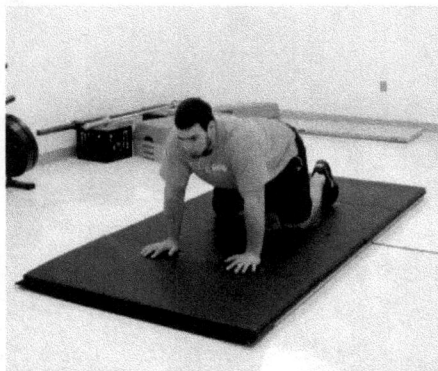

Wide Base Quad Bottom Position   Wide Base Quad Top Position Picture

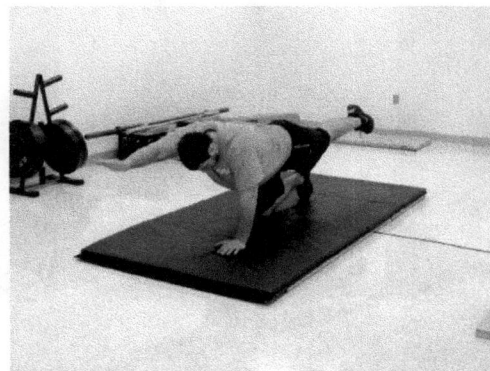

Medium Base Quad

- Starting Position – on hands and knees with back flat
- Place hands and knees 3-6 inches (10 cm) apart
- Elevate one arm and opposite leg so that a straight line can be drawn from toes to fingertips
- Do not raise arms and legs too high causing back to arch
- Can be performed as repetitions (with a short hold) or as a prolonged hold
- Alternate combination of arms and legs raised each repetition

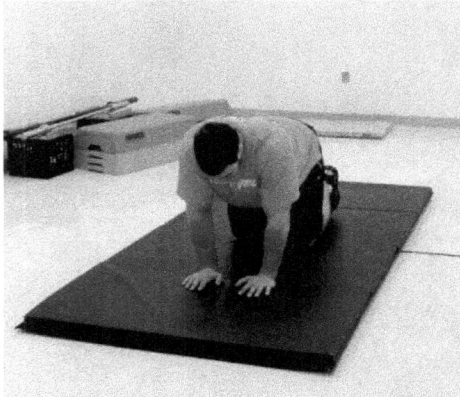

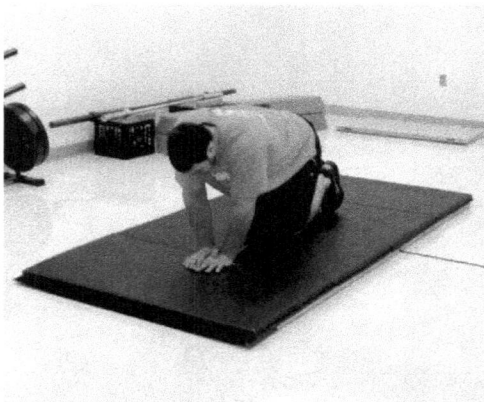

Medium Base Quad Bottom Position   Medium Base Quad Top Position

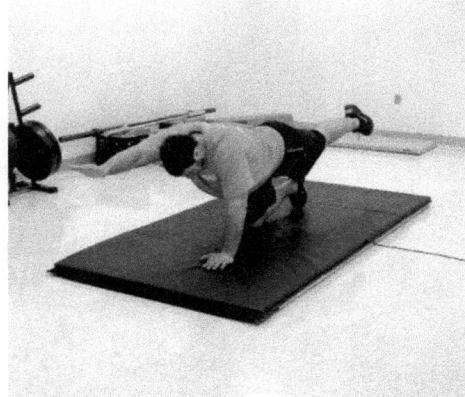

Narrow Base Quad

- Starting Position – on hands and knees with back flat
- Place hands together and knees together
- Elevate one arm and opposite leg so that a straight line can be drawn from toes to fingertips
- Do not raise arms and legs too high causing back to arch
- Can be performed as repetitions (with a short hold) or as a prolonged hold
- Alternate combination of arms and legs raised each repetition

Narrow Base Quad Bottom Position   Narrow Base Quad Top Position

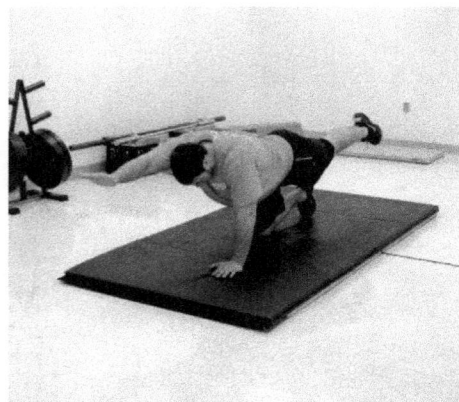

Front Plank Series

<u>Wide Base Front Plank</u>

- Starting Position – four points of contact, toes and elbows/forearms (both shoulder width apart)
- Body should form straight line from shoulders through ankles
- Draw in abdominals (pulling belly button to spine)
- Can be performed as repetitions (with a short hold) or as a prolonged hold
- Transfer from toes to knees for rest position

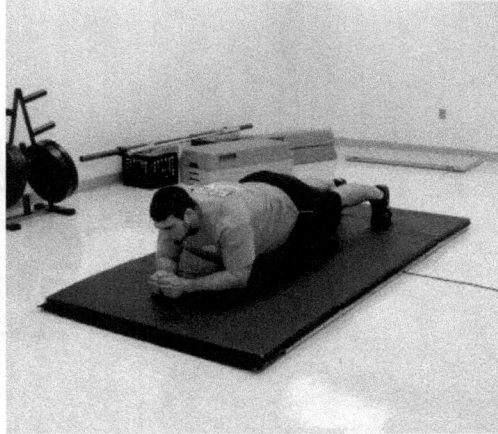

<u>Medium Base Front Plank</u>

- Starting Position – four points of contact, toes and elbows/forearms (both elbows and toes 3-6 inches or 10 cm apart)
- Body should form straight line from shoulders through ankles
- Draw in abdominals (pulling belly button to spine)
- Can be performed as repetitions (with a short hold) or as a prolonged hold
- Transfer from toes to knees for rest position

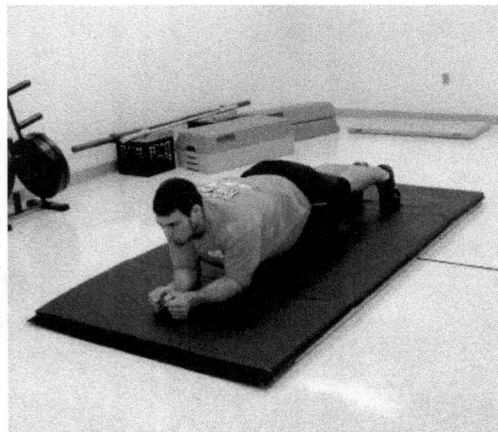

Arm or Leg Raise Front Plank

- Starting Position – four points of contact, toes and elbows/forearms (both elbows and toes 3-6 inches or 10 cm apart)
- Raise either one arm or one leg
- Body should form straight line from shoulders through ankles
- Draw in abdominals (pulling belly button to spine)
- Can be performed as repetitions (with a short hold) or as a prolonged hold
- Transfer from toes to knees for rest position

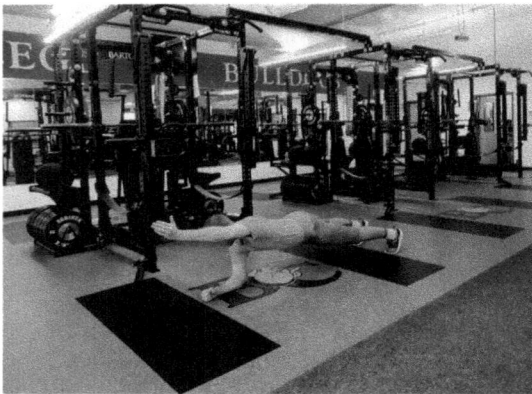

One Arm Raise Front Plank

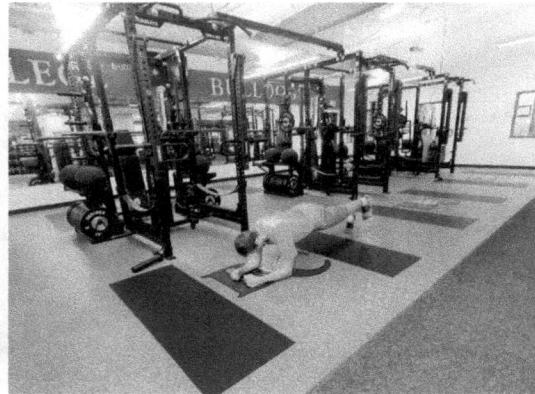

One Leg Raise Front Plank

Arm / Leg Raise Front Plank

- Starting Position – four points of contact, toes and elbows/forearms (elbows narrow as possible and toes together)
- Raise one arm and opposite leg (like in quad exercise)
- Body should form straight line from shoulders through ankles
- Draw in abdominals (pulling belly button to spine)
- Can be performed as repetitions (with a short hold) or as a prolonged hold
- Transfer from toes to knees for rest position

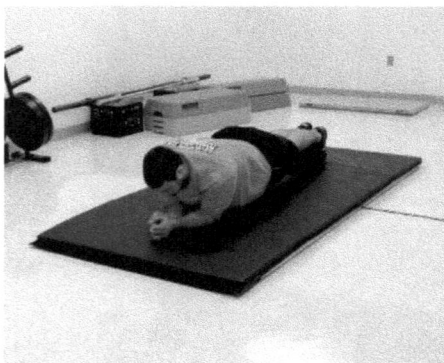

Narrow Base Plank

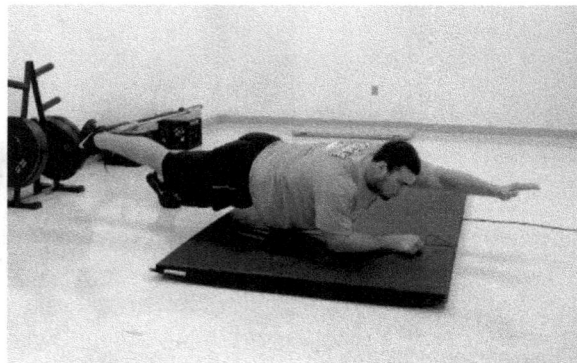

Arm/Leg Raise Front Plank with Narrow Base

Side Plank Series

<u>Side Plank</u>

- Starting Position – two points of contact one forearm and side of one foot (feet stacked position)
- Elevate hips, bringing body into a straight line
- Can be performed as repetitions (with a short hold) or as a prolonged hold
- Drop hips down for rest position

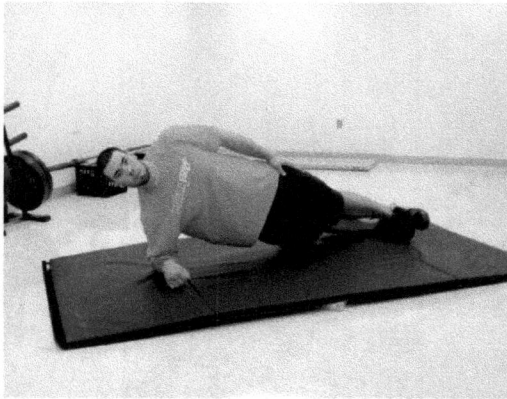

Side Plank front view

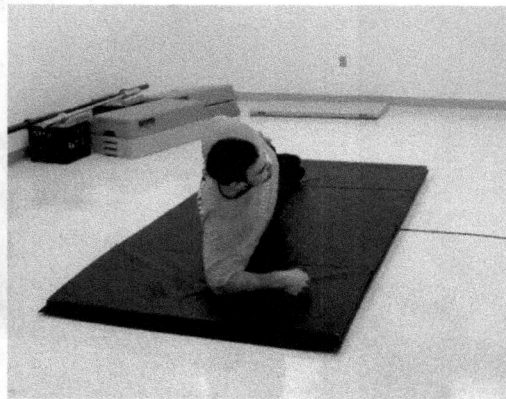

Side Plank side view

<u>Bottom Leg Lift Side Plank</u>

- Starting Position – two points of contact one forearm and side of one foot
- Rest on side of top foot, bending bottom leg out of the way
- Elevate hips, bringing body into a straight line
- Lift bottom leg up
- Can be performed as repetitions (with a short hold) or as a prolonged hold
- Drop hips down for rest position

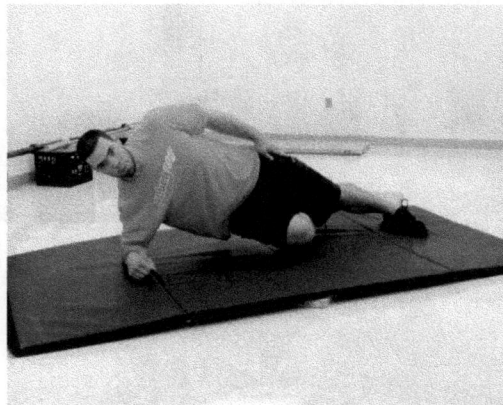

Top Leg Raise (Low) Side Plank

- Starting Position – two points of contact one forearm and side of one foot (feet stacked position)
- Elevate hips, bringing body into a straight line
- Lift top leg up 6-12 inches (or about 20 cm apart)
- Can be performed as repetitions (with a short hold) or as a prolonged hold
- Drop hips down for rest position

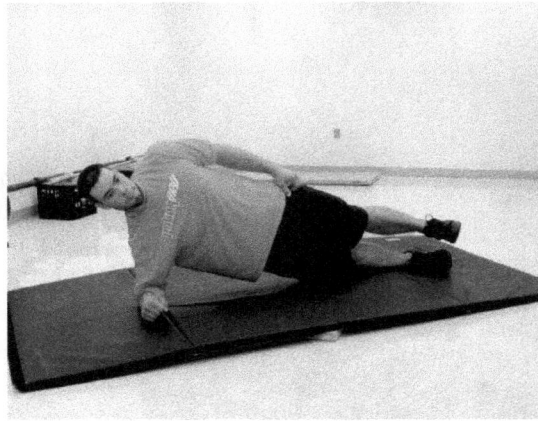

Top Leg Raise (high) Side Plank

- Starting Position – two points of contact one forearm and side of one foot (feet stacked position)
- Elevate hips, bringing body into a straight line
- Lift top leg up as high as you can
- Can be performed as repetitions (with a short hold) or as a prolonged hold
- Drop hips down for rest position

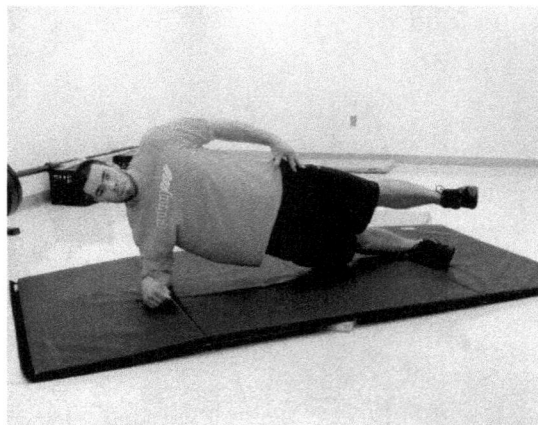

Traditional Body Weight Exercises

Back Extension

- Using a glute ham bench (like the one in the pictures below) or back extension bench, position the hip pad so that the end of the pad is placed on the top of the leg below where the hip bends
- With arms placed across your chest, flex trunk to lower the upper body to the 90 degree starting position
- Using the muscles in the lower back, extend the trunk and bring upper body up to the straight (180 degree) top position
- Do not place excess pressure on lower back by hyper extending past the straight (180 degree) top position

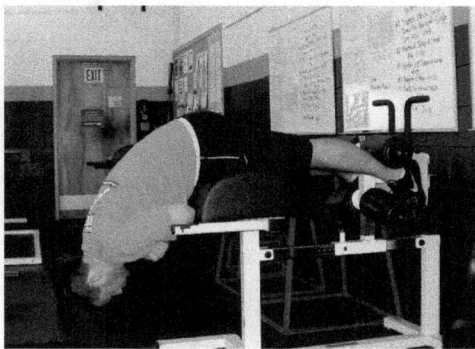

Back Extension Bottom Position

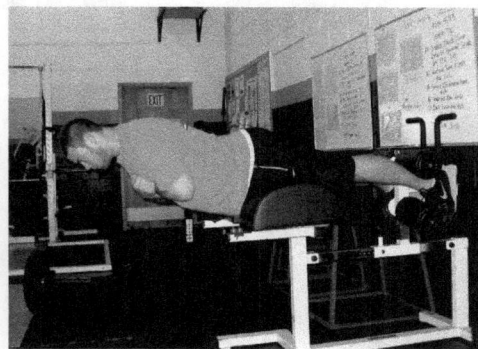

Back ExtensionTop Position

Knee-Ups/Leg Curl on Ball

- Start face up, with shoulders on the ground and arms stretched out to the sides at a 45 degree angle
- Dig heels into the ball as hips lift up forming a straight line from the shoulders to the ankles
- Keeping hips up, lift knees and pull the ball and heels towards hamstrings
- Keeping abdominal and gluteus maximus muscles tight in a slow and controlled manner, extend legs out (straight back) to the starting position

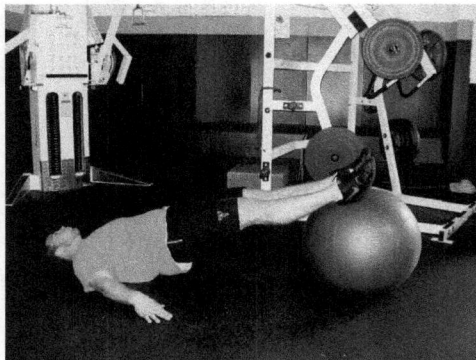

Ball Leg Curl Starting Position

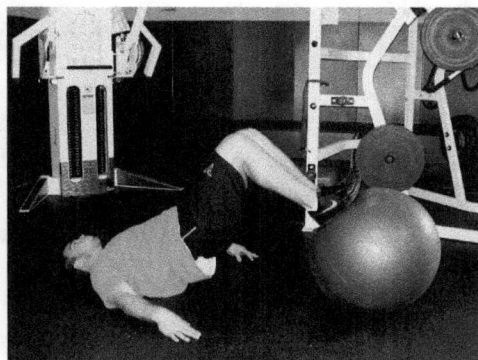

Ball Leg Curl Finishing position

Knees to Elbows

- Start face down in a push-up position with arms extended
- Place toes on top of ball, keeping body straight from the ankles through the shoulders
- Bend knees and bring the ball and knees forward towards elbows as knees are tucked into chest
- Extend legs straight back to the starting position
- Keeping abdominal and gluteus maximus muscles tight, tuck knees forward and then extend legs out straight in a slow and controlled manner

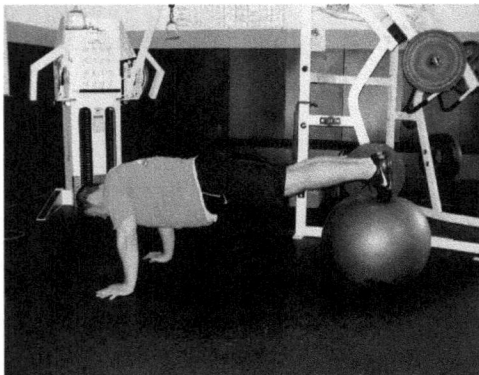

Knees to Elbows Starting Position

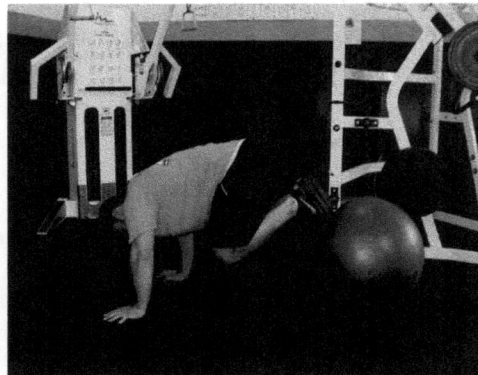

Knees to Elbows Finishing Position

Rotational Push-ups

- Start in a push-up position with arms extended
- Lower chest so that elbows are bent at 90 degrees
- Press up and rotate body to form a "T" while in an extended arm front plank
- Feet stacked on top of each other, body forms a straight line from between the feet to nose
- Reach top arm straight up to complete the "T"
- Rotate body back to the starting position

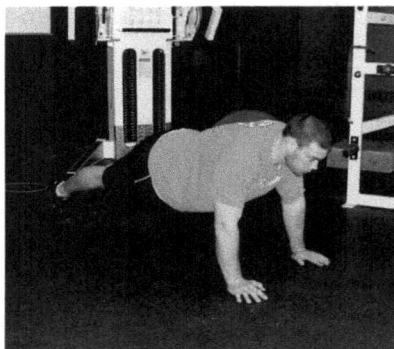

Rotational Push Up Starting Position

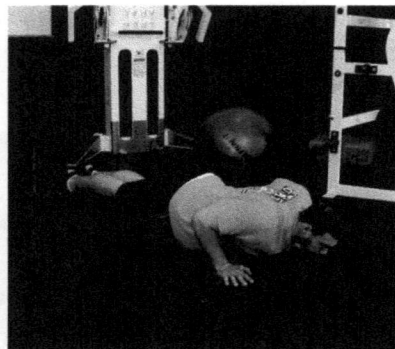

Rotational Push Up Middle Position

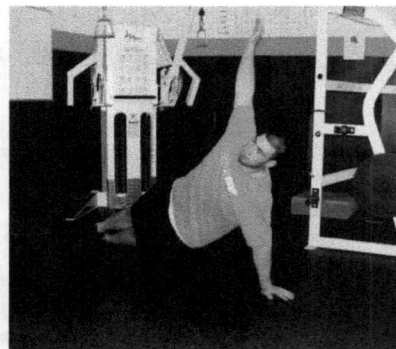

Rotational Push Up Finishing Position

Medicine Ball Slam

- Using a medicine ball for resistance, raise the ball above head, fully extending the body to engage the back and core muscles
- Forcefully throw the ball straight down in front of feet as hard as possible
- Repeat for the desired number of repetitions

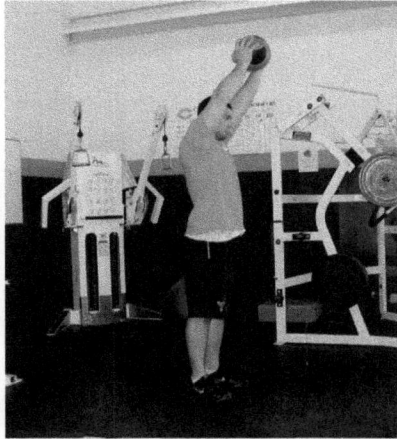

Slam Starting Position

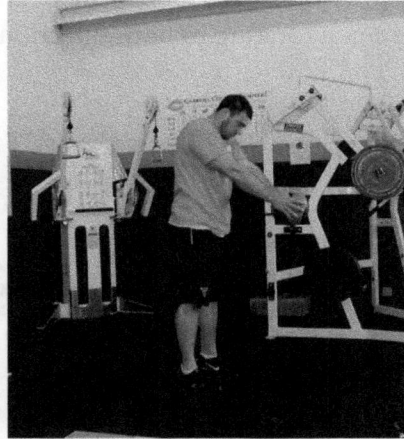

Slam Finishing Position

Overhead Medicine Ball Throw

- Using a medicine ball for resistance, raise the ball above head, fully extending the body to engage the back and core muscles
- The throwing mechanics are similar to the medicine ball slam, except that instead of throwing the ball straight down the goal is to throw the ball as far forward as possible
- Forcefully throw the ball forward as hard as possible
- Repeat for the desired number of repetitions

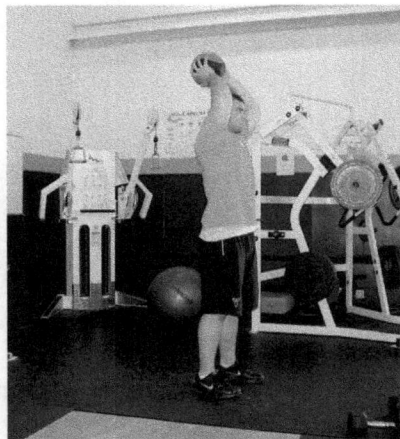

Overhead Ball Starting Position

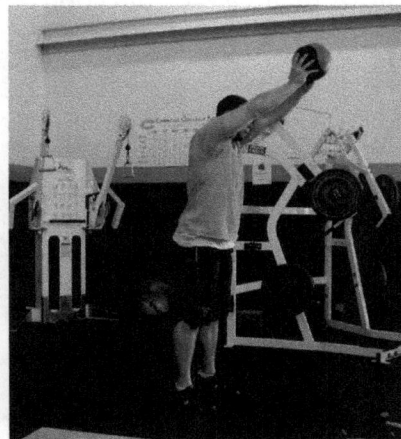

Overhead Ball Finishing Position

Rotational Core Exercises

<u>Medicine Ball Partner Rotation</u>

- Start standing back to back with a partner with feet shoulder width apart
- Keeping feet in the same spot, twist upper body to the left to receive the ball from partner
- Take the ball on the left side, twist torso and bring the ball to the right side
- Pass the ball off to partner so that they can complete their repetition
- Perform exercise rotating to both directions

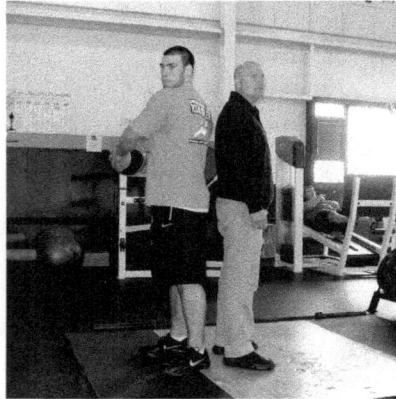

Partner Rotation Starting Position

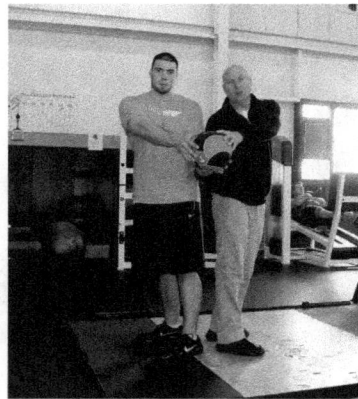

Partner Rotation Finishing Position

<u>Rotational Medicine Ball Throw</u>

- Start with feet shoulder width apart and knees bent (in good athletic position)
- Holding the ball with two hands, extend arms to one side with the ball at hip height
- Load body weight more towards the side of the ball
- Shift body weight while rotating torso and bring the ball diagonally across body
- Release the ball when arms are fully extended
- Perform throws rotating each direction

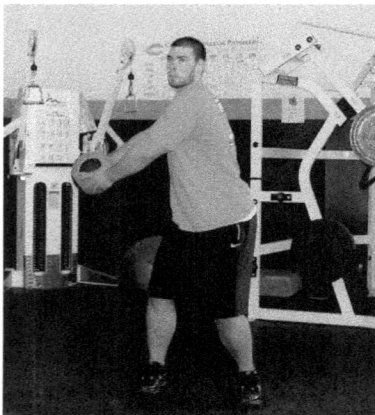

Rotational MB Throw Starting Position

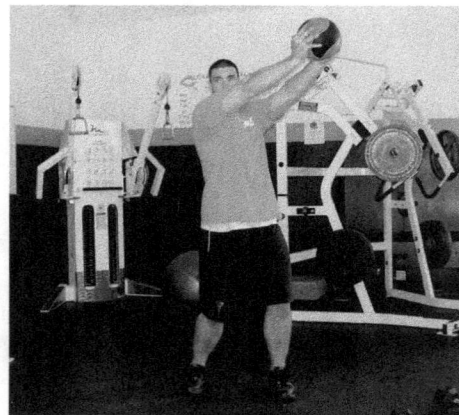

Rotational MB Throw Finishing Position

One Arm Rotational Row

- Start standing perpendicular to the attachment with knees slightly bent
- Reach across body with arm farthest away grabbing the handle at chest height
- Pull the band handle across body until hand is outside of the hip on the same side as the arm you are pulling with
- Inside arm swings and extends over the top while rotating
- Then rotate feet and hips 90 degrees
- Rotate back to the starting position
- Repeat movement with other side

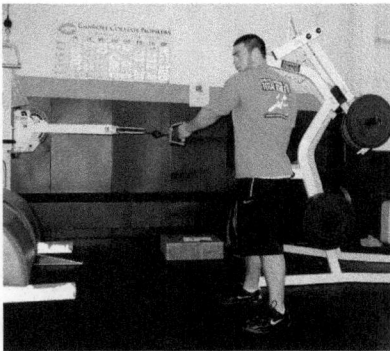

One Arm Rotational Row
Starting Position

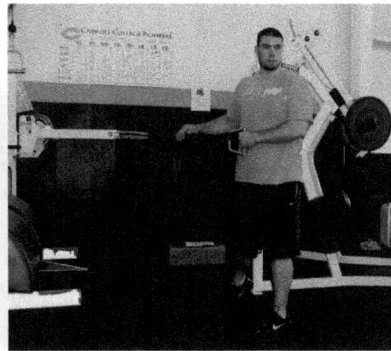

One Arm Rotational Row
Middle Position

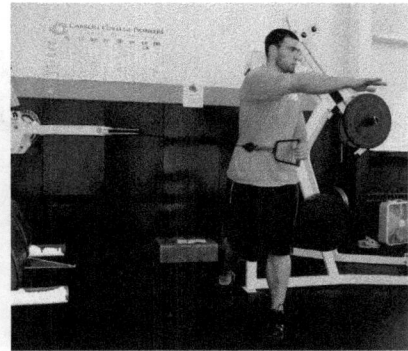

One Arm Rotational Row
Finishing Position

Lateral Chop

- Start standing perpendicular to the cable attachment (adjusted to about chest height) with knees slightly bent
- Reach across body with both hands grabbing the handle with both hands at chest height
- Pull the handle while rotating hips and feet 90 degrees
- When finished rotating hips and feet, extend arms out in front as if chopping wood with an ax
- Rotate back to the starting position
- Repeat movement with other side

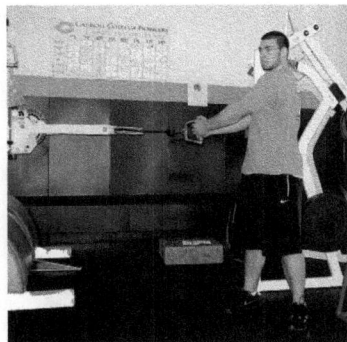

Lateral Chop Starting Position

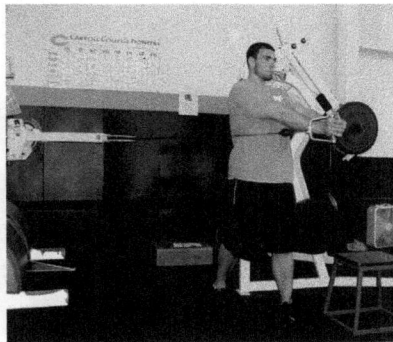

Lateral Chop Finishing Position

High/Low Chop

- Start standing perpendicular to the high cable attachment with knees slightly bent
- Reach up and across body with both hands grabbing the handle with both hands at about a height slightly higher than head
- Pull the handle down on an angle while rotating hips and feet 90 degrees
- When finished rotating hips and feet, extend your arms out in front maintaining the same angle as the initial pull down as if chopping wood with an ax
- Rotate back up to the starting position
- Repeat movement with other side

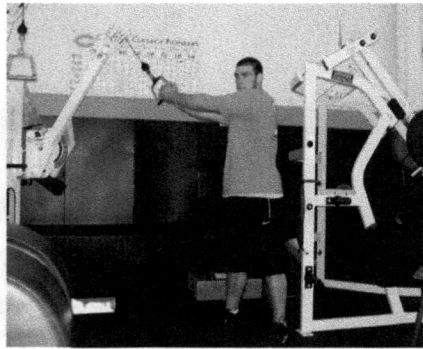

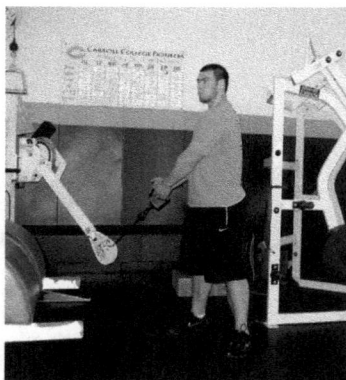

High low Starting Position   High low Finishing Position

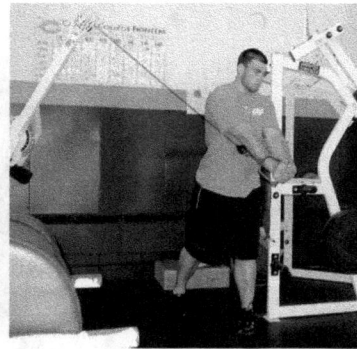

Low / High Chop

- Start standing perpendicular to the low cable attachment with knees slightly bent
- Reach up and across body with both hands grabbing the handle below hip height
- Pull the handle up on an angle while rotating hips and feet 90 degrees
- When finished rotating hips and feet, extend arms out in front maintaining the same angle as the initial pull up as if chopping wood with an ax
- Rotate back up to the starting position
- Repeat movement with other side

Low high Starting Position   Low high Finishing Position

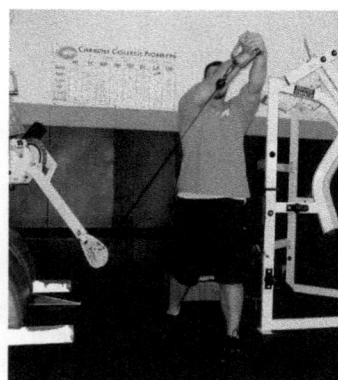

References: Chapter 5

Sections in this chapter are adapted from a previously published book by Dornemann:

1. Dornemann, T. M. PowerRev "Four Laws of Victory" Character Development Program: Build successful teams and athletes by teaching lessons that transcend sports, 2016, Ronkonkoma, NY: Linus

6
STRENGTH DEVELOPMENT & LIFTING TECHNIQUES

By: Tim Dornemann, Ed. D., CES, PES, CSCS, OS Pro

Exercise Science Program & Kinesiology Director, Barton College
Associate Professor of Exercise Science, Barton College

Part 1: Lower Body Exercises

SQUATS ARE A primary lower body exercise. Lunge variations, deadlift and lower level squat variations can be used as secondary lower body movements. The Romanian deadlift and good morning exercises are used to train posterior chain musculature.

Squat Series

Body Weight Squat

- Start with feet slightly wider than shoulder width, toes angled slightly out and arms extend in front at shoulder height for balance
- Push the hips back sticking the butt out, keeping chest forward to balance out body
- Lower the hips down and back with the feet flat and the pressure on the heels
- Lower the hips down and back until the hips are lower than the knees (or top of the thigh parallel to the ground)
- Upon reaching the lower point of the descent, drive back up through the heels while also driving the hips forward to keep the chest up

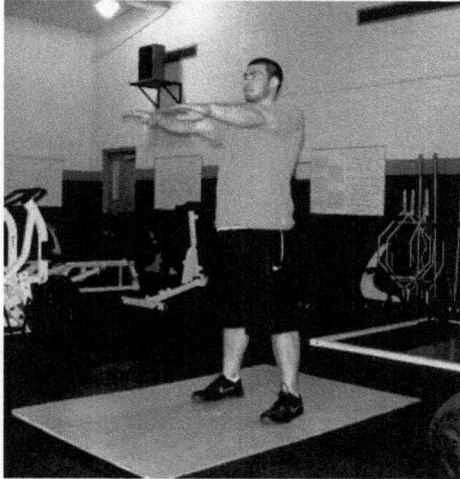

Body Weight Squat Top Position

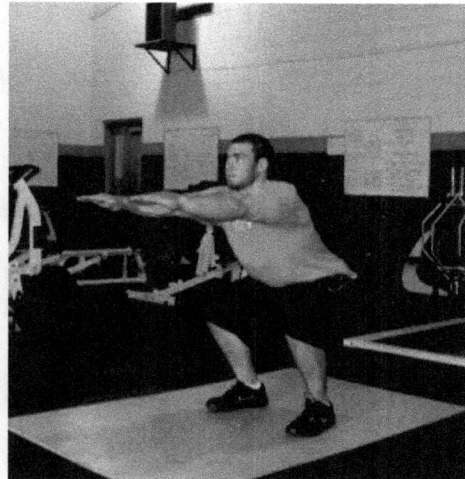

Body Weight Squat Bottom Position

Overhead Squat

- Start with dowel, stick or light weight bar to learn and practice good form
- With a snatch width grip, place the bar overhead slightly behind or directly above the ears
  - Raise arms to shoulder height
  - Bend elbows to 90-degrees
  - Maintaining that hand width, grab bar with over hand grip
  - Extend arms as bar is raised overhead
- While performing the lower body squatting movement, gradually rotate the bar back as you go down
- Overhead squat can build flexibility and reveal tightness in shoulder, ankle and hip joints

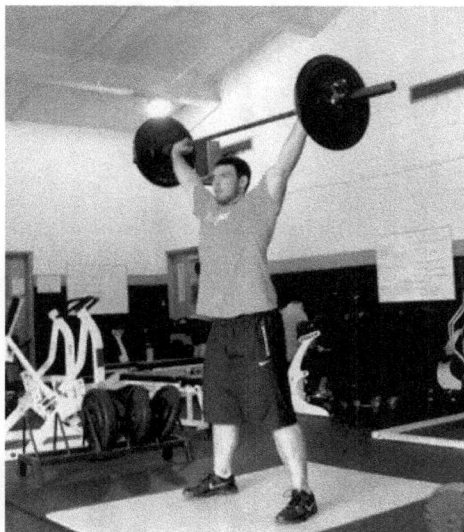

Overhead Squat Top Position

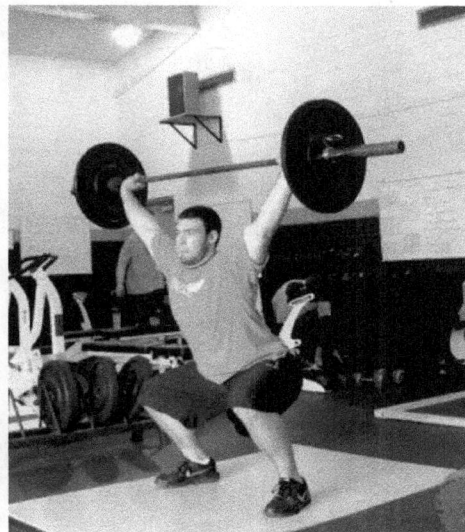

Overhead Squat Bottom Position

Front Squat

- Hands are placed with a grip slightly wider than shoulder width
- Barbell should rest on the upper chest and shoulders
- Pushing the elbows up and inward will form a rack on which the bar will rest while also keeping the chest up during the movement
  - Clean grip or crossover grip
- While performing the lower body squatting movement, focus on keeping the elbows up the entire time and therefore keeping the chest up.

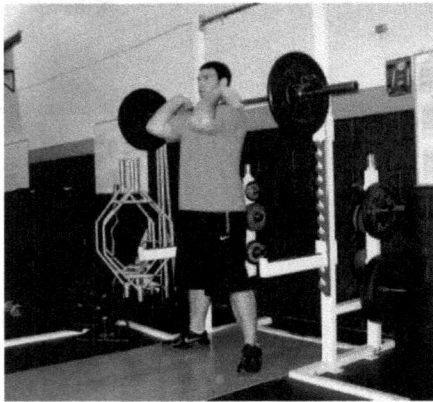

Clean Grip Front Squat Top Position

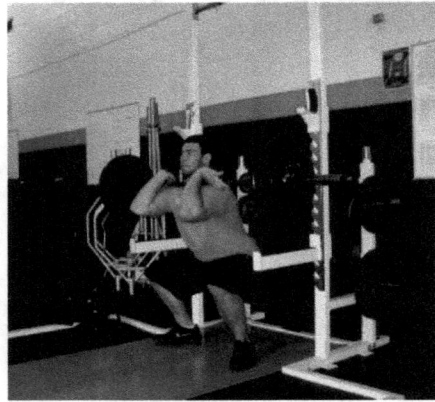

Clean Grip Front Squat Bottom

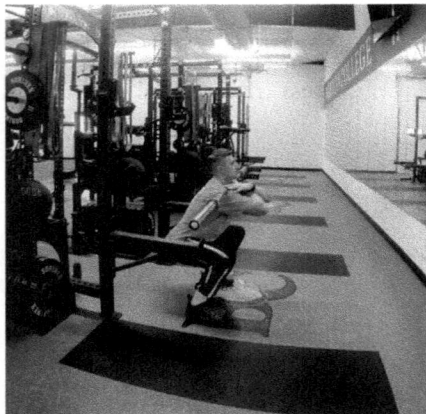

Crossover Grip Front Squat
Top Position

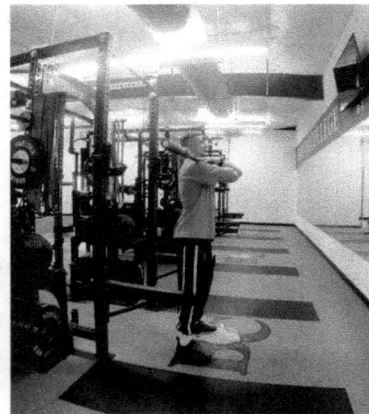

Crossover Grip Front Squat
Bottom Positio

Back Squat

- Squeeze the shoulders back and place the bar high on top of the shoulder muscles
- Perform the squatting movement
- While coming up, push through the heels and drive the hips forward, keeping the chest up

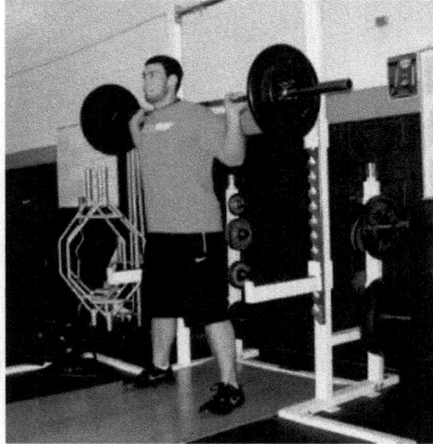

Back Squat Top Position

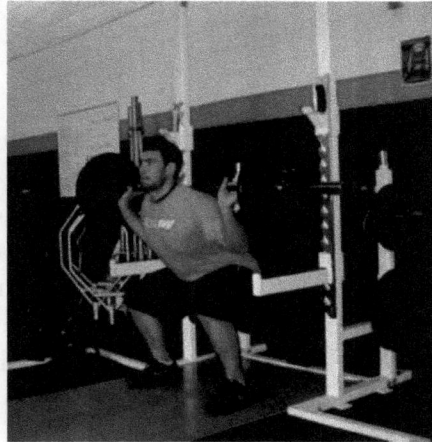

Back Squat Bottom Position

Deadlift

Clean Deadlift (Deadlift from Clean starting position)

- Feet at hip width, hands should be placed on the bar just outside of legs (using overhand or alternating grip)
- Barbell in close to the body with arms straight and elbows rotated out
- Shoulder blades should be squeezed back with the chest as high as possible
- Hips are higher than the knees, but lower than the shoulders
- Eyes straight ahead
- Raise up hips slowly, pulling bar off ground
- Maintain consistent back angle as you extend your hips and legs, pulling the bar to hip height
- Finish lift with slight back hyperextension and shoulders pulled back (retracted)

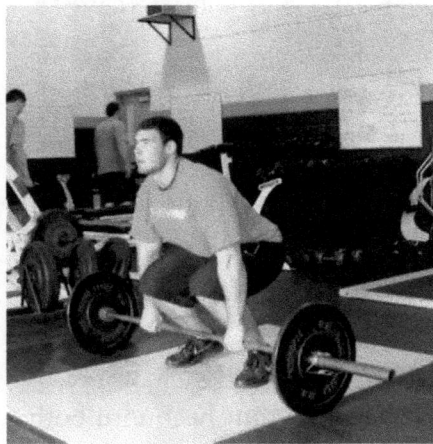

Deadlift Bottom Position

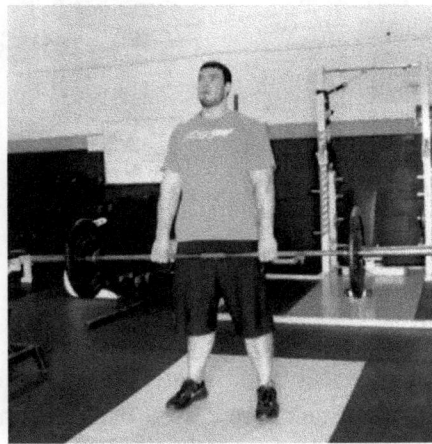

Deadlift Top Position

Lunge Series

Front Lunge

- Start with the feet underneath the hips and lined up evenly with each other
- Take an over-exaggerated step forward
- Drop the hips straight down into 90-degree bend of both front and back legs
    - Proper stride length places front knee over the ball of the foot
    - Too long of a stride places knee over heel or back leg is extended past 90 degrees
    - Too short of a stride places front knee in front of toes
- Drive through the front heel and pull with the back foot to return to the starting position
- Alternate legs throughout the set

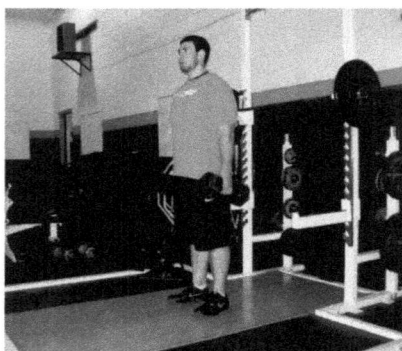

Front Lunge (DB) Top Position

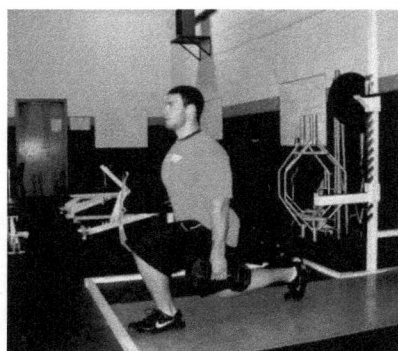

Front Lunge (DB) Bottom Position

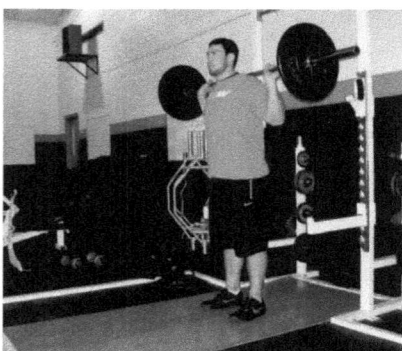

Front Lunge (Bar) Top Position

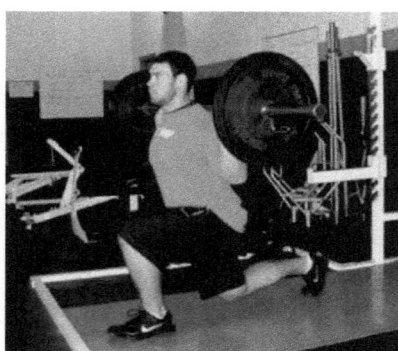

Front Lunge (Bar) Bottom Position

Back Lunge

- Start with the feet underneath the hips and lined up evenly with each other
- Take an over-exaggerated step back, sitting back into the front heel until both front and back knees are bent at 90 degrees
- Same stride length cues apply as front lunge
- Push through the front heel driving the hips forward and returning the back foot to the starting position

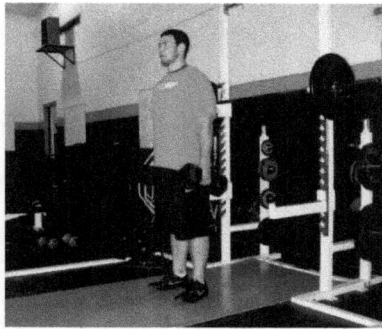

Back Lunge (DB) Top Position

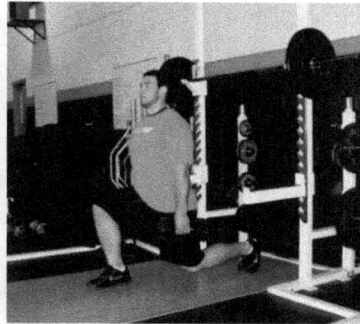

Back Lunge (DB) Bottom Position

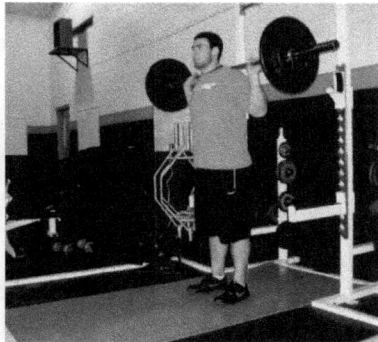

Back Lunge (Bar) Top Position

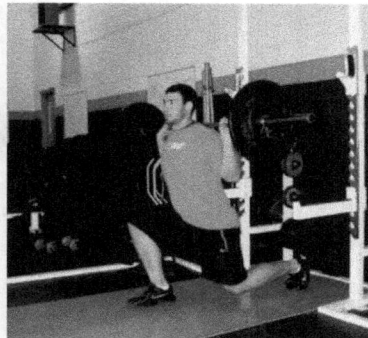

Back Lunge (Bar) Bottom Position

Side Lunge

- Start with feet shoulder width apart
- Take an exaggerated step out to the side keeping toes pointed forward
- Drop hips down bending knee of lead leg to 90 degrees
- As you drop down, sit hips back, leaning chest forward to balance body
- Trail leg is extended with slight knee bend
- Push off lead leg back to standing position
- Alternate movement to both sides

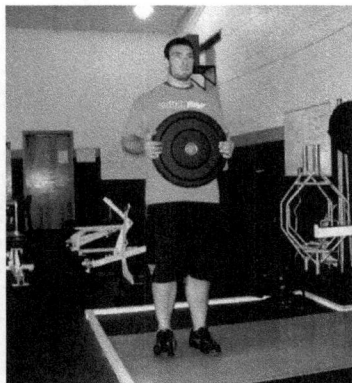

Side Lunge Top Position

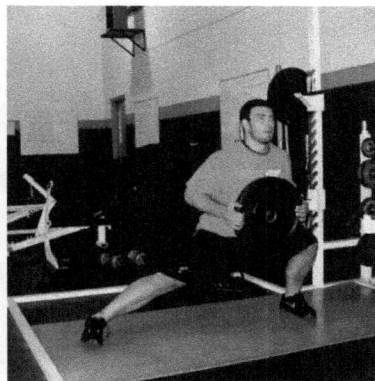

Side Lunge Bottom Position

Posterior Leg Exercises

Romanian Deadlift (RDL)

- Stand upright, holding the barbell with the hands at the hip width
- Place a slight bend in the knees (knees straight but not locked)
- Stick chest out and squeeze the shoulders back with an over-exaggerated posture
- In a controlled manner, lower the bar down, keeping the bar behind the toes
- When lowering the bar, keep the shoulders squeezed back (with over-exaggerated posture) and the knees straight but not locked, lowering the bar by sticking the butt out (NOT bending the knees or rounding the back)

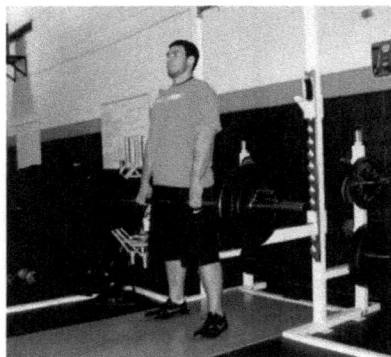

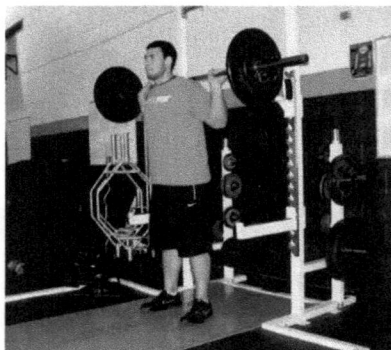

Romanian Deadlift Top Position   Romanian Deadlift Bottom Position

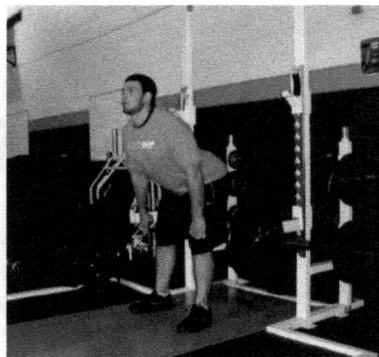

Good Morning Exercise

- Squeeze the shoulders back and place the barbell high on top of shoulders
- Place a slight bend in the knees (knees straight but not locked)
- Squeeze the shoulders back with an over-exaggerated posture
- In a controlled manner, lower the bar down, keeping the bar behind the toes
- When lowering the bar, keep the shoulders squeezed back (with over-exaggerated posture) and the knees straight but not locked, lowering the bar by sticking the butt out (NOT bending the knees or rounding the back)

Good Morning Top Position   Good Morning Bottom Position

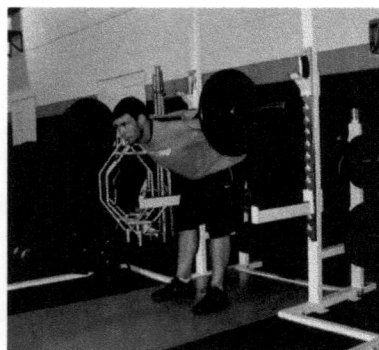

Calf Raise

- Use a step or platform, feet shoulder width apart (can use a stable block of wood that allows your heel to be off the ground, if no step or platform)
- Place balls of feet securely on edge
  - Placing too much of foot on edge limits range of motion
  - Putting too little of foot on edge increases risk of slipping off edge
- Use a wall or railing for balance (in front with two hands or to the side with one hand)
- Dorsiflex, dropping heels down
- Then plantarflex, raising up on balls of feet
- To add resistance, work one leg at a time or balance with one hand and hold a dumbbell or weight in the other hand

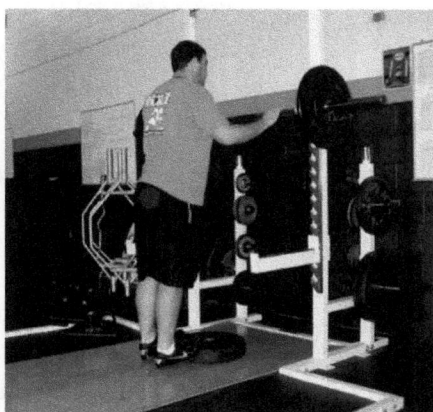

Calf Raise Top Position   Calf Raise Bottom Position

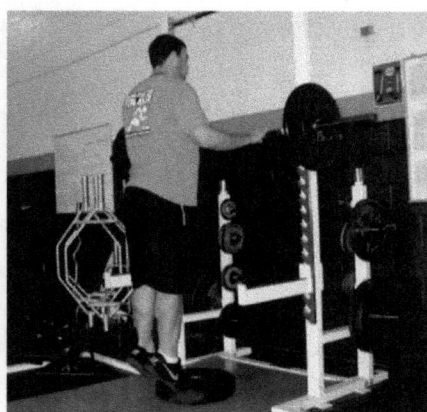

Calf Raise Variation Pictures

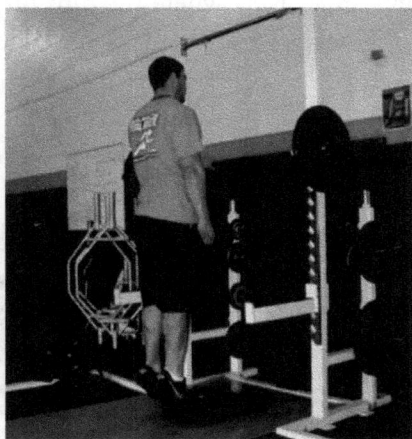

Two Leg DB Calf Raise (Top)   Two Leg DB Calf Raise (Bottom)

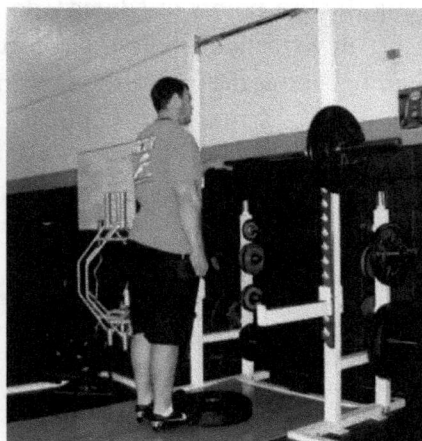

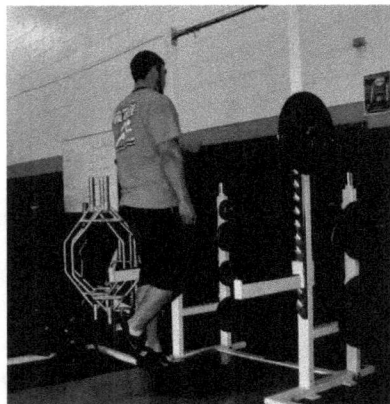

Single Leg DB Calf Raise (Top)

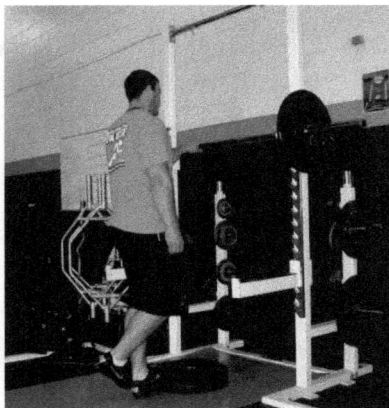

Single Leg DB Calf Raise (Bottom)

Part 2: Upper Body

The larger upper body muscle groups of the back and chest are targeted as primary areas.

Chest Exercises

Bench Press

- Lie back on bench establishing five points of contact (head, shoulders/back and buttocks) on the bench and right and left feet flat on floor
- Position body so that eyes are directly below the racked bar
- Using an overhand, closed grip, place your hands wide enough that your forearms are perpendicular to the floor in the bottom position of the lift
- With help of a spotter, lift the bar off the rack so that the bar is above the shoulders
- Slowly and under control, lower the bar to the chest, touching the chest in line with the nipples
- Maintaining the five points of contact (do not arch excessively where the hips lift off the bench), press the bar upwards and slightly back to the original position over the shoulders, keeping the elbows slightly bent at the top of the movement

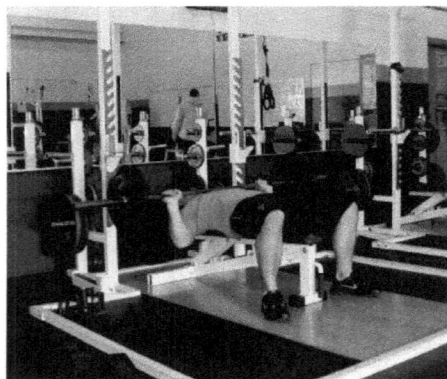

Bench Press Bottom Position

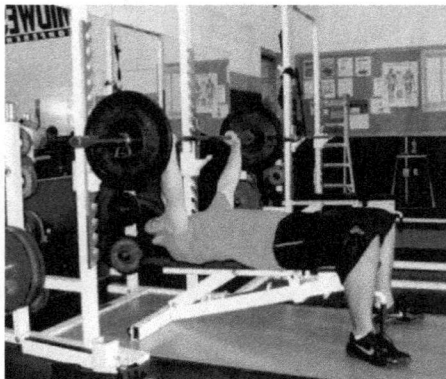

Bench Press Top Position

Dumbbell Chest Press

- Lie back on bench establishing five points of contact (head, shoulders/back and buttocks) on the bench and right and left feet flat on floor
- Starting with the dumbbell in your hands, start with hands just outside your chest, just above chest height
- Maintaining the five points of contact (do not arch excessively where the hips lift off the bench), press the dumbbell upwards and slightly back to over the shoulders, keeping the elbows slightly bent at the top of the movement
- Slowly and under control, lower the dumbbell to the chest, touching the side of the chest in line with the nipples

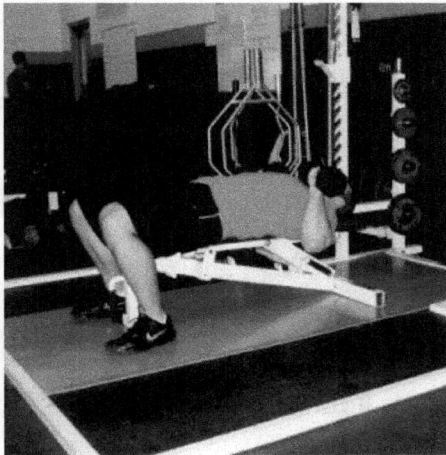

Dumbbell Chest Press Bottom Position   Dumbbell Chest Press Top Position

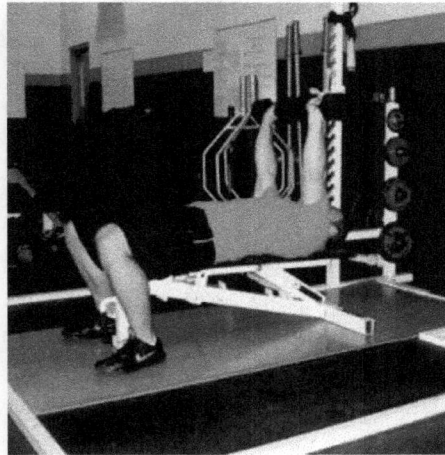

Incline Bench Press

- Sit down at the incline bench (positioned at a 45- to 60-degree angle), position your feet flat on the ground with thighs parallel to the floor
- Lean back on bench establishing five points of contact (head, shoulders/back and buttocks) on the bench and right and left feet on floor
- Grip the bar with an overhand, closed grip, slightly wider than shoulder width (a narrower grip than the bench press grip increases the focus on the upper chest)
- Starting with the bar above your eyes, lower the bar slowly, under control, touching the bar to your upper chest
- Maintaining the five points of contact (do not arch excessively where the hips lift off the bench), press the bar upwards and slightly back to the original position, keeping the elbows slightly bent at the top of the movement

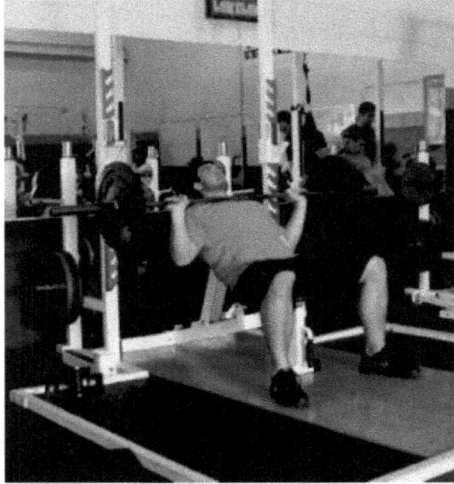

Incline Bench Press Bottom

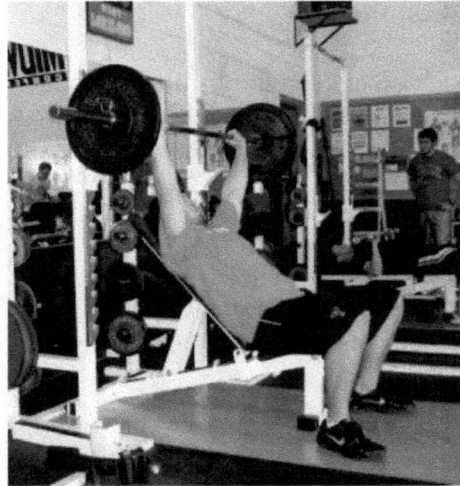

Incline Bench Press Top

Incline Dumbbell Chest Press

- Sit down at the incline bench (positioned at a 45- to 60-degree angle) position your feet flat on the ground with thighs parallel to the floor
- Lean back on bench establishing five points of contact (head, shoulders/back and buttocks) on the bench and right and left feet on floor
- With the dumbbell in your hands, start with hands just outside your chest, even with your upper chest
- Maintaining the five points of contact (do not arch excessively where the hips lift off the bench), press the dumbbell upwards and slightly back to over the eyes, keeping the elbows slightly bent at the top of the movement
- Slowly and under control, lower the dumbbell to the upper chest, touching the side of the upper chest

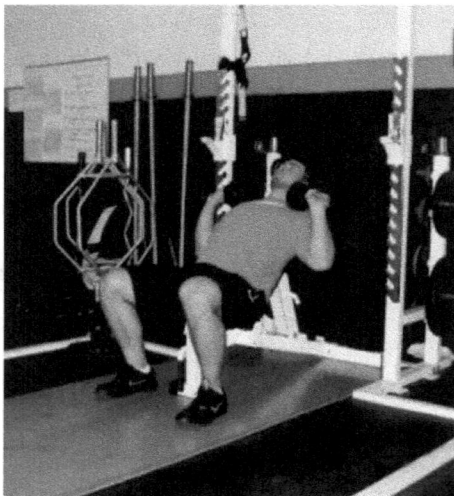

Incline Dumbbell Chest Press Bottom

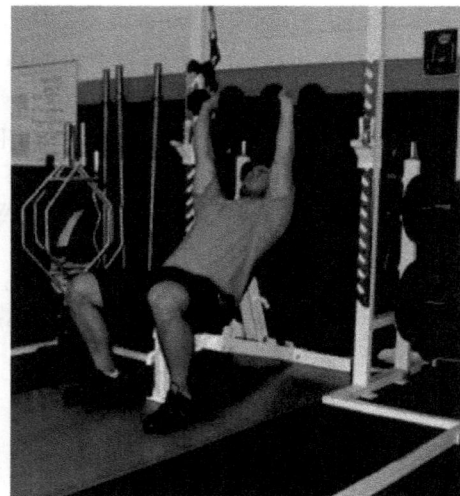

Incline Dumbbell Chest Press Top

Flat Dumbbell Fly

- Lie back on bench establishing five points of contact (head, shoulders/back and buttocks) on the bench and right and left feet flat on floor
- Starting with your arms extended (with slight bend in the elbows) with the dumbbell over your chest and palms facing together
- With elbows staying bent at the same angle all the way through the movement, slowly and under control, lower the arms directly out to the sides in an arcing pattern
- When hands are even with the chest, maintain the five points of contact (do not arch excessively where the hips lift off the bench) and in the same arcing pattern raise the back up to the starting position

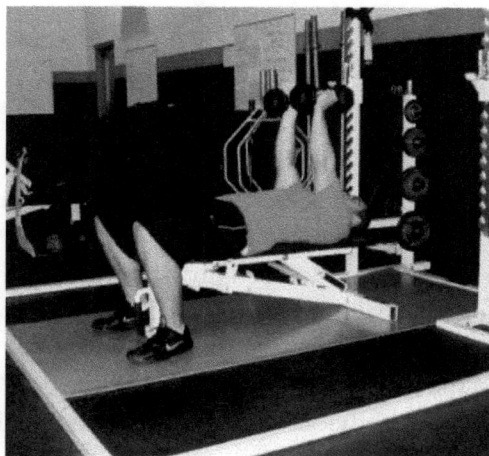

Dumbbell Fly Starting Position

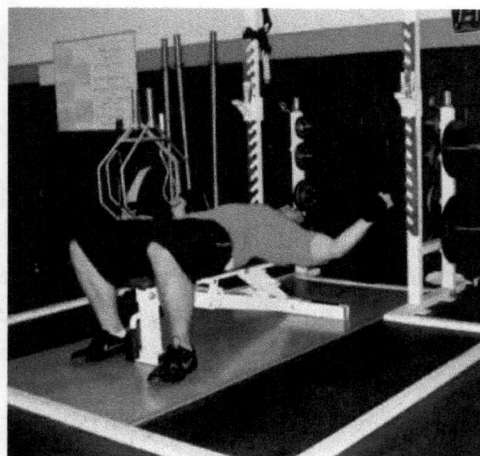

Dumbbell Fly Bottom Position

Back Exercises

Wide Grip Lat Pulldown

- From a seated position with thighs parallel to the floor and feet flat on the floor, grab the bar with an overhand, closed grip with hands evenly spaced wider than shoulder width
- Lean back slightly, with arms extended and elbows slightly bent
- Keeping your upper body stable, pull the bar down, leading with your elbows to the clavicles/upper chest
- Under control, slowly guide the bar back to the starting position
- Do not let the bar jerk you up, maintain your upper body position and maintain a slight bend in the elbows are the top of the movement

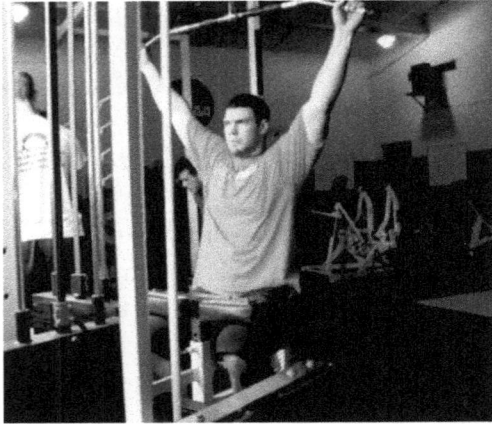

Wide Grip Lat Pulldown Top

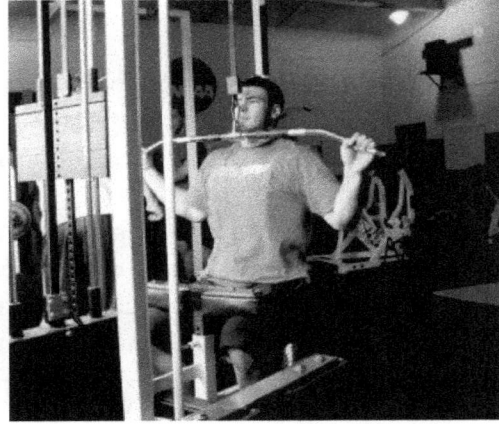

Wide Grip Lat Pulldown Bottom

Narrow Grip Lat Pulldown

- From a seated position with thighs parallel to the floor and feet flat on the floor, grab the bar with an underhand, closed grip using a narrow grip (hands 6-10 inches apart)
- Keep the upper body straight in line, arms extended with elbows slightly bent
- Keeping your upper body stable, pull the bar down, leading with your elbows to the clavicles/upper chest
- Under control, slowly guide the bar back to the starting position
- Do not let the bar jerk you up. Maintain your upper body position and maintain a slight bend in the elbows are the top of the movement

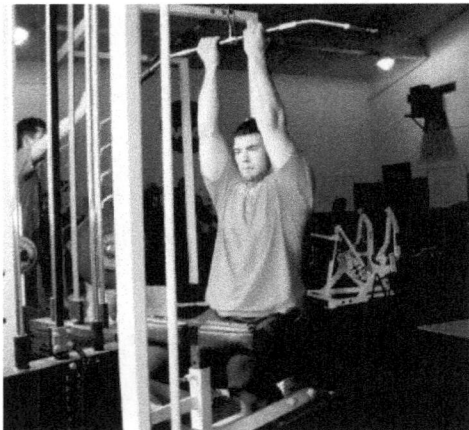

Narrow Grip Lat Pulldown Top

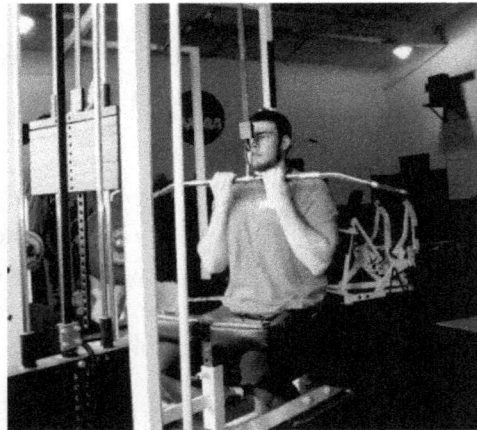

Narrow Underhand Grip Lat Pulldown

Bent-Over Row

- With feet shoulder width apart (or slightly wider) and keeping legs straight (with slight bend in knees) bend your upper body forward so that your back is parallel to the ground
- Grip the bar with either an overhand (pronated) or underhand (supinated) closed grip
- As you pull the bar up to just below your chest, maintain your back position, while pulling the shoulders back as the elbows flex upwards and away from the body (the underhand grip will keep the elbows tighter to the body)
- Pull the bar all the way up to your body, then slowly and under control lower the bar back down extending your arms
- Maintain a slight bend in the elbows at the bottom position and do not let the weight touch the ground between repetitions so that the muscles remain under resistance during the whole set

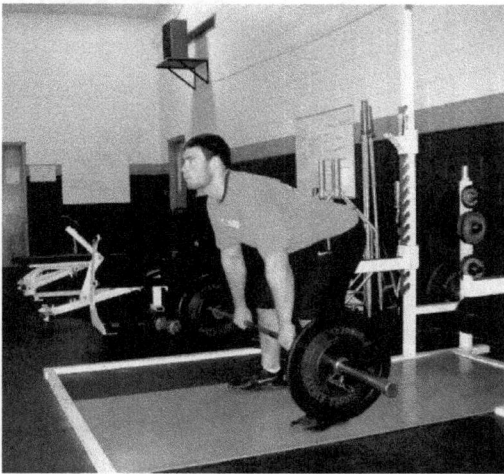

Pronated Grip Bent-Over Row Bottom

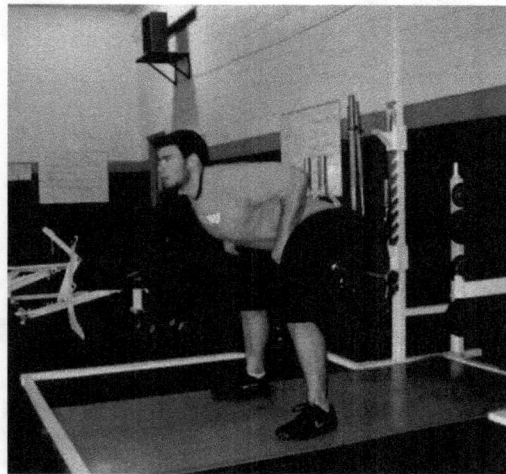

Pronated Grip Bent-Over Row Top

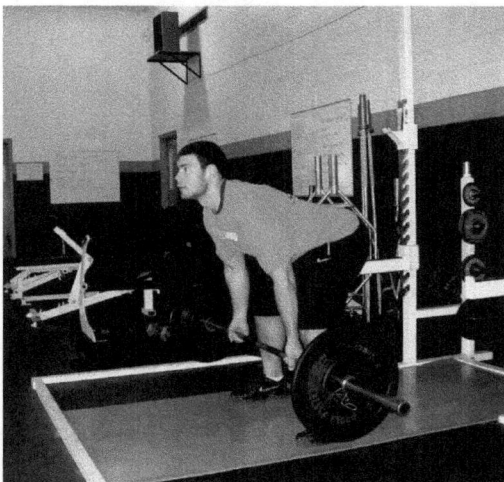

Supinated Grip Bent-Over Row Bottom

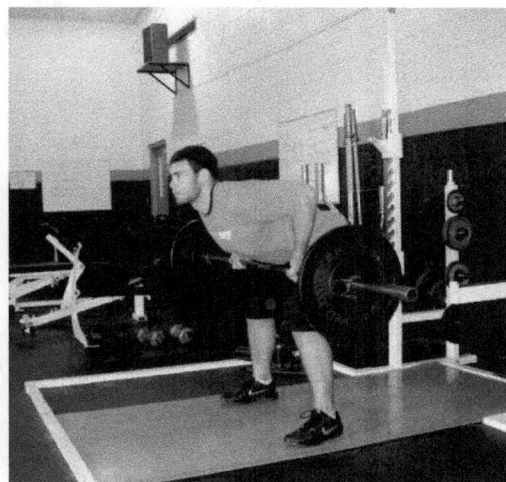

Supinated Grip Bent-Over Row Top

Dumbbell Variations

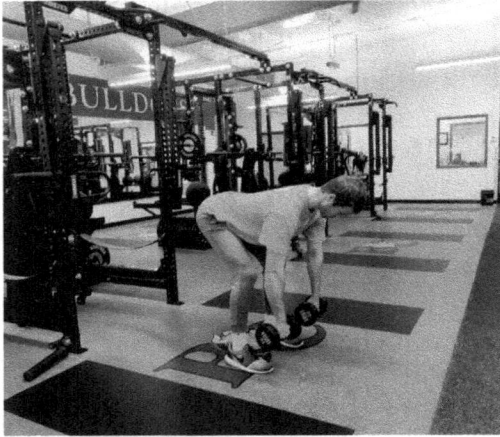

Pronated Grip Bent-Over Row
Bottom with Dumbbell

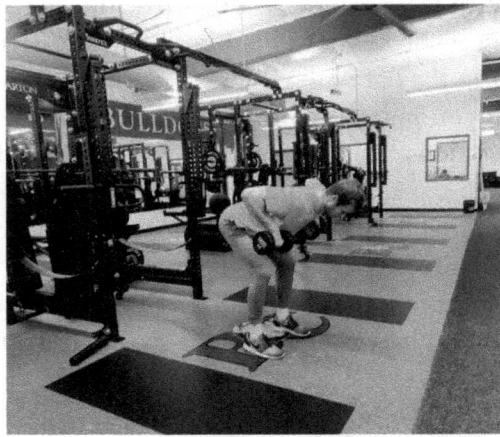

Pronated Grip Bent-Over Row
Top with Dumbbell

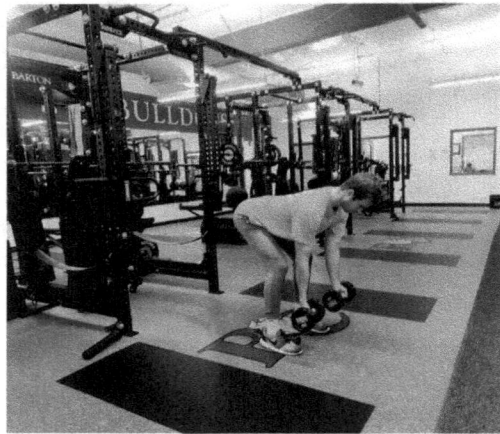

Supinated Grip Bent-Over Row
Bottom with Dumbbell

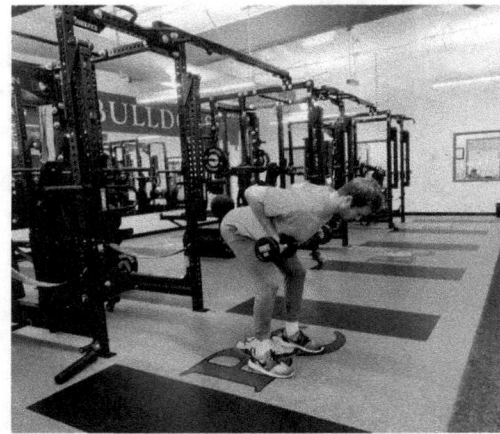

Supinated Grip Bent-Over Row
Top with Dumbbell

One-Arm Dumbbell Row

- Stand to the right side of a flat bench, place your left hand on the bench in line with your shoulder and place your left knee on the bench in line with your hip
- With your left hand and left knee on the bench, keep your upper body parallel to the floor maintaining a flat back
- Your right leg should be close to the side of the bench with a slight bend in the right knee and your foot flat on the floor
- Grasping a dumbbell in your right hand extend your arm in line with your chest, keeping a slight bend in your elbow at the bottom position

- Maintaining a flat back position, pull the dumbbell up, leading with your elbow, until your elbow is slightly higher than your back and your hand is just below your chest
- Lower the dumbbell in a slow, controlled manner back to the starting position
- Repeat with the other side

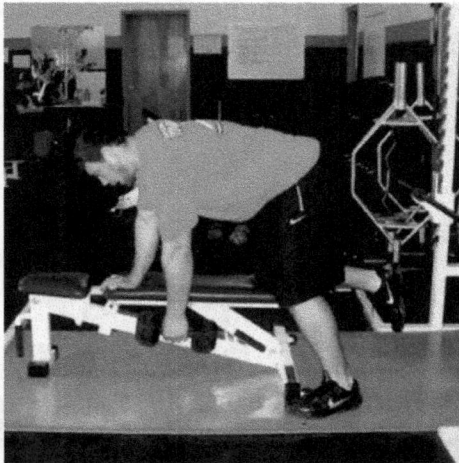

One-Arm Row Bottom

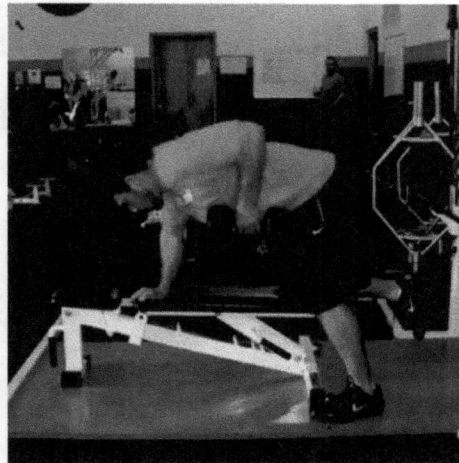

One-Arm Row Top

Three-Point Stance Row

- The Three-Point Stance Row is performed the same way as the One-Arm Row. The only difference is that the lifter uses his/her own body for support instead of a bench
- Take a staggered stance with knees slightly bent, bending at the hips so that your upper body is parallel to the floor with your back flat
- Place the hand opposite the DB on your knee to stabilize your position

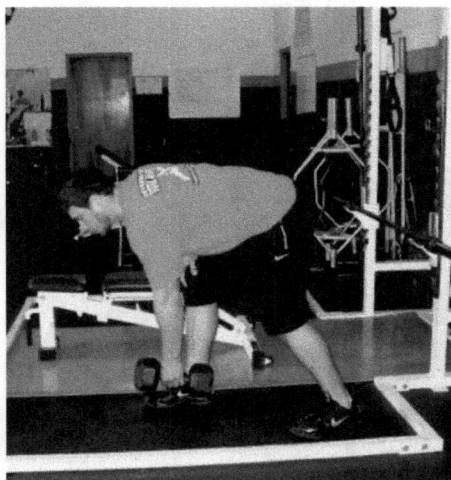

Three-Point Stance Row Bottom

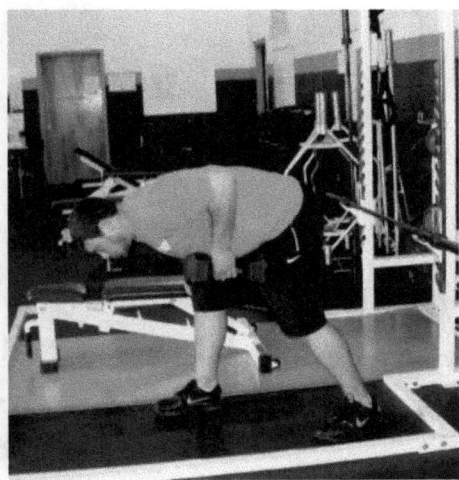

Three-Point Stance Row Top

Upright Row

- Standing with feet shoulder width apart and knees slightly bent, grip the bar using an overhand, closed grip with hands narrower than shoulder width
- With the bar hanging at hip height and with arms extended (maintaining a slight bend in the elbows), keep your body stable as you pull the bar up until your hands are at shoulder height
- As you raise the bar close to your body leading with your elbows, keep the elbows above the wrists throughout the whole movement
- Maintaining a stable body position, lower the bar as you slowly extend your arms back to the starting position

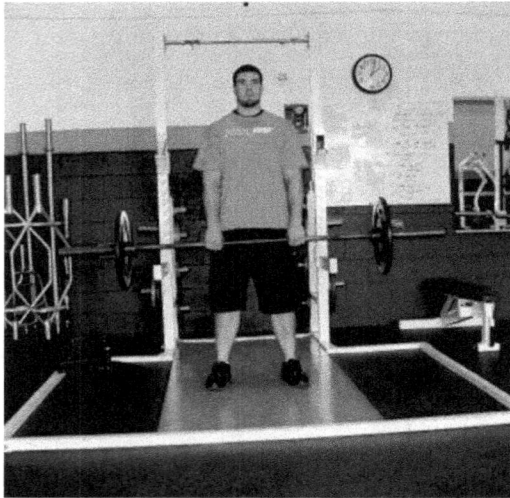

Upright Row Bottom (front view)

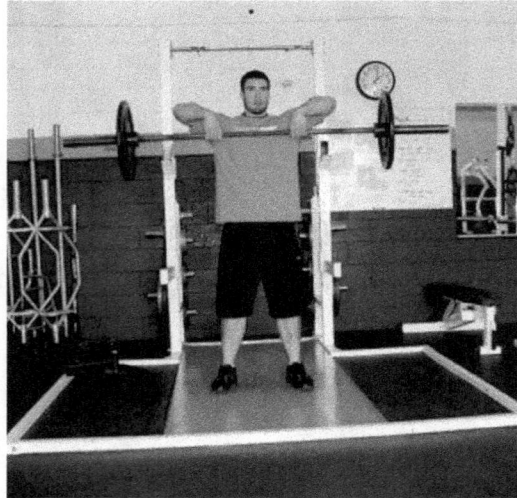

Upright Row Top (front view)

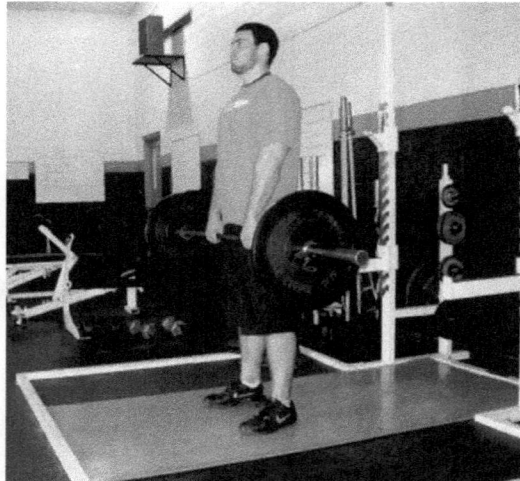

Upright Row Bottom (side view)

Dumbbell Variations

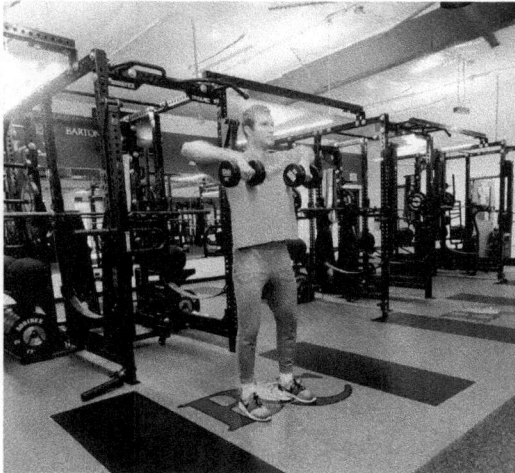

Upright Row Top with Dumbbell

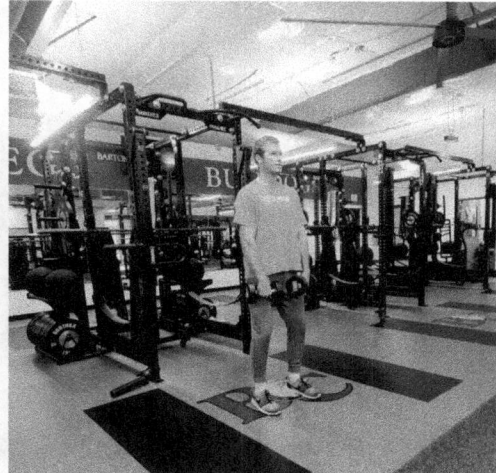

Upright Row Bottom with Dumbbell

Shoulder Exercises

Shoulder Press

- Can be performed in either a seated or standing position
  - Standing: stand up straight with feet shoulder width apart and knees slightly bent
  - Seated: sit with feet firmly on the floor, shoulder width apart, keeping back straight (if bench has a back pad, rest back against pad for support)
- Start holding dumbbells with an overhand grip, with hands at shoulder height
- Press the weight straight up, stopping just short of fully extending the elbows
- Under control, lower the weight back to shoulder height

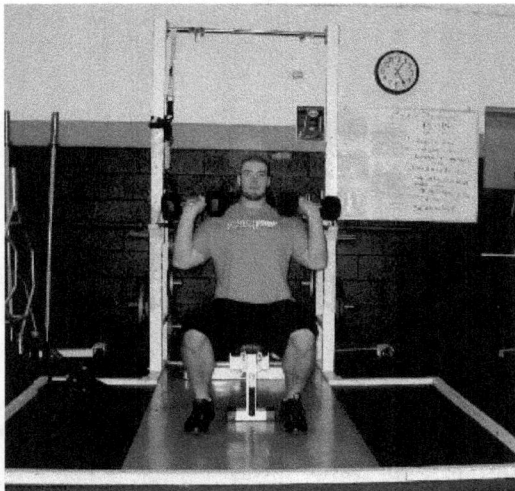

Shoulder Press (seated) Bottom Position

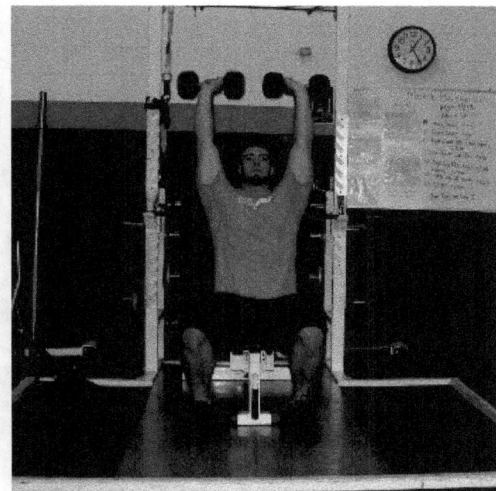

Shoulder Press (seated) Top Position

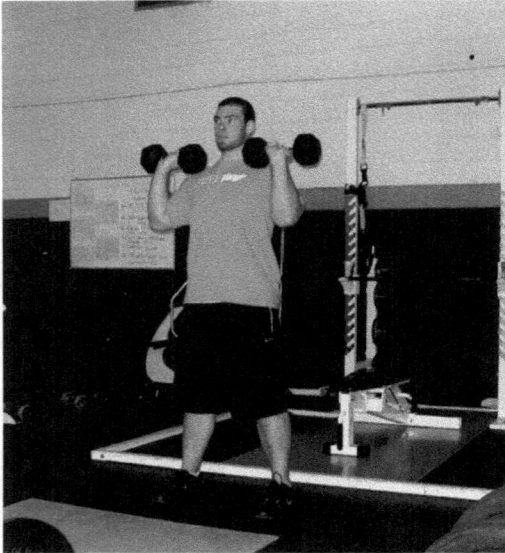

Shoulder Press (standing) Bottom Position

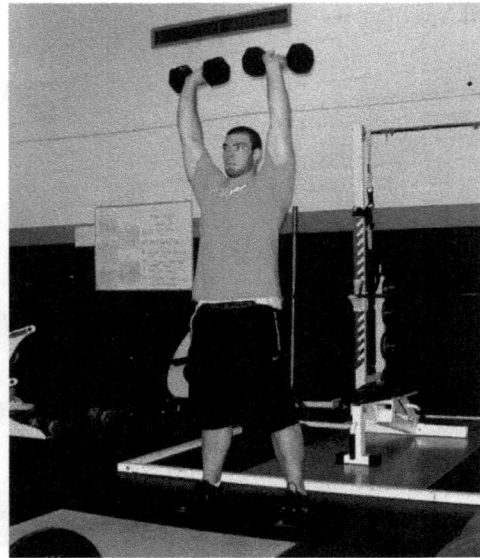

Shoulder Press (standing) Top Position

Front Raise

- Start in a standing position with knees slightly flexed and with hands placed in front of thighs using an overhand close grip (hands facing thighs)
- Body should remain stable throughout movement with knees slightly flexed (to take pressure off the lower back)
- Pull hands and weight vertically, raising the arms to shoulder height leading with the hands/wrist
- Pause briefly, and then lower arms down, keeping elbows slightly flexed, back to starting position

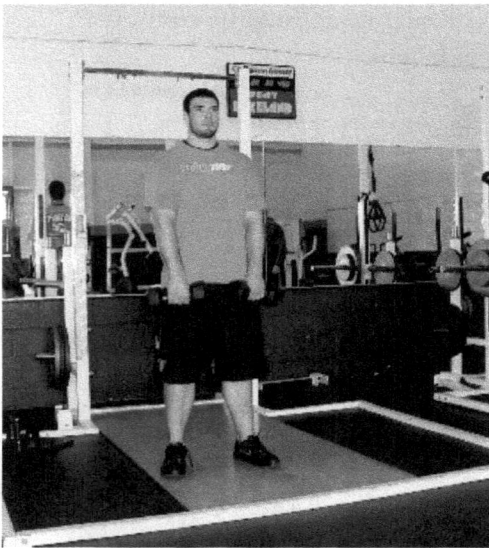

Front Raise Bottom Position

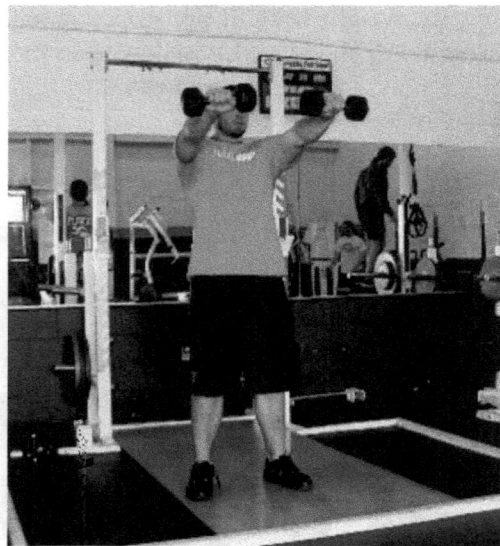

Front Raise Top Position

Side Raise

- Start in a standing position with knees slightly bent
- Hands placed in on the side of thighs using an overhand close grip (hands facing in)
- Body should remain stable throughout movement with knees slightly flexed (to take pressure off the lower back)
- Pull hands and weight vertically raising/abducting the arms to shoulder height leading with the hands/wrist
- Pause briefly, and then lower arms down, keeping elbows slightly flexed, back to starting position
- Always keep elbows slightly flexed and at the same angle all the way through the movement

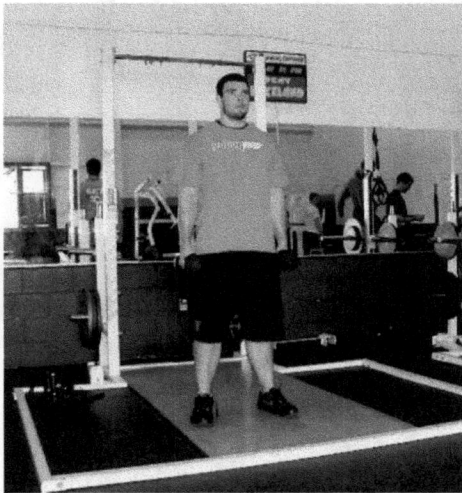

Side Raise Bottom Position

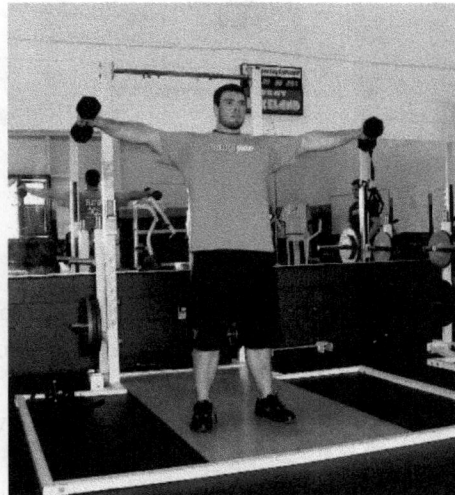

Side Raise Top Position

Posterior Raise

- Bending at the waist, lower your upper body to parallel with the floor
  - In a standing position, place feet shoulder width apart with knees slightly bent
  - In a seated position, keep feet firmly on the ground shoulder width apart and lower your chest to your knees
- Keeping back straight, let your arms be extended towards the ground with elbows bent slightly and the top of your hands even with your ears (to align line of pull with the posterior deltoid)
- Maintain the same elbow angle as you raise your arms up to shoulder height, keeping the hands forward so that tension remains on the targeted muscle
- Under control, lower your arms / hands back to the starting position

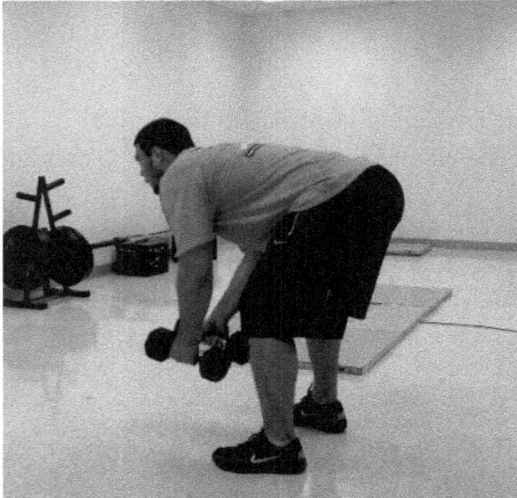

Posterior Raise Bottom Position

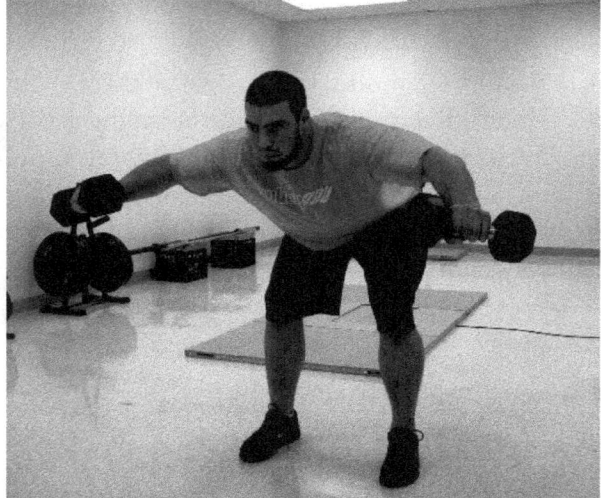

Posterior Raise Top Position

Internal Rotation

- Tubing or cable height should be placed at elbow height
- Using an adequate resistance, step far enough from the machine or anchor so that the cable or tube is tight without slack
- Holding elbow steady at your side, start with your hand reaching out while your elbow is bent at 90 degrees
- Keeping elbow stationary, internally rotate your shoulder to pull the cable or tube across your body
- Externally rotate your shoulder to return to starting position

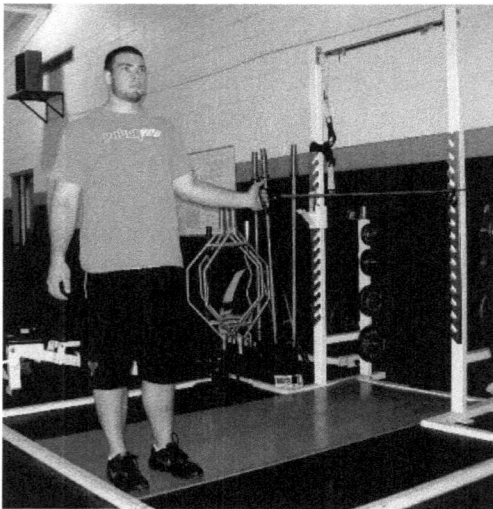

Internal Rotation Starting Position

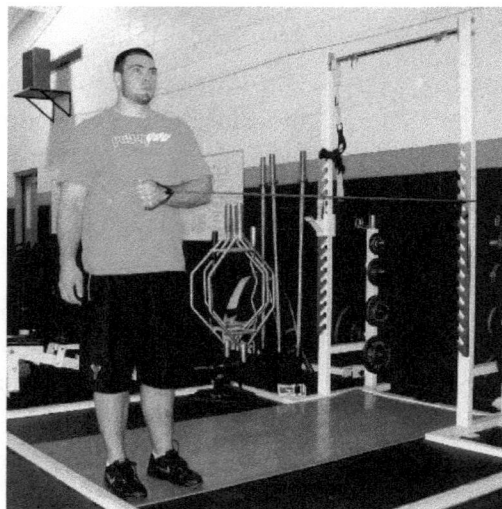

Internal Rotation Finishing Position

External Rotation

- Tubing or cable height should be placed at elbow height
- Using an adequate resistance, step far enough from the machine or anchor so that the cable or tube is tight without slack
- Holding elbow steady at your side, start with your hand across your body while your elbow is bent at 90 degrees
- Keeping elbow stationary, externally rotate your shoulder to pull the cable or tube across your body until your hand is extended away from your body
- Internally rotate your shoulder to return to starting position

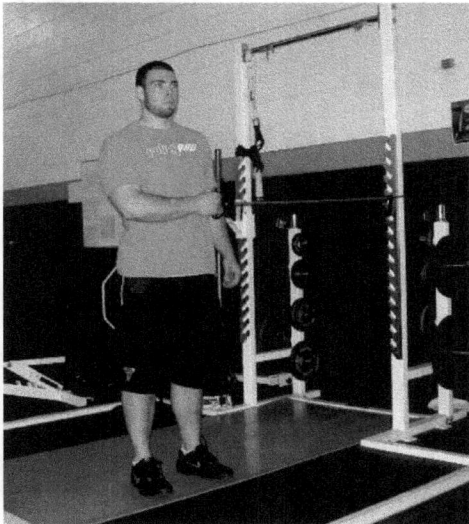

External Rotation Starting Position   External Rotation Finishing Position

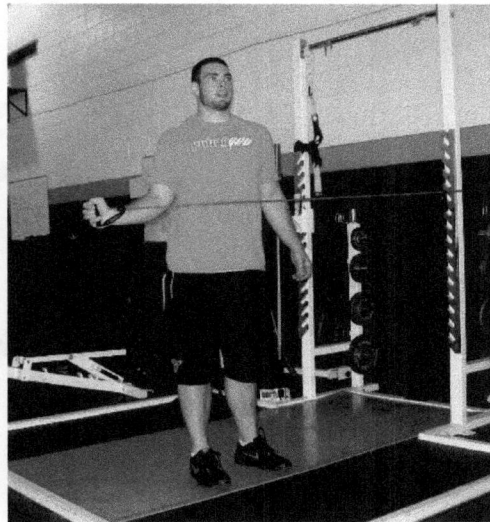

Straight Bar Curl

- Start in a standing position with knees slightly flexed, with feet shoulder width apart, arms extended, with hands to the side of your thighs shoulder width apart using an underhand grip
- Upper body should remain upright and stable throughout movement, with knees slightly flexed (to take pressure off the lower back)
- Pull bar up to shoulder height, flexing only at the elbow joint (keeping elbows steady and in tight throughout movement)
- Pause briefly then return hands back down to starting position

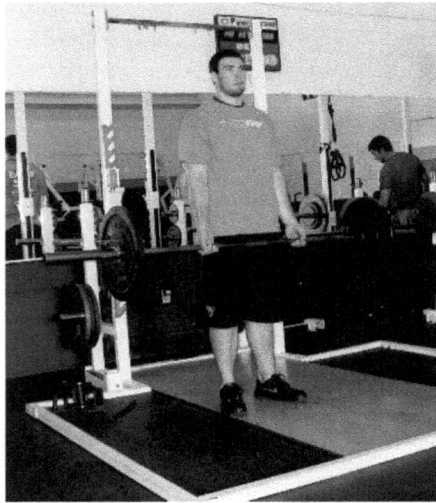

Straight Bar Curl Bottom Position   Straight Bar Curl Top Position

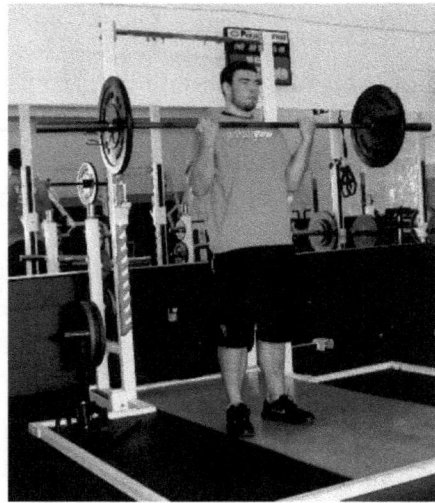

Standing Dumbbell Curl

- Start in a standing position with knees slightly flexed, with feet shoulder width apart, arms extended, with hands to the side of your thighs shoulder width apart using an underhand grip
- Upper body should remain upright and stable throughout movement with knees slightly flexed (to take pressure off the lower back)
- Pull dumbbells up to shoulder height, flexing only at the elbow joint (keeping elbows steady and in tight throughout movement)
- Pause briefly then return hands back down to starting position

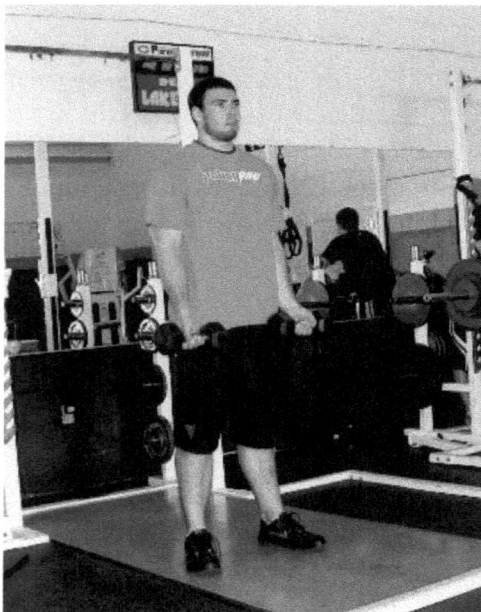

Standing Dumbbell Curl Bottom Position   Standing Dumbbell Curl Top Position

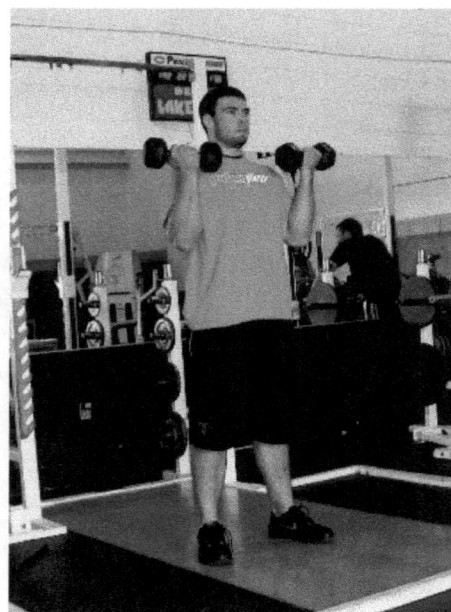

Hammer Curl

- Start in a standing position with knees slightly flexed, with feet shoulder width apart, arms extended, with hands to the side of your thighs shoulder width apart using an underhand grip
- Grip the dumbbells as you would grip a hammer so that your palms face your thighs
- Use of the hammer grip shifts more emphasis to the forearm muscles
- Upper body should remain upright and stable throughout movement with knees slightly flexed (to take pressure off the lower back)
- Pull dumbbells up to shoulder height, flexing only at the elbow joint (keeping elbows steady and in tight throughout movement)
- Pause briefly then return hands back down to starting position

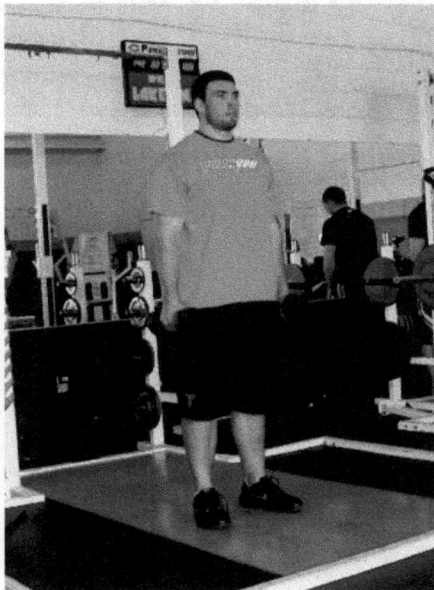

Hammer Curl Bottom Position   Hammer Curl Top Position

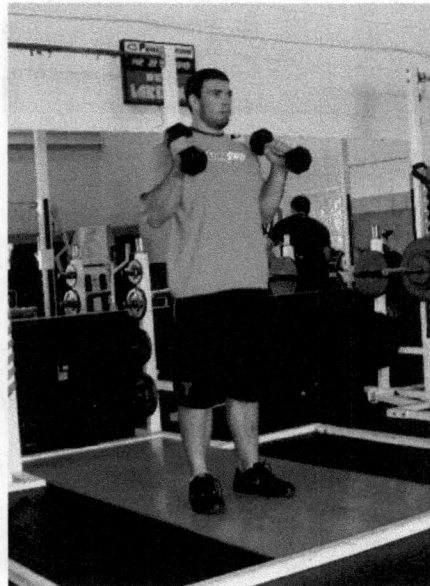

Overhead Triceps Extensions (Two Hands)

- Position one dumbbell overhead with both hands under inner plate (heart shaped grip)
- With elbows overhead, lower weight behind the head by flexing elbows
- Flex wrists at bottom to avoid hitting dumbbell on back of neck
- Raise dumbbell overhead by extending elbows
- Keep elbows tight to the ears/head to keep resistance focused on the triceps
- Slowly lower the dumbbell back to the starting position

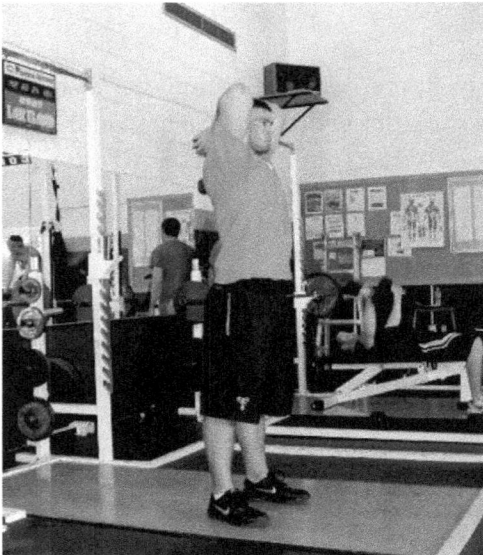

Overhead Triceps Extensions (Two Hands)
Bottom Position

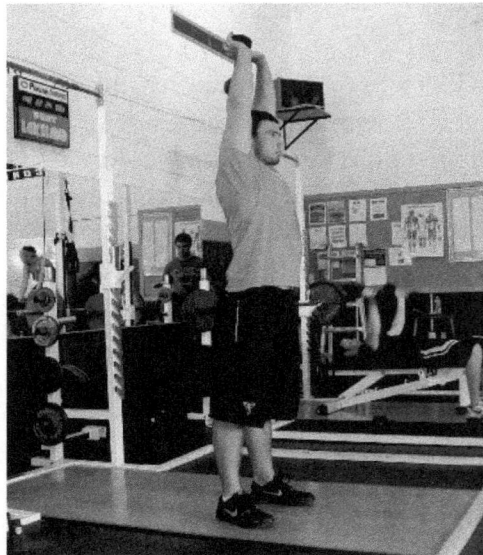

Overhead Triceps Extensions (Two Hands)
Top Position

Overhead Triceps Extensions (Single Arm)

- Position dumbbell over head with arm straight up or slightly back
- Lower dumbbell behind neck or shoulder while maintaining upper arm's vertical position throughout exercise
- Extend arm until almost straight
- Slowly lower the dumbbell back to the starting position
- Continue with opposite arm

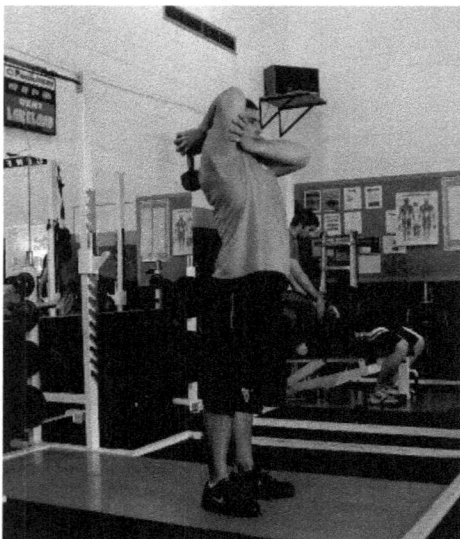

Overhead Triceps Extensions (Single Arm)
Bottom Position

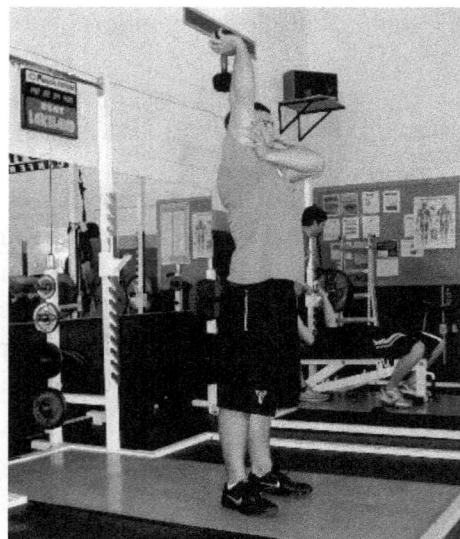

Overhead Triceps Extensions (Single Arm)
Top Position

Lying Triceps Extensions

- Lie on bench maintaining five points of contact (head, shoulders, hips and feet) with narrow overhand grip on barbell or heart-shaped grip with a dumbbell (like in the two arm overhead extension)
- Position barbell over shoulders with arms extended
- With a bar: lower bar to forehead by bending elbows
- With a dumbbell: lower the dumbbell behind your head till hands are at forehead height
- Keeping elbows in tight, extend arms just short of full extension

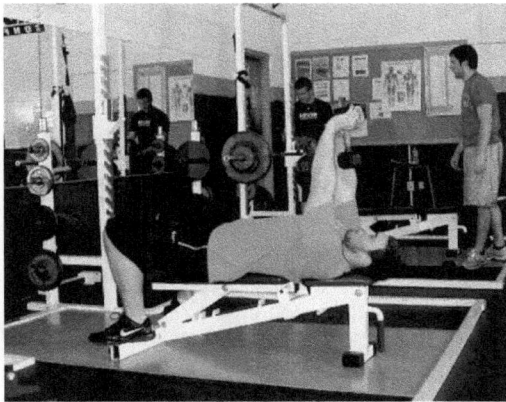

Laying Triceps Extensions Starting Position

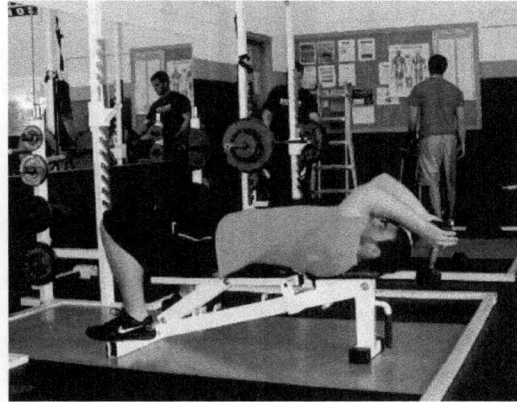

Laying Triceps Extensions Bottom Position

Triceps Kickback

- Kneel on bench with one knee and with arm of the same side supporting body, keeping back flat
- Other foot is firmly on the floor next to the bench
- Grasp dumbbell with other hand, position upper arm parallel to floor
- Extend arm until it is almost straight
- Continue with opposite arm

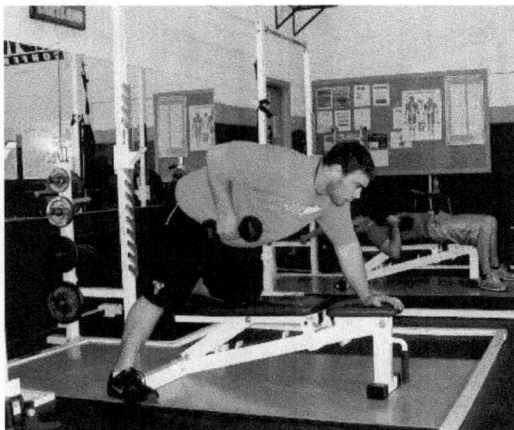

Triceps Kickback Starting Position

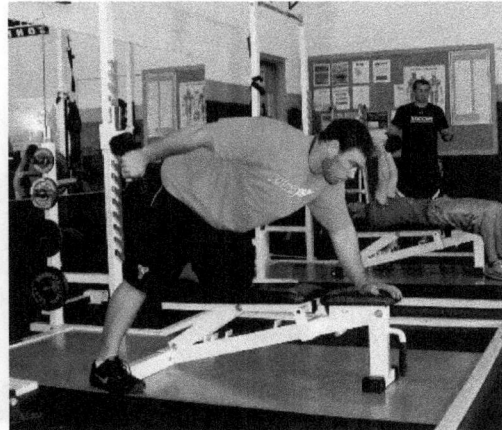

Triceps Kickback Finishing Position

Triceps Pushdowns

- Stand close to the high pulley station of the machine
- Start in a standing position with feet shoulder width apart and knees slightly flexed
- Hands placed just above chest height using an overhand close grip with elbows firmly tucked in against sides
- Body should be upright, remaining stable throughout movement with knees slightly flexed (to take pressure off the lower back)
  - Be careful of leaning upper body forward and shifting emphasis to the chest
- Push handles down just short of full extension, keeping elbows close to sides. Pause briefly, then raise hands back to starting position.
  - A rope attachment can be used in place of the handle to put more emphasis on the triceps by spreading the hands apart at the bottom of the movement.

Triceps Pushdowns with Bar

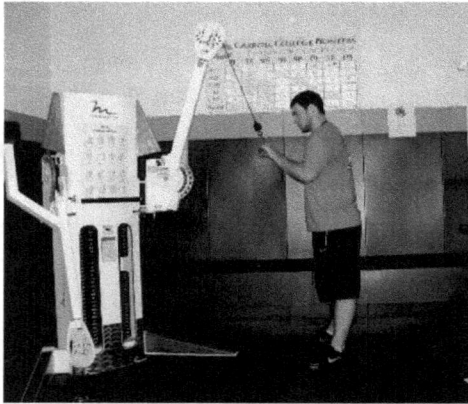

Triceps Pushdowns (Bar) Starting Position

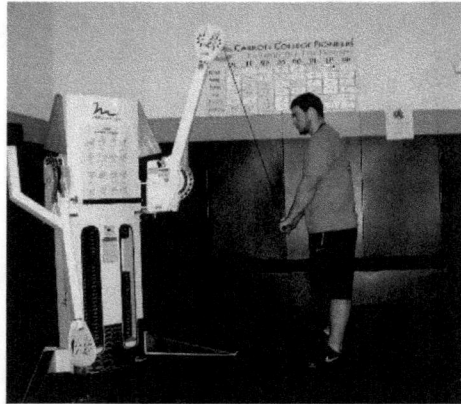

Triceps Pushdowns (Bar) Finishing Position

Triceps Pushdowns with Rope

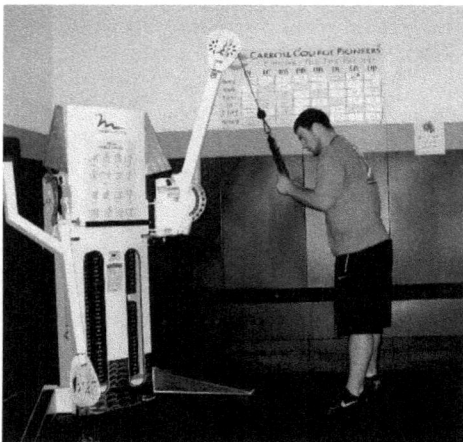

Triceps Pushdowns (Rope) Starting Position

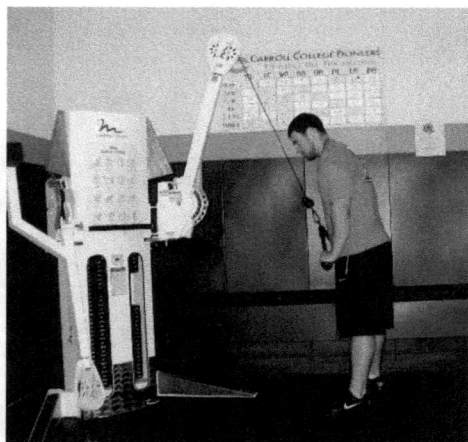

Triceps Pushdowns (Rope) Finishing Position

Forearm Extension

- Sit on bench and grip dumbbell with overhand grip
- Rest forearm on thigh with wrist just beyond knee
- Raise dumbbell by pointing knuckles upward as high as possible
- Return until knuckles are pointing downward as far as possible
- Keep elbow approximately wrist height to maintain resistance through full range of motion
- Can be done with both sides at one time, or one arm can be done at a time with other hand helping support the wrist to help isolate the movement (perform one arm version for both sides)

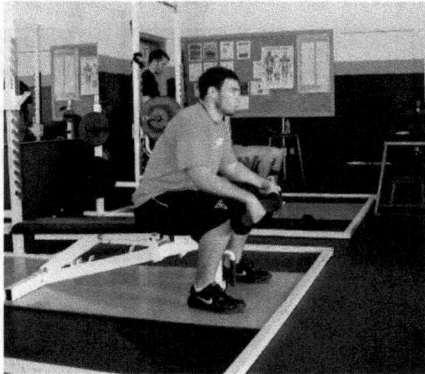

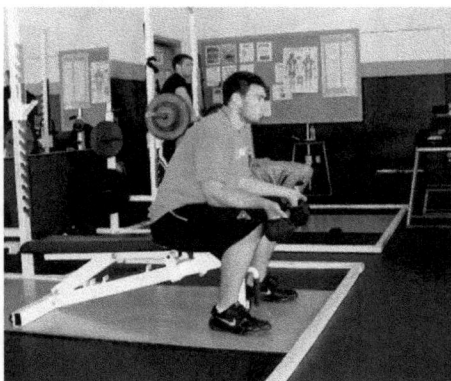

Forearm Extension Starting Position   Forearm Extension Finishing Position

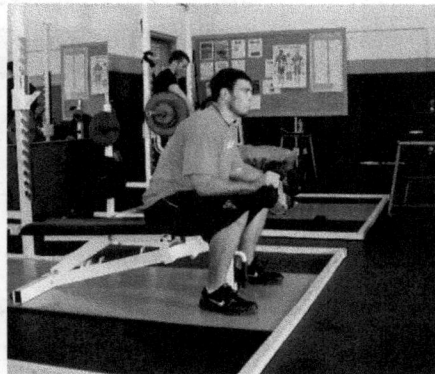

Forearm Flexion

- Sit and grasp dumbbell with underhand grip
- Rest forearm on thigh with wrist just beyond knee
- Allow dumbbell to roll out of palm down to fingers
- Raise dumbbell back up by gripping and pointing knuckles up as high as possible
- Keep elbow approximately wrist height to maintain resistance through full range of motion
- Can be done with both sides at one time, or one arm can be done at a time with other hand helping support the wrist to help isolate the movement (perform one arm version for both sides)

Forearm Flexion Starting Position   Forearm Flexion Finishing Position

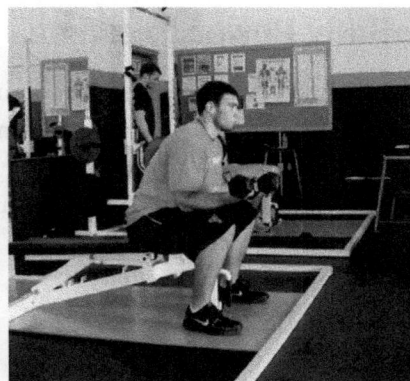

Part 3: Sport-Specific Exercises

The sport-specific exercises are special auxiliary exercises that are designed to add a sport-specific element to your program and aid in injury prevention. Below is a chart that provides examples of sports-specific exercises that can be inserted into your program. For multi-sport athletes, the sport-specific exercise can be based on their primary sport or exercises can be rotated using the exercises for the sports the athlete participates in.

Suggested Sport-Specific Exercises			
Sport	**Exercise**	**Sport**	**Exercise**
Football	4-Way Neck	**Volleyball**	External Rotation Ex./Jump Landing Drills
Basketball	Lateral Hops	**Ice Hockey**	4-Way Neck
Tennis	External Rotation Ex./Wrist Flexion/Extension	**Soccer**	Lateral Hops
Golf	Wrist Flexion/Extension	**Baseball**	External Rotation Ex.
Softball	External Rotation Ex.	**Wrestling**	4-Way Neck

For alternative exercise selections or suggestions for additional sports, contact your local sports medicine resources.

Part 4: Full-Body Power Exercises

PowerRev full-body exercises are explosive lifts that feature triple extension of the hips, knees, and ankles. These are the program's primary power development exercises. The primary core lifts in the program are the Power Clean and Snatch movements. Both these lifts are taught using a progressive series of exercises. The Push Jerk and any of the Clean or Snatch progression exercises can be used as secondary full body movements in the program.

Power Clean Progression Series

Box/Rack Pull

- Use rack or box to elevate bar off the floor to above the knees (feet shoulder width, hands placed on bar at side of legs)
- Bend knees so that bar is aligned with middle of upper thigh
- Lean trunk forward so that chest is over bar (cover bar)
- Explosively pop hips forward as you triple extend

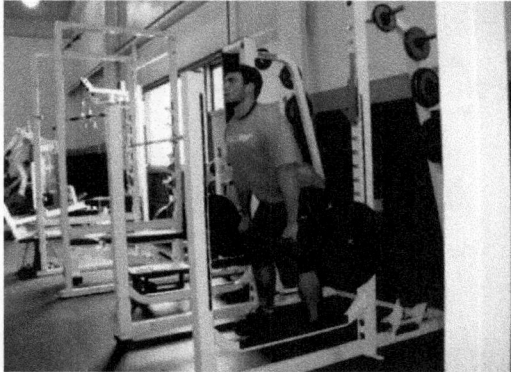

Box/Rack Pull Start Position

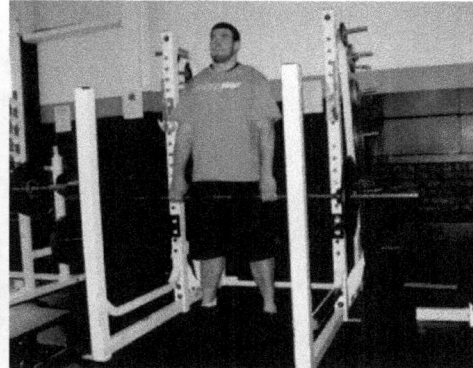

Box/Rack Pull Top Position

Box/Rack Shrug

- Use rack or box to elevate bar off the floor to above the knees (feet shoulder width, hands placed on bar at side of legs)
- Bend knees so that bar is aligned with middle of upper thigh
- Lean trunk forward so that chest is over bar (cover bar)
- Explosively pop hips forward as you triple extend
- Continue to accelerate the bar (introducing the upper body) by aggressively shrugging the shoulders

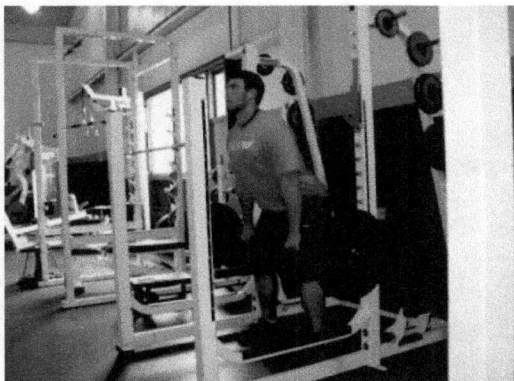

Box/Rack Shrug Start Position

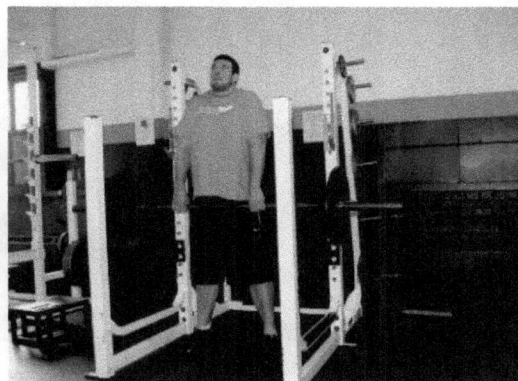

Box/Rack Shrug Top Position

Box/Rack High Pull

- Use rack or box to elevate bar off the floor to above the knees (feet shoulder width, hands placed on bar at side of legs)
- Bend knees so that bar is aligned with middle of upper thigh
- Lean trunk forward so that chest is over bar (cover bar)
- Explosively pop hips forward as you triple extend
- Continue to move bar upwards, keeping elbows above wrists
- Pull bar as high as possible (as weight is increased, ability to pull bar up high decreases)

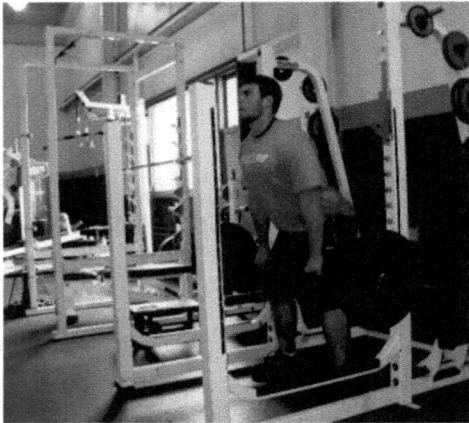

Box/Rack High Pull Start Position   Box/Rack High Pull Top Position

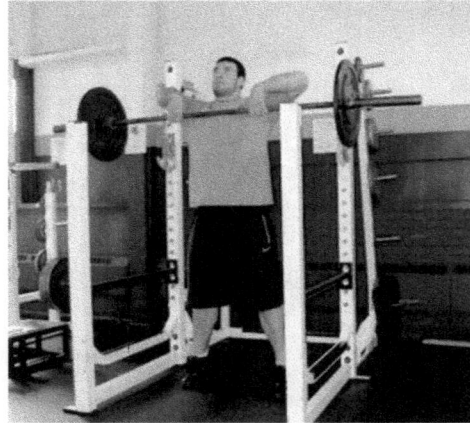

Hang Pull

- Picking up bar from floor, lift bar above knees and bend knees so that bar is aligned with middle of upper thigh (feet shoulder width, hands placed on bar at side of legs) - hang position
- Flex at the hips, slightly leaning trunk forward so that chest is over bar - cover bar (power position)
- Immediately from power position, explosively pop hips forward as you triple extend

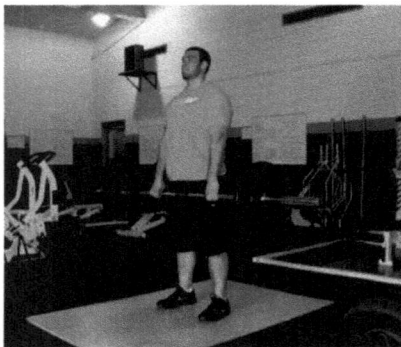

Hang Pull Start Position   Hang Pull Power Position   Hang Pull Top Position

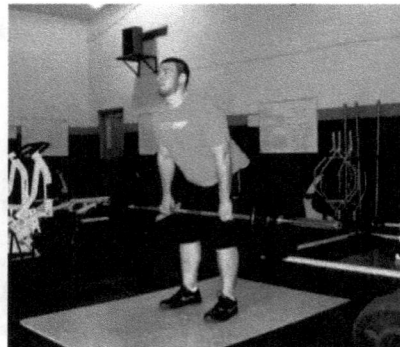

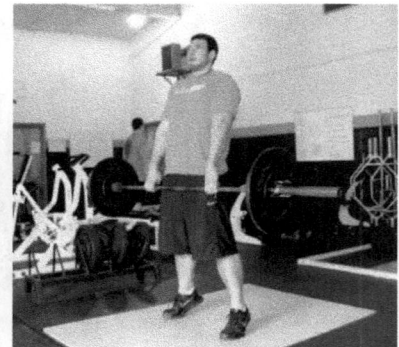

Hang Shrug

- Picking up bar from floor, lift bar above knees and bend knees so that bar is aligned with middle of upper thigh (feet shoulder width, hands placed on bar at side of legs) - hang position
- Flex at the hips, slightly leaning trunk forward so that chest is over bar - cover bar (power position)
- Immediately from power position, explosively pop hips forward as you triple extend
- Continue to accelerate the bar (introducing the upper body) by aggressively shrugging the shoulders

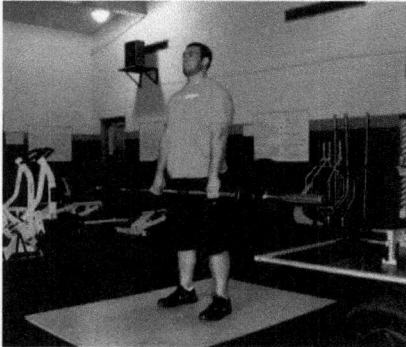

Hang Shrug Start Position   Hang Shrug Power Position   Hang Shrug Top Position

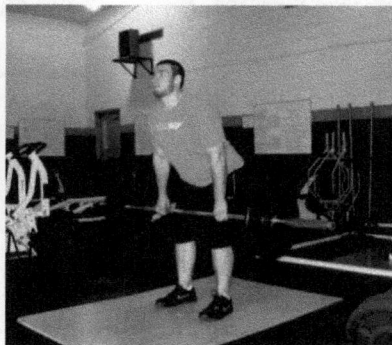

Hang High Pull

- Starting with bar in hang position
- Perform same movement as hang shrug
  - Explosively extend hips forward
  - Complete triple extension
  - Aggressively shrug shoulders upwards
- Continue to move bar upwards, keeping elbows above wrists
- Pull bar as high as possible (as weight is increased, ability to pull bar up high decreases)

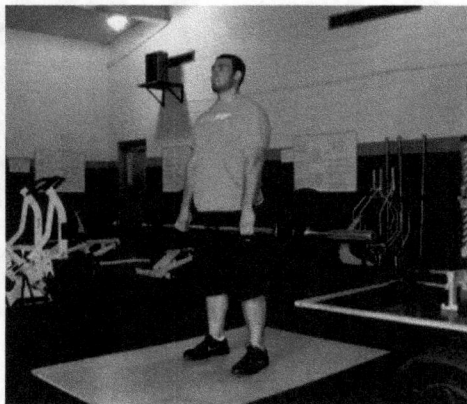

Hang High Pull Start Position   Hang High Pull Power Position

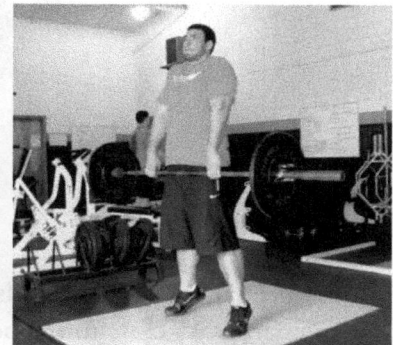

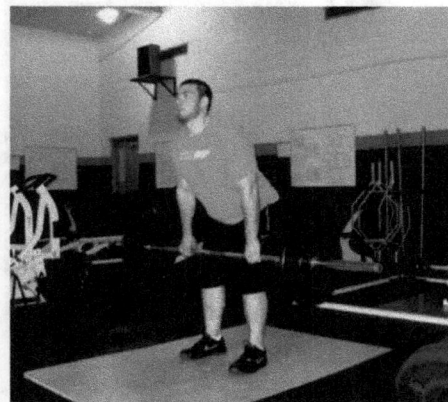

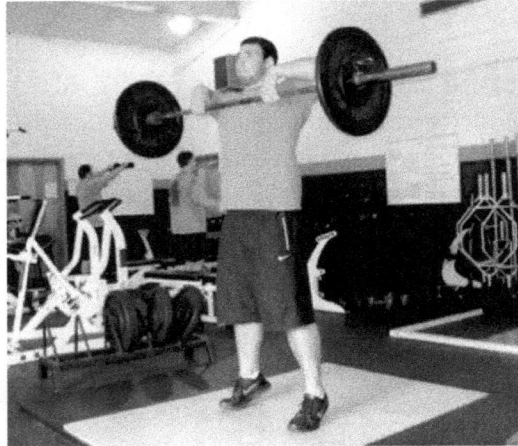

Hang High Pull Top Position

Floor Initial Pull

- Feet at hip width, hands should be placed on the bar just outside of legs
- Barbell in close to the body with arms straight with the elbows rotated out
- Shoulder blades should be squeezed back with the chest as high as possible
- Hips are higher than the knees but lower than the shoulders
- Eyes straight ahead
- Raise up hips slowly, pulling bar off ground
- Maintain consistent back angle
- As soon as the bar gets to above the knees, initiate a violent, explosive hip extension
- Complete triple extension rising up on toes
- Return weights to the ground

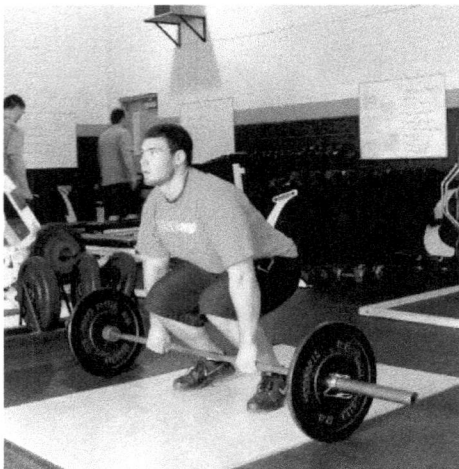

Clean Start Position

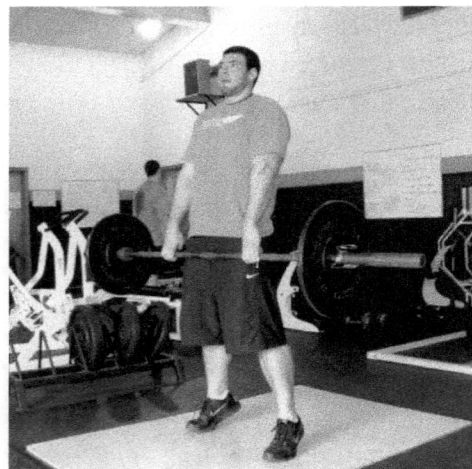

Floor Pull Top Position

Floor Shrug

- Perform same steps as Floor Pull
- Add in aggressive shoulder shrug by lifting/shrugging shoulders up towards ears

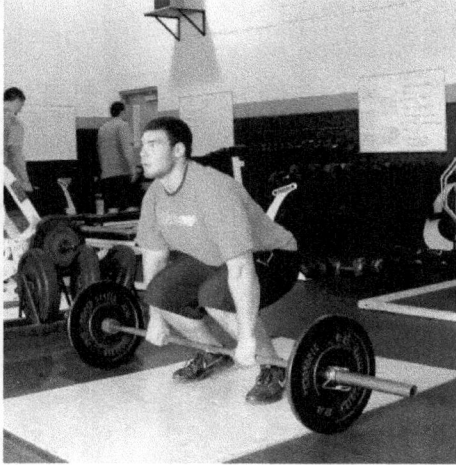

Clean Start Position

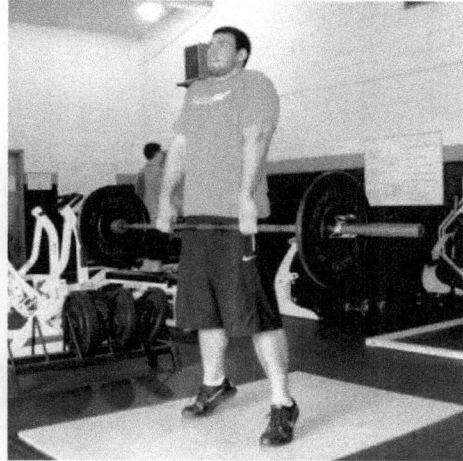

Floor Shrug Top Position

Floor High Pull

- Perform same movement as Floor Shrug
  - o Explosively extend hips forward once bar passes above knees
  - o Complete triple extension
  - o Aggressively shrug shoulders upwards
- Continue to move bar upwards, keeping elbows above wrists
- Pull bar as high as possible (as weight is increased, ability to pull bar up high decreases)

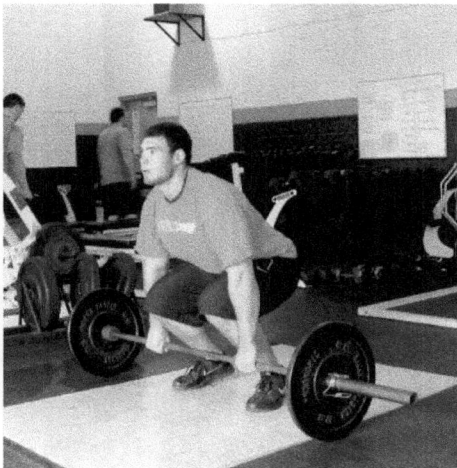

Clean Start Position

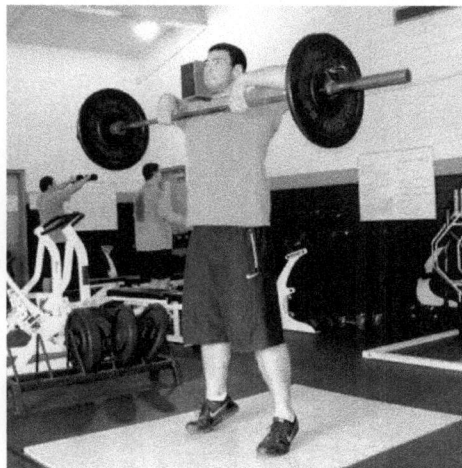

Floor High Pull Top Position

Power Clean

- Perform the Floor High Clean Pull
- Spread the feet to squat width (heels under the shoulders with the toes pointed slightly out)
- At the same time, violently force the elbows forward and up while dropping the hips down and back
- Catch bar in a Front Squat (Clean Grip) position and stand up with it

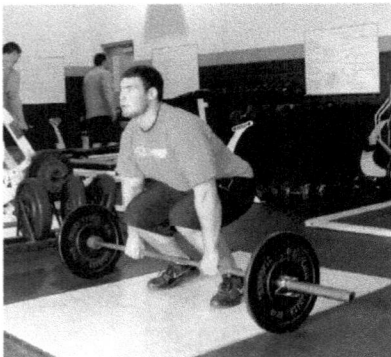

Clean Start Position   Clean Catch Position   Clean Finish Position

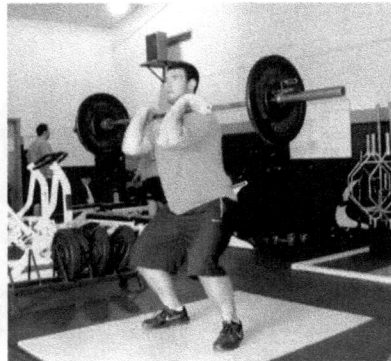

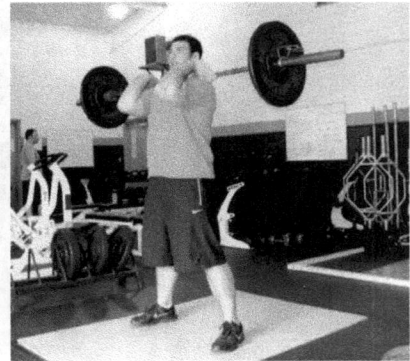

Snatch Progression Series

Box/Rack Pull

- Use rack or box to elevate bar off the floor above the knees (feet shoulder width, using a snatch width grip – overhead squat grip)
- Bend knees so that bar is aligned with middle of upper thigh
- Lean trunk forward so that chest is over bar (cover bar)
- Explosively pop hips forward as you triple extend

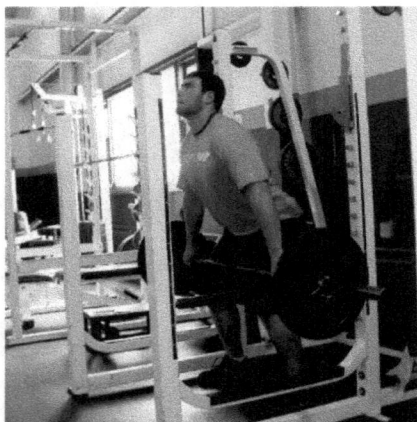

Box/Rack Snatch Start Position   Box/Rack Snatch Pull Top Position

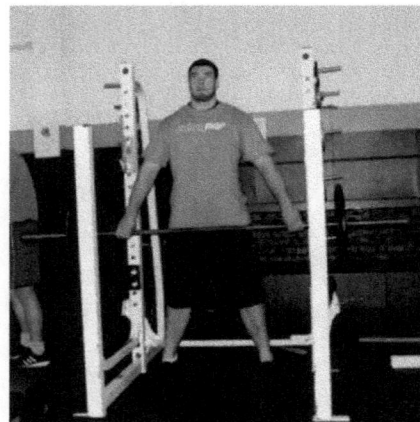

Box/Rack Shrug

- Use rack or box to elevate bar off the floor to above the knees (feet shoulder width, using a snatch width grip – overhead squat grip)
- Bend knees so that bar is aligned with middle of upper thigh
- Lean trunk forward so that chest is over bar (cover bar)
- Explosively pop hips forward as you triple extend
- Continue to accelerate the bar (introducing the upper body) by aggressively shrugging the shoulders

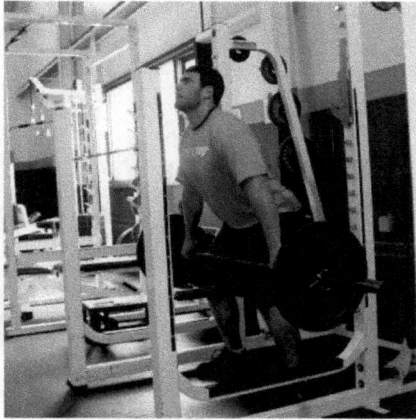

Box/Rack Snatch Start Position   Box/Rack Snatch Shrug Top Position

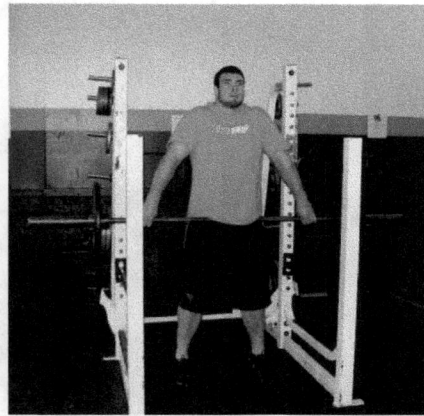

Hang Snatch

- Picking up bar from floor, lift bar above knees and bend knees so that bar is aligned with middle of upper thigh (feet shoulder width, using a snatch width grip – overhead squat grip) - hang position
- Flex at the hips, slightly leaning trunk forward so that chest is over bar - cover bar (power position)
- Immediately from power position, explosively pop hips forward as you triple extend

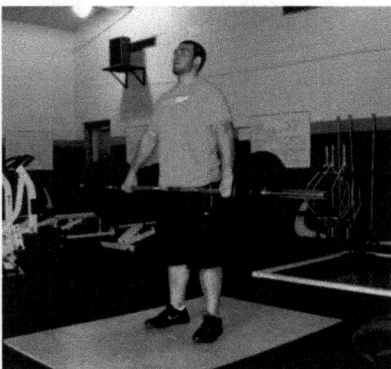

Hang Snatch Start Position   Hang Snatch Power Position   Hang Snatch Pull Position

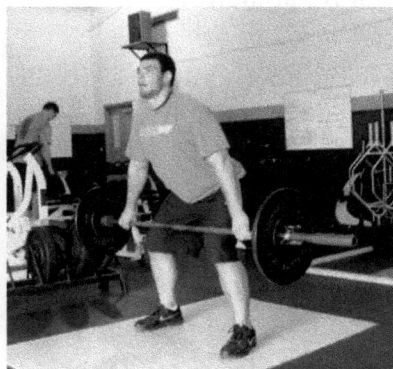

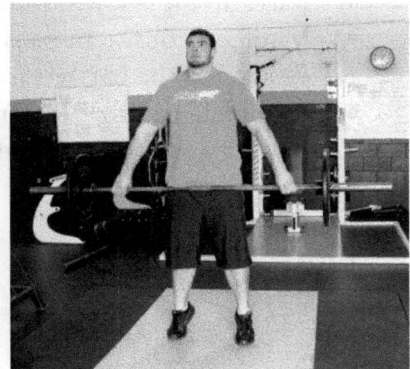

Hang Shrug

- Picking up bar from floor, lift bar above knees and bend knees so that bar is aligned with middle of upper thigh (feet shoulder width, using a snatch width grip – overhead squat grip) - <u>hang position</u>
- Flex at the hips, slightly leaning trunk forward so that chest is over bar - cover bar (<u>power position</u>)
- Immediately from power position, explosively pop hips forward as you triple extend
- Continue to accelerate the bar (introducing the upper body) by aggressively shrugging the shoulders

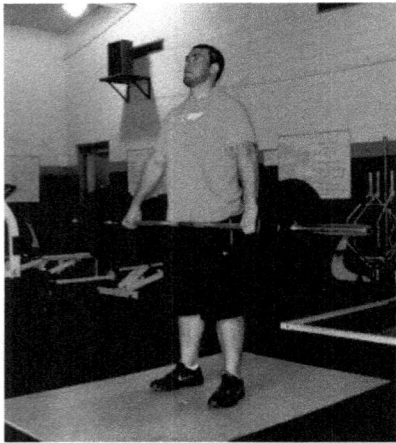

Hang Snatch Start Position   Hang Snatch Power Position   Hang Snatch Shrug Position

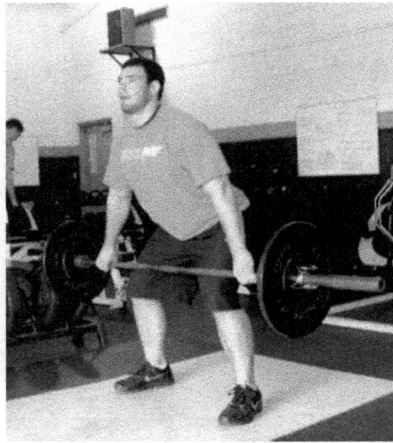

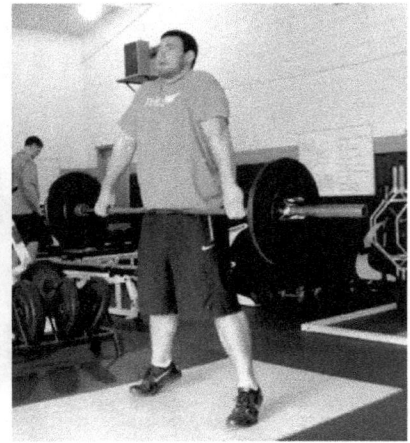

Floor Initial Pull

- Feet at hip width, using a snatch width grip – overhead squat grip
- Barbell in close to the body with arms straight and with the elbows rotated out
- Shoulder blades should be squeezed back with the chest as high as possible
- Hips are higher than the knees but lower than the shoulders
- Eyes straight ahead
- Raise up hips slowly, pulling bar off ground
- Maintain consistent back angle
- As soon as the bar gets to above the knees, initiate a violent, explosive hip extension
- Complete triple extension, rising up on toes
- Return weights to the ground

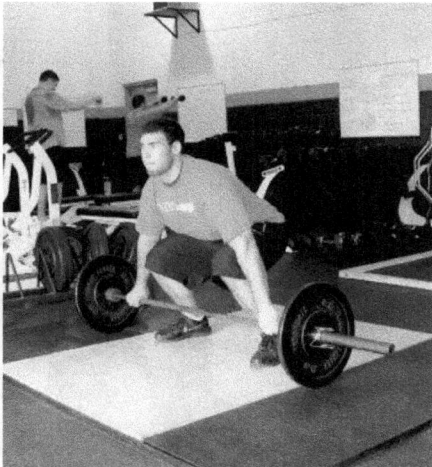

Snatch Start Position

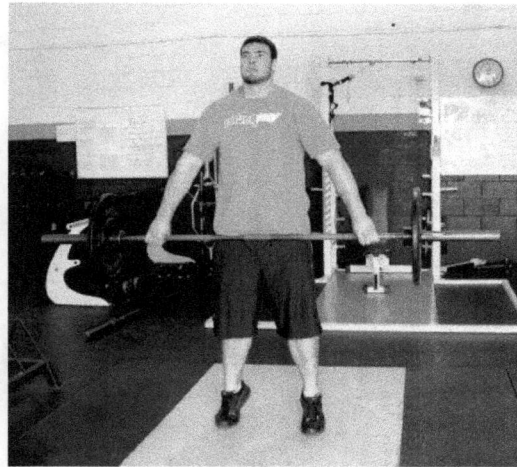

Floor Initial Snatch Pull Top Position

Floor Shrug

- Perform same steps as Floor Initial Pull
- Add in aggressive shoulder shrug
- Lifting / shrugging shoulders up towards ears

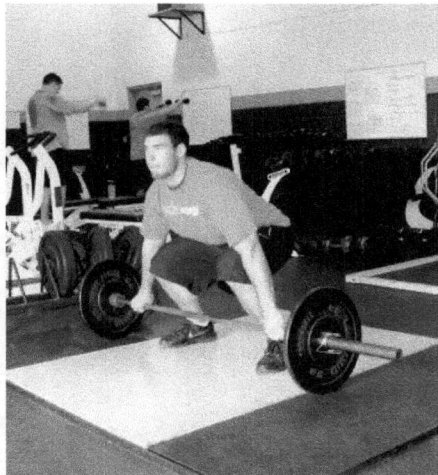

Snatch Start Position

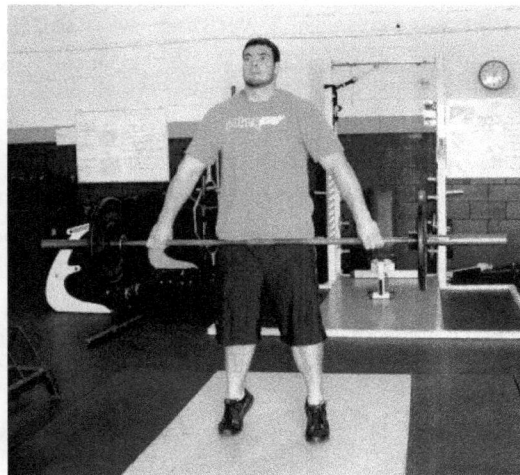

Floor Snatch Shrug Top Position

Snatch

- Perform the Snatch Shrug continuing to accelerate the bar upwards
- Spread the feet to squat width (heels under the shoulders with the toes pointed out)
- At the same time, allow the bar to fly right by the lifter's nose while dropping the hips down and back to catch the bar in an Overhead Squat position
- Stand up with the bar overhead

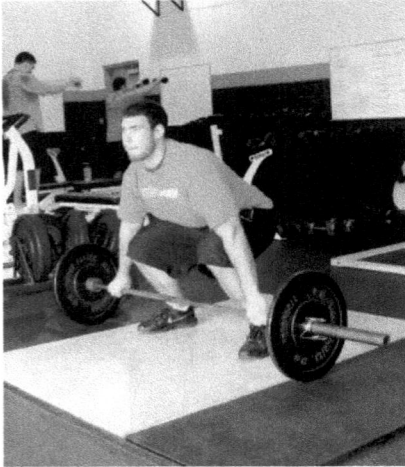

| Snatch Start Position | Snatch Catch Position | Snatch Finish Position |

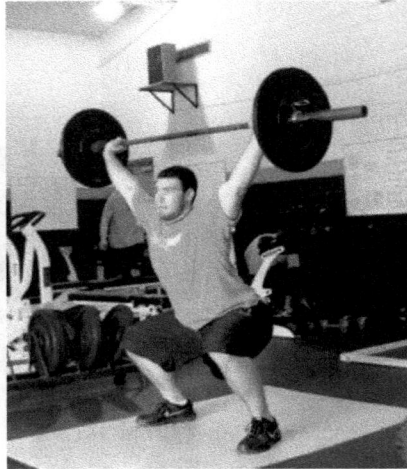

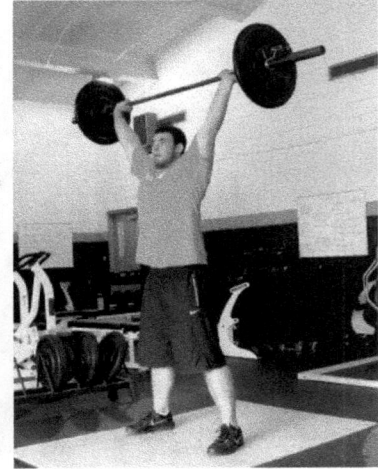

Secondary Full Body Movements

Pressing Continuum

- Shoulder Press – all upper body and no help from the lower body
- Push Press – primarily upper body with some help from the legs
- Push Jerks – primarily lower body with some help from the upper body

Push Press

- The Push Press and Push Jerk are very similar movements (see Push Jerk teaching points)
- The difference is in the use of the arms and the legs
  - In the Push Press emphasizes the upper body, using more force production from the upper body and shoulders, with some help from the legs
  - The Push Jerk emphasizes the lower body, using more explosive force production from the lower body with some help from the upper body

Push Jerk

- Starting position - Shoulder Press-In Front
- Slightly dip the hips down and back while slightly bending the knees
- Immediately extend the legs, explosively pushing the bar upward and slightly back, tucking the chin out of the way
- Once the bar passes the head, return the head to its original position
- Finishing the lift by pressing the bar with the shoulders
  - Allow the heels to return to the ground
  - Dip with knees slightly bent to absorb impact of bar coming down (getting under bar)
  - Lock the elbows out with the bar right behind the ears and straighten legs out to standing position

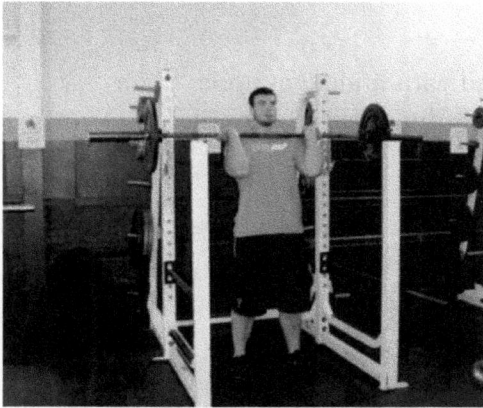

Push Jerk Starting Position

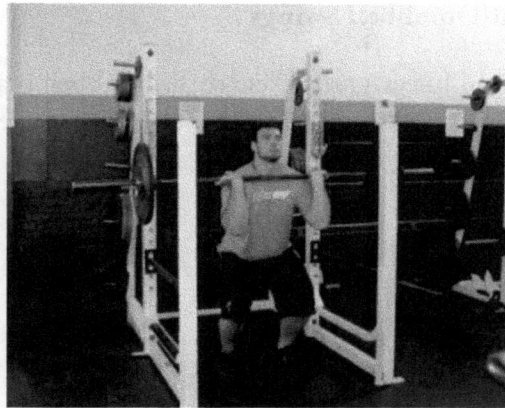

Push Jerk Hip Dip Position

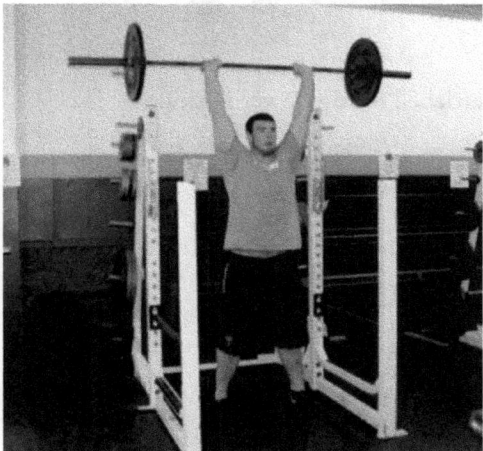

Jerk Extension Position

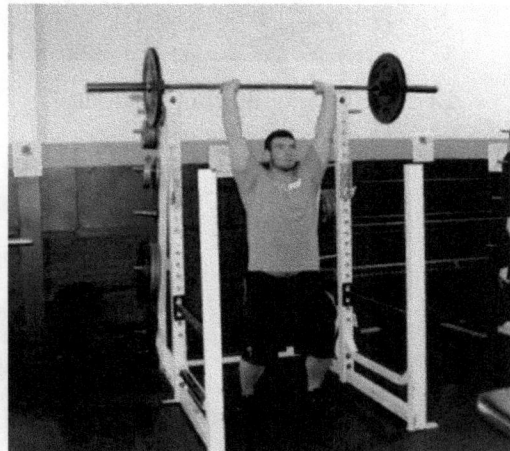

Push Jerk Catch Position

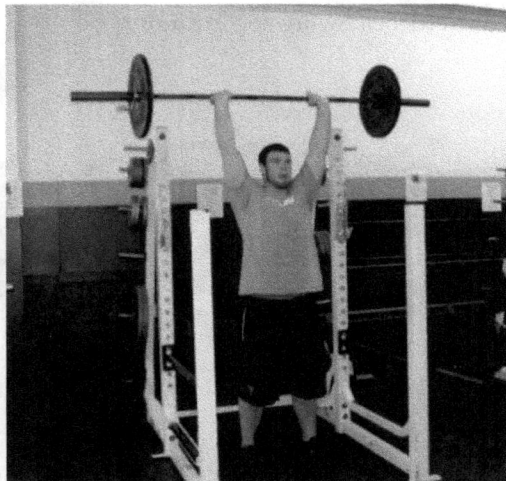

Push Jerk Finish Position

Kettlebell/Dumbbell Swings

- Bend knees so that kettlebell/dumbbell is aligned with middle of upper thigh
- Lean trunk forward so that chest is over kettlebell/dumbbell (cover weight)
- Explosively pop hips forward as you triple extend

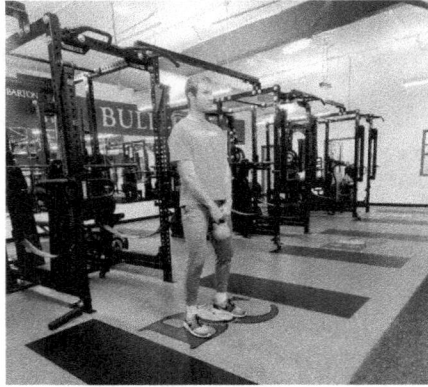

Kettlebell Swing Bottom Position

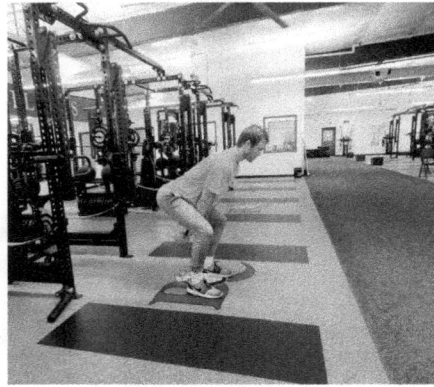

Kettlebell Swing Power Position

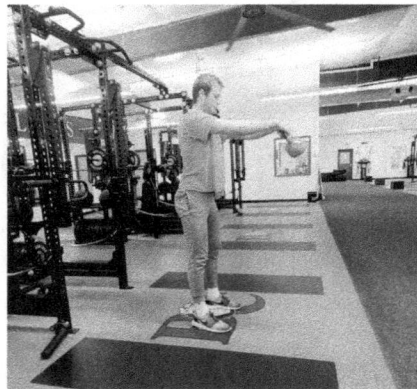

Kettlebell Swing Top Position

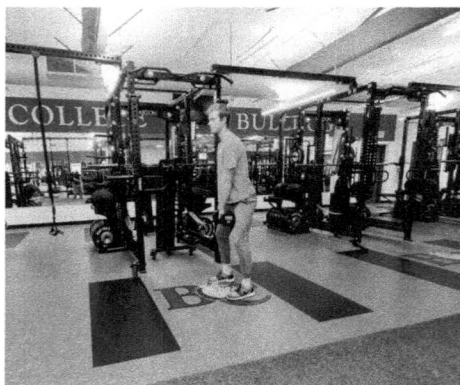

Dumbbell Swing Starting Position

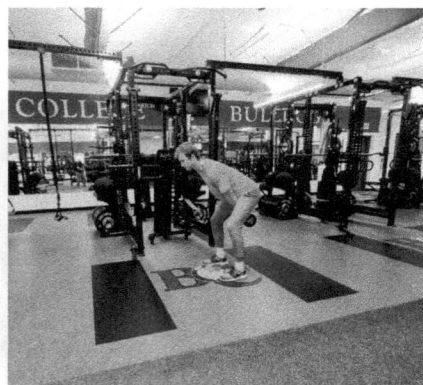

Dumbbell Swing Power Position

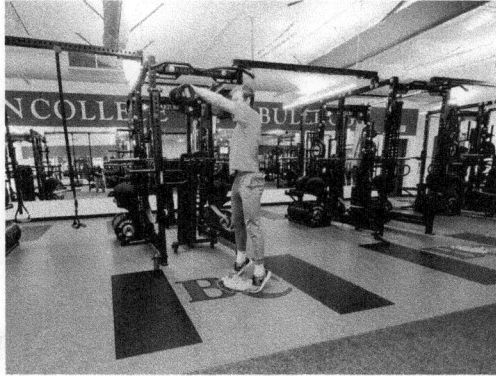

Dumbbell Swing Triple Extension Position

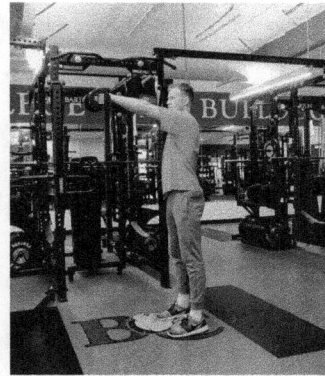

Dumbbell Finishing Position

Kettlebell/Dumbbell Clean

- Lean trunk forward so that chest is over kettlebell/dumbbell (cover weight)
- Explosively pop hips forward as you triple extend
- Continue to accelerate (introducing the upper body) the kettlebell/dumbbell by aggressively shrugging the shoulders

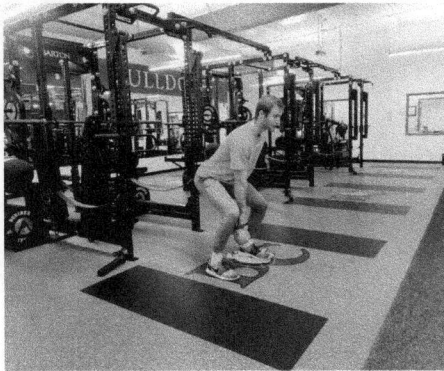

Kettlebell Clean Bottom Position

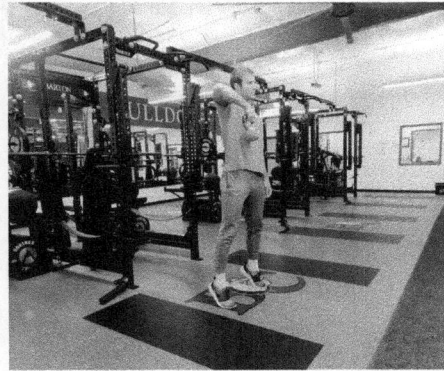

Kettlebell Clean Pull Position

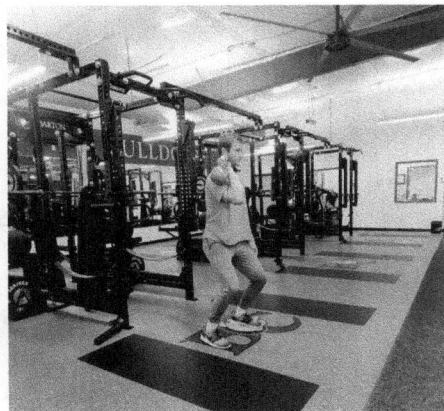

Kettlebell Clean Receiving Position

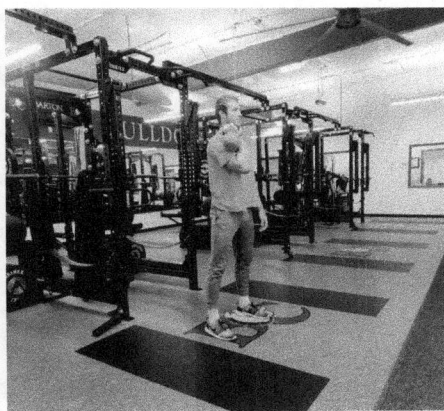

Kettlebell Clean Top Position

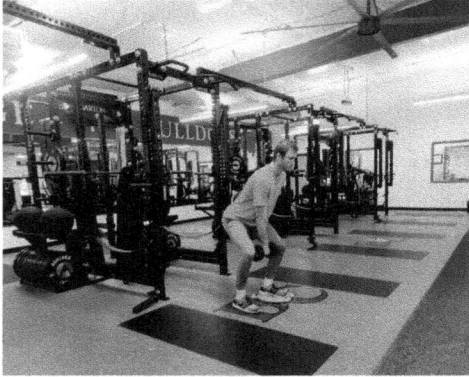

Dumbbell Clean Bottom Position

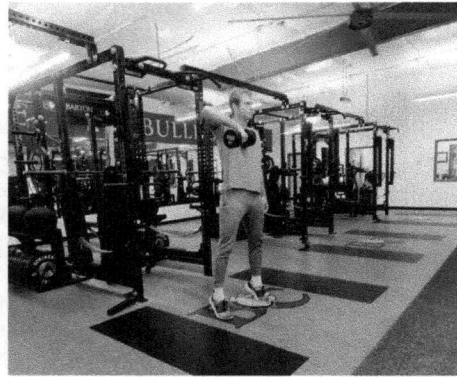

Dumbbell Clean Pull Position

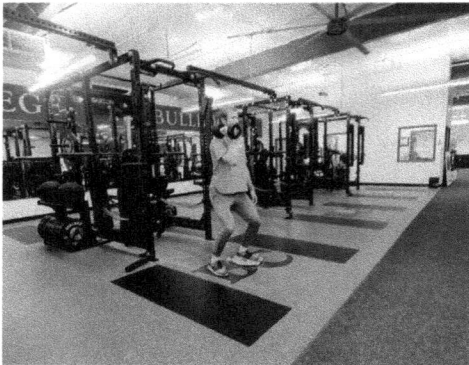

Dumbbell Clean Receiving Position

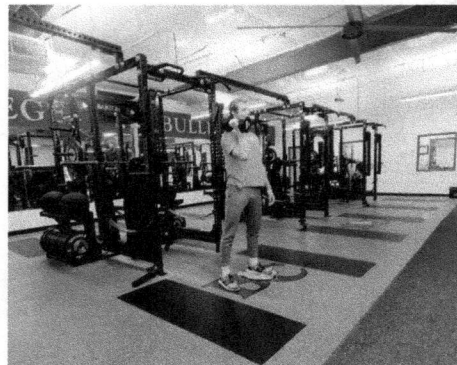

Dumbbell Clean Top Position

Kettlebell/Dumbbell Snatch

- Bend knees so that kettlebell/dumbbell is aligned with middle of upper thigh
- Lean trunk forward so that chest is over kettlebell/dumbbell (cover weight)
- Explosively pop hips forward as you triple extend

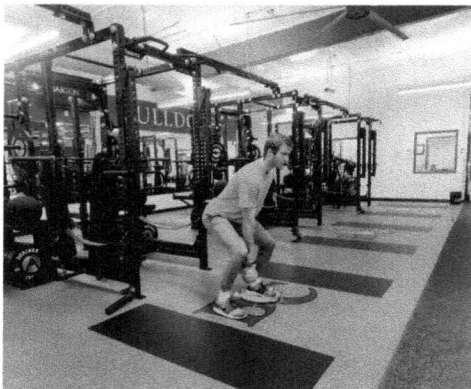

Kettlebell Snatch Bottom Position

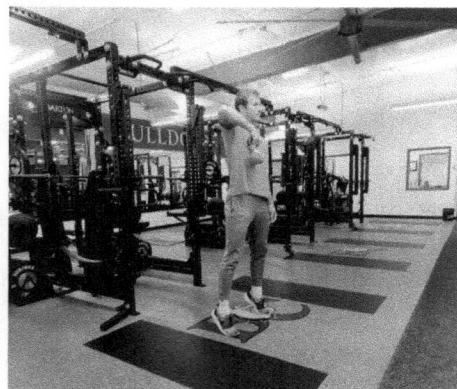

Kettlebell Snatch Pull Position

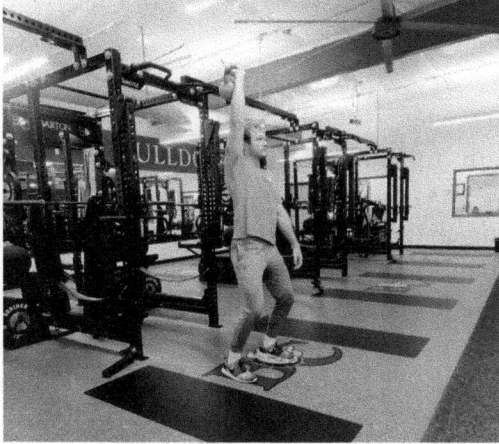

Kettlebell Snatch Receiving Position

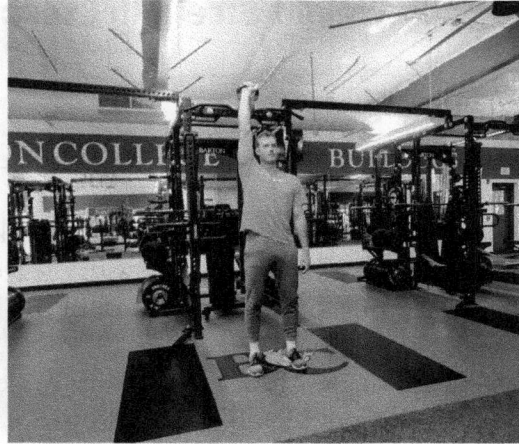

Kettlebell Snatch Top Position

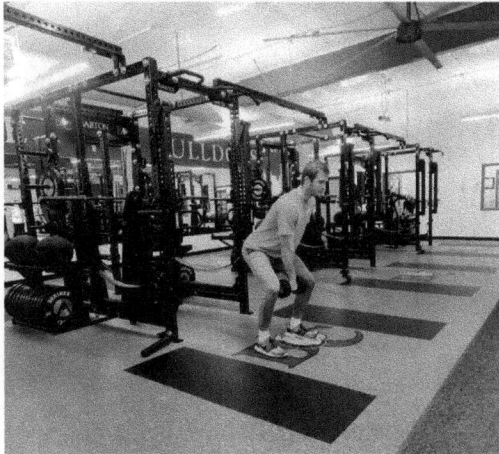

Dumbbell Snatch Bottom Position

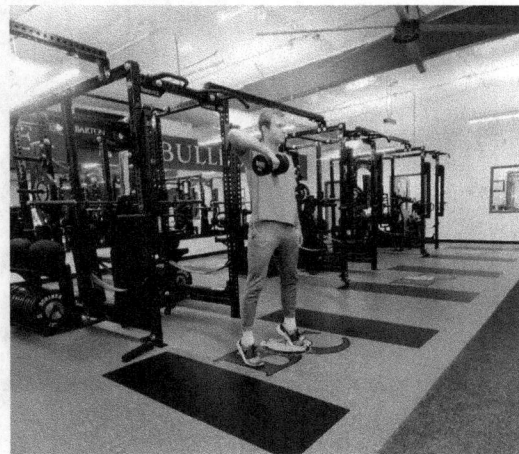

Dumbbell Snatch Pull Position

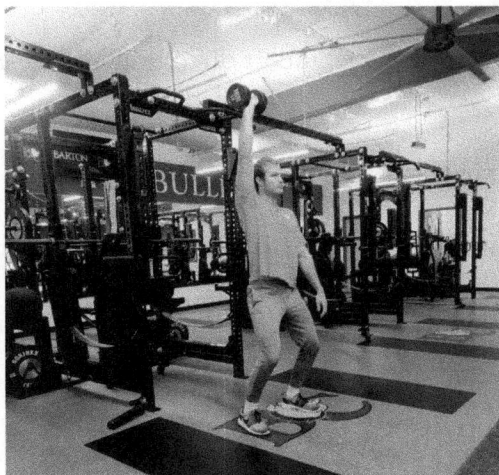

Dumbbell Snatch Receiving Position

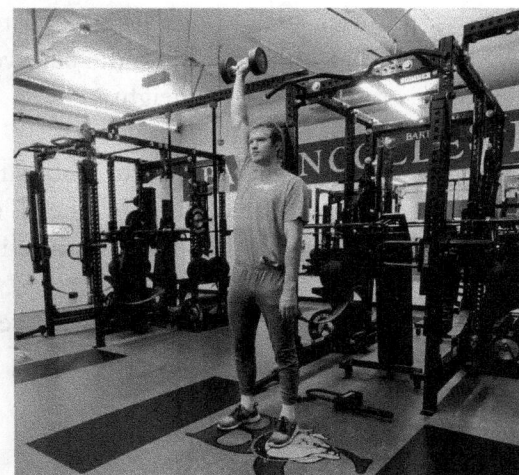

Dumbbell Snatch Top Position

Part 5 : Body Weight Strength Exercises

Body Weight Squat

- Start with feet slightly wider than shoulder width, toes angled slightly out and arms extend in front at shoulder height for balance
- Push the hips back, sticking the butt out, keeping chest forward to balance out body
- Lower the hips down and back with the feet flat and the pressure on the heels
- Lower the hips down and back until the hips are lower than the knees (or top of the thigh is parallel to the ground)
- Upon reaching the lower point of the descent, drive back up through the heels while also driving the hips forward to keep the chest up

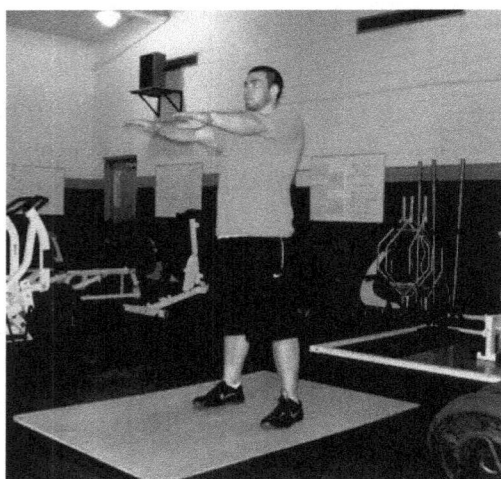

Body Weight Squat Top Position

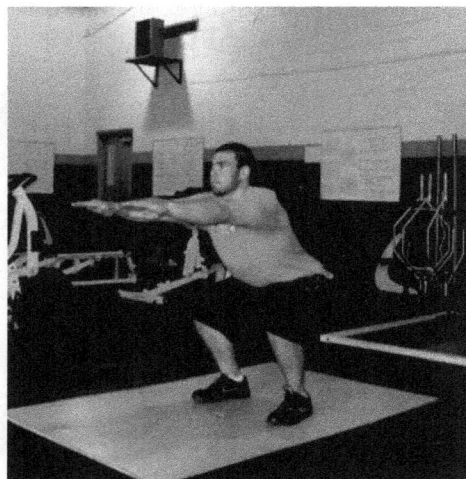

Body Weight Squat Bottom Position

Overhead Squat

- Start with dowel, stick or lightweight bar to learn form
- With a snatch-width grip, place the bar overhead, slightly behind or directly above the ears
  - Raise arms to shoulder height
  - Bend elbows to 90 degrees
  - Maintaining that hand width, grab bar with over and grip
  - Extend arms as bar is raised overhead, cock wrist back
- While performing the lower body squatting movement, gradually rotate the bar back as you go down
- Overhead squat can build flexibility and reveal tightness in shoulder, ankle and hip joints

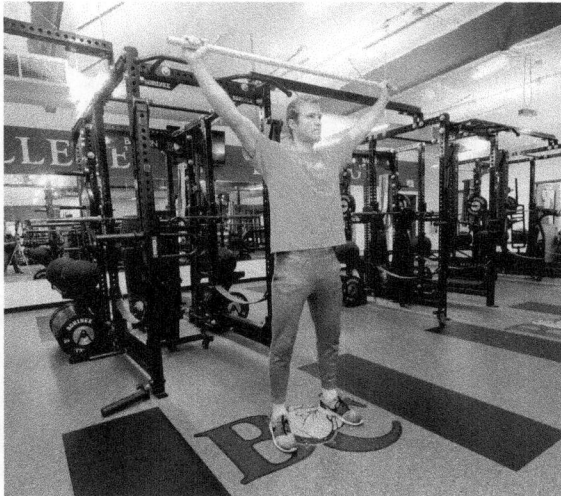

Body Weight Overhead Squat Top Position

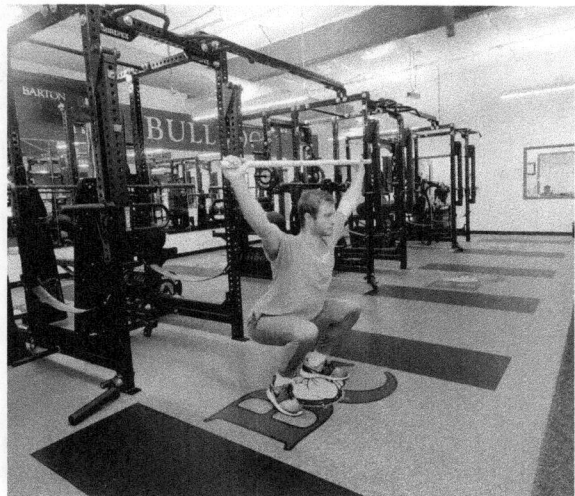

Body Weight Overhead Squat Bottom Position

Rear Leg Elevated Split Squat

- Support the rear leg on something like a bench in a comfortable position off the ground
- With the rear leg supported, position the front foot far enough forward that when the back leg is lowered to the floor, the front knee does not extend out in front of the toes
- Bending the front knee, drop the hips straight down into 90-degree bend of both front and back legs
- Push up on the front leg, extending the knees and hips back to the starting position
- If needed, something like a wooden dowel can be used for balance; just be sure to keep the emphasis on the leg muscle

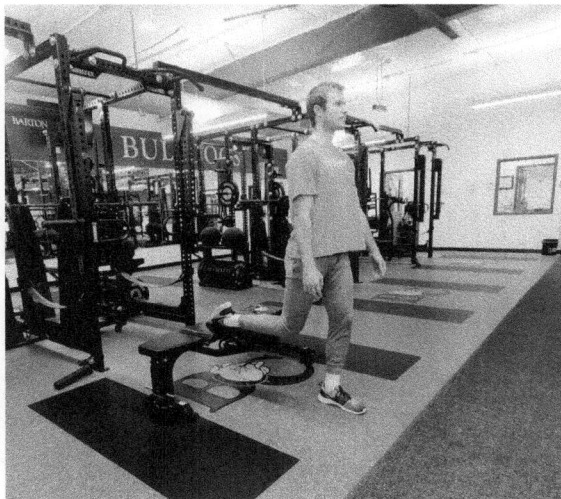

Body Weight Rear Elevated Squat Top Position

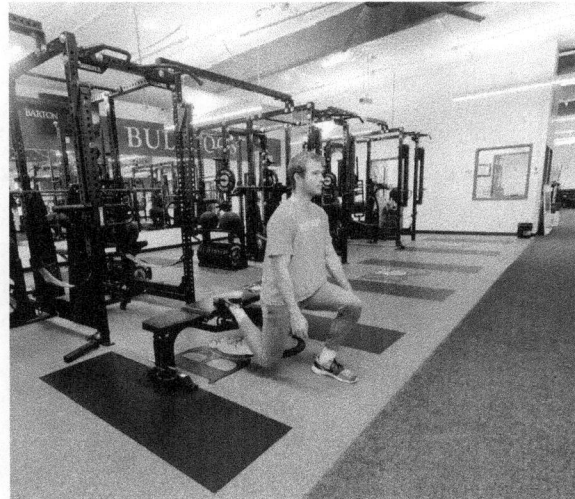

Body Weight Rear Elevated Squat Bottom Position

Front Lunge

- Start with the feet underneath the hips and lined up evenly with each other
- Take an exaggerated step forward
- Drop the hips straight down into 90- degree bend of both front and back legs
- Proper stride length places front knee over the ball of the foot
  - Too long a stride places knee over heel or back leg is extended past 90 degrees
  - Too short a stride places front knee in front of toes
- Drive through the front heel and pull with the back foot to return to the starting position
- Alternate legs throughout the set

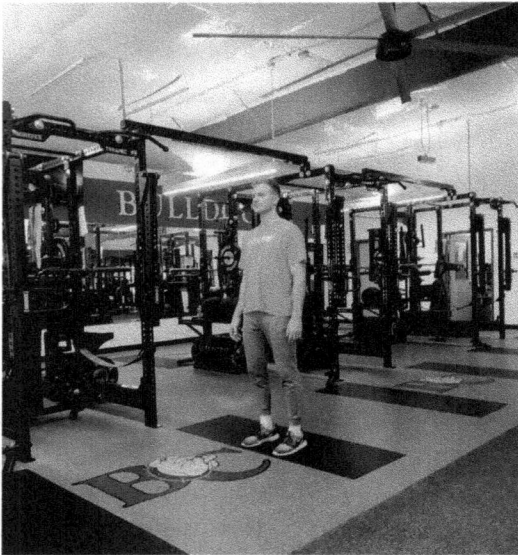

Body Weight Front Lunge Starting Position

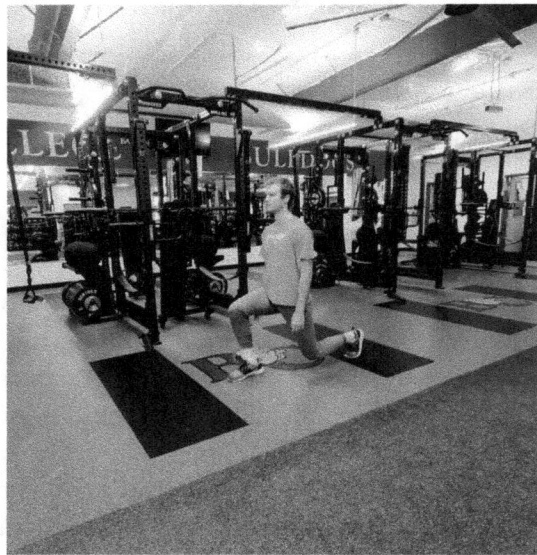

Body Weight Front Lunge Finishing Position

Side Lunge

- Start with feet shoulder width apart
- Take an exaggerated step out to the side, keeping toes pointed forward
- Drop hips down, bending knee of lead leg to 90 degrees
- As you drop down, sit hips back, leaning chest forward to balance out body
- Trail leg is extended with slight knee bend
- Push back off lead leg back to standing position
- Alternate movement to both sides

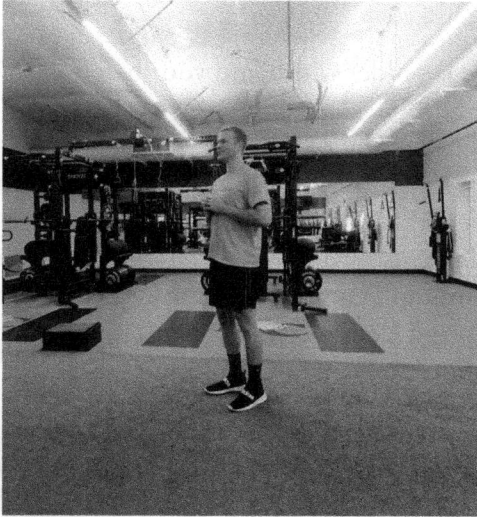

Body Weight Side Lunge Starting Position

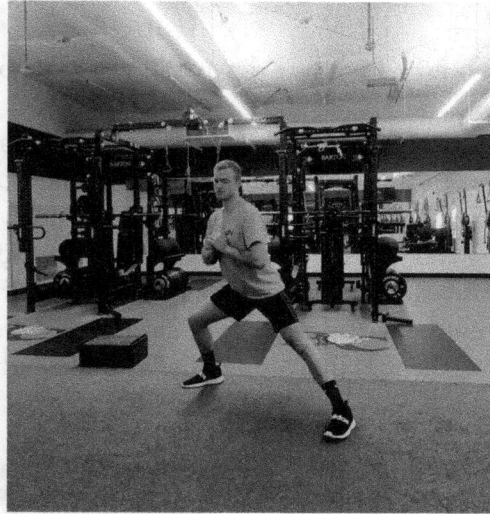

Body Weight Side Lunge Finishing Position

Back Lunge

- Start with the feet underneath the hips and lined up evenly with each other
- Take an over-exaggerated step back, sitting back into the front heel until both front and back knees are bent at 90 degrees
- Same stride length cues apply as front lunge
- Push through the front heel, driving the hips forward and returning the back foot to the starting position

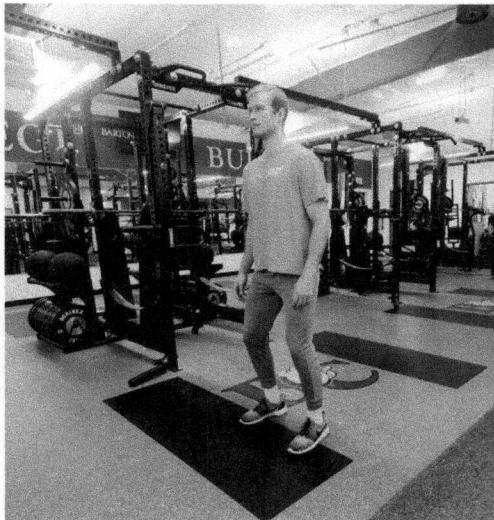

Body Weight Back Lunge Starting Position

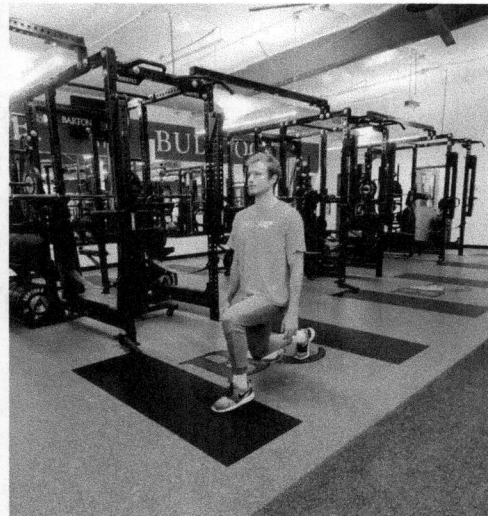

Body Weight Back Lunge Finishing Position

Push Up

- Lie on the floor face down and place just outside shoulder width and your hands even with your chest.
- Feet should be shoulder width apart, pressing through the toes.
- Now breathe out and press your upper body up to almost full extension (keep a slight bend in your elbows to avoid locking out joints) while squeezing your chest.
- After a brief pause, lower yourself downward until your chest almost touches the floor as you inhale.
- Pause without relaxing, then press yourself upwards and complete as many repetitions as desired. Keep the core engaged by maintaining proper plank body position, maintaining a straight line from the toes up through the shoulders, throughout movement.

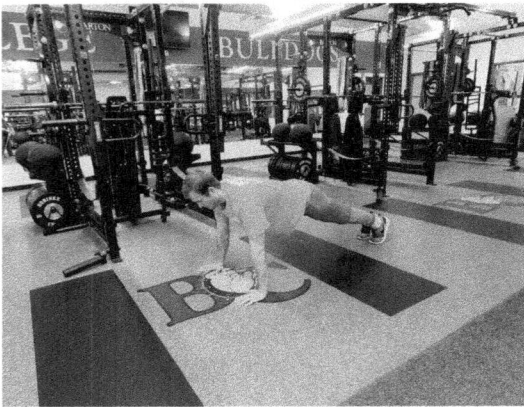

Body Weight Push Up Starting Position

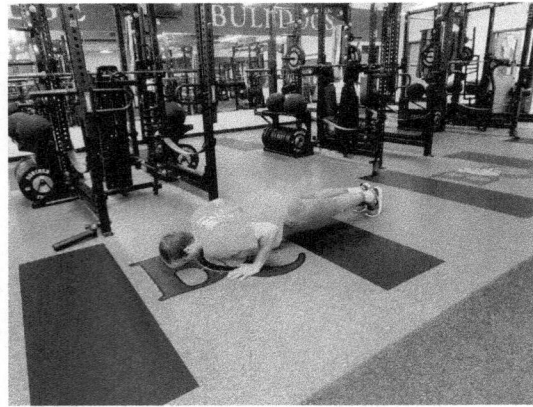

Body Weight Push Up Starting Position

Basic Variations

- Wall Push Up (lower strength option)
  - Place hands at chest height and perform push-ups at a comfortable body angle (less of an angle reduces the body weight being worked against)

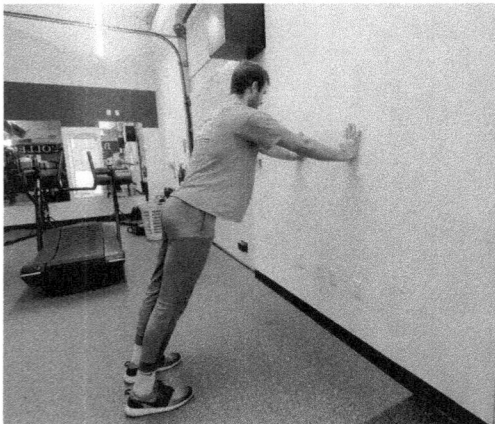

Body Weight Wall Push Up Starting Position

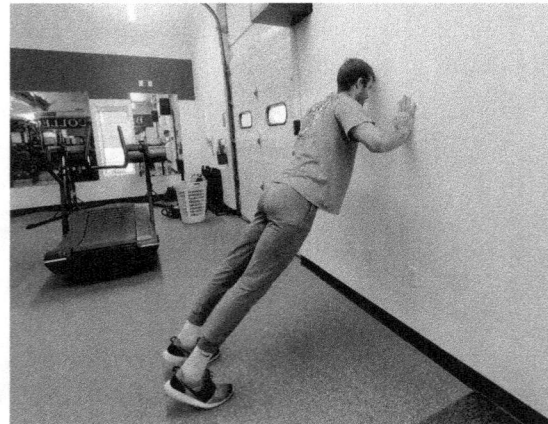

Body Weight Wall Push Up Bottom Position

- Modified Push Up (lower strength option)
  - ○ Instead of using the toes as an anchor point, use the knees as the back pivot/anchor point. Keep the rest of the body in a good plank position maintaining a straight line from the knees up through the shoulders

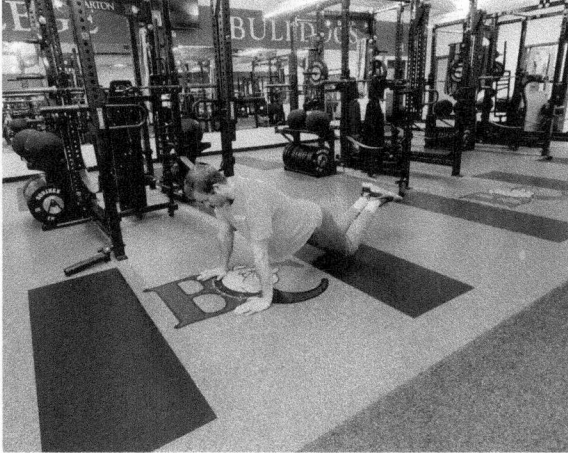

Body Weight Modified Push Up Starting Position

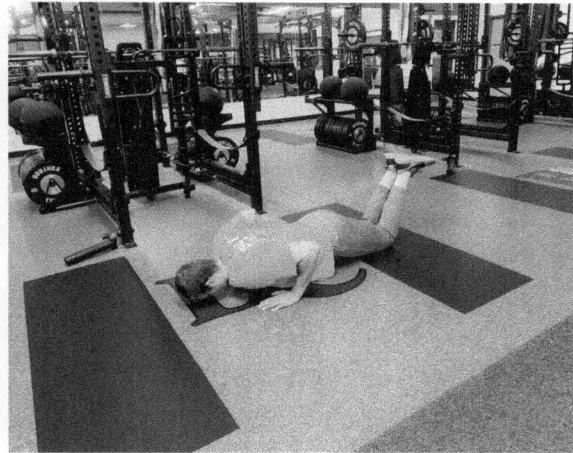

Body Weight Modified Push Up Bottom Position

- Incline Push Up (increased strength option)
  - ○ Elevate the feet and maintain a good plank body position as you perform push-ups.
  - ○ The higher the feet are, the more body weight resistance is pushed against. Highest level is the wall pushup where full body weight resistance is provided (body position also transfers emphasis to the shoulders, like a body weight shoulder press).

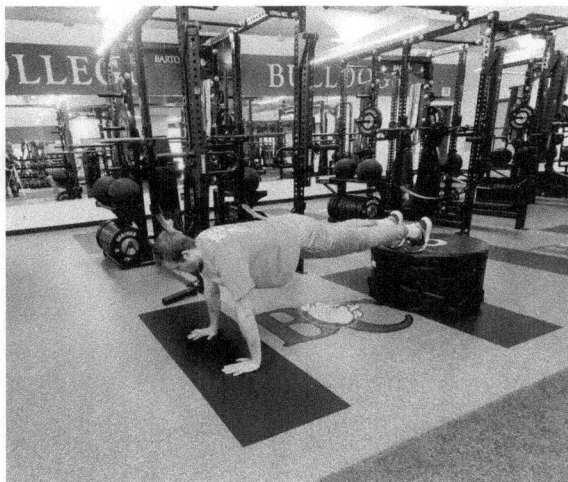

Body Weight Incline Push Up Starting Position

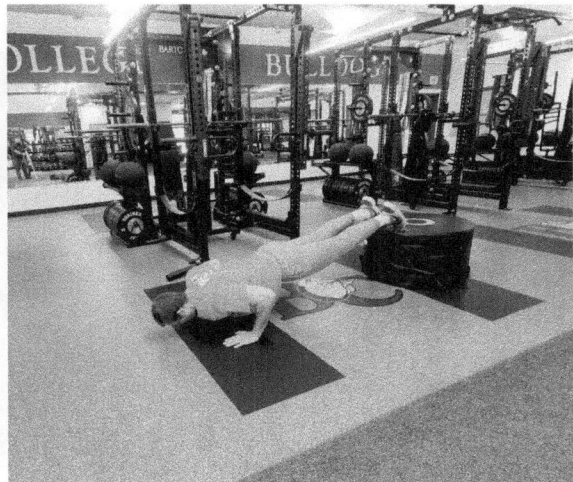

Body Weight Incline Push Up Bottom Position

- Hands Elevated Push Up (reduced strength option)
  - Place hands on object and perform push-ups at a comfortable body angle (as you reduce the incline, getting closer to a push up on the ground, the more body weight being worked against)

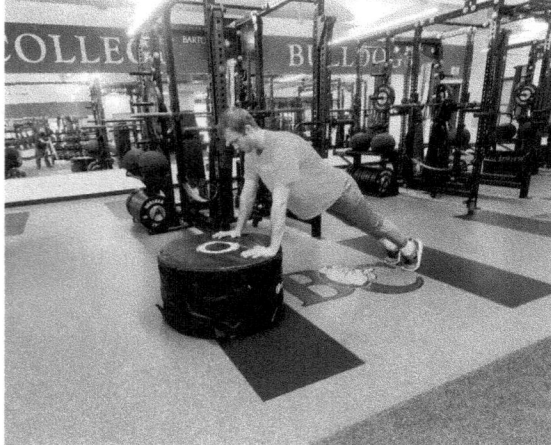

Body Weight Hands Elevated Starting Position

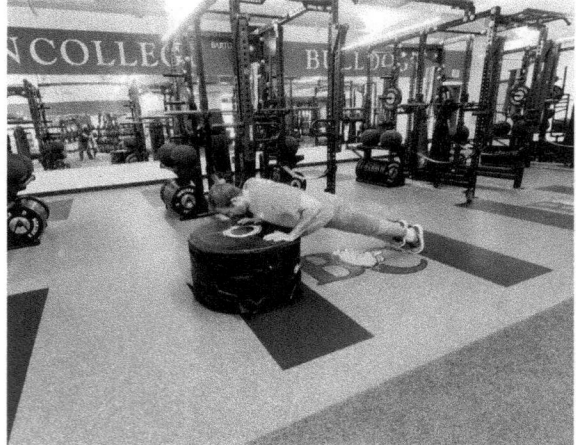

Body Weight Hands Elevated Bottom Position

- Bar Incline Push Up
  - Place hands on bar and perform push-ups at a comfortable body angle (as you reduce the incline, getting closer to a push up on the ground, the more body weight being worked against)

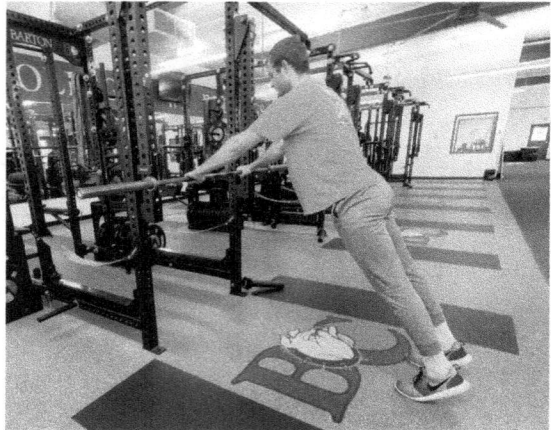

Body Weight Bar Incline Starting Position

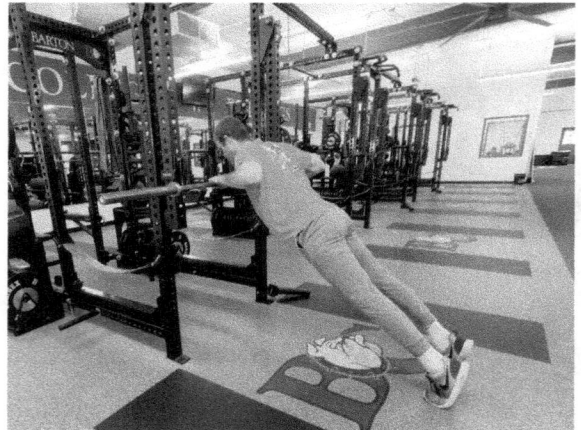

Body Weight Bar Incline Bottom Position

- Diamond Push Up
  - Start with hands close together, with thumbs and index fingers touching to create a "diamond"
  - Narrowing the width of the hands places greater emphasis on the triceps as you lower the body down and press back up

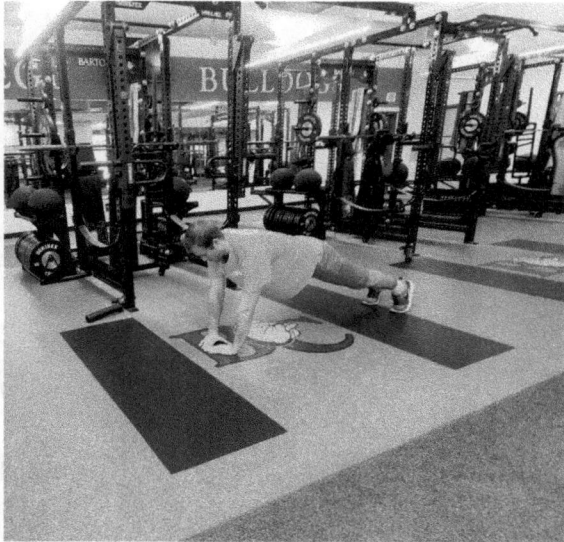

Body Weight Diamond Push Up Starting Position

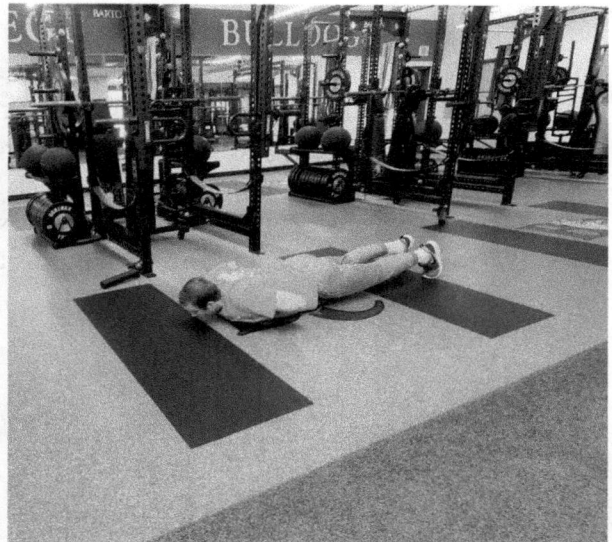

Body Weight Diamond Push Up Bottom Position

- Dive Bomber Push Up (Rocking Push Up)
  - Start in a modified push up position with feet wide and hips raised to place the upper body at a forward incline.
  - As you lower yourself, rock your upper body forward in a curved pattern bringing your chest close to the ground.
  - Reverse the pattern to rock yourself back to the starting position.

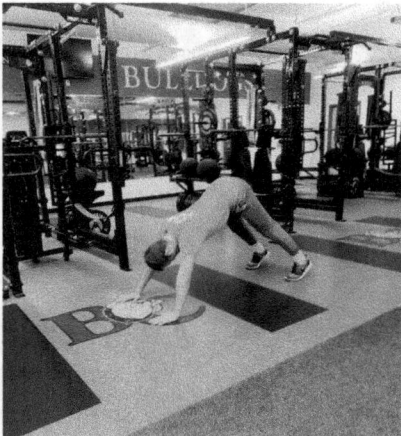

Body Weight Dive Bomber
Push Up Starting Position

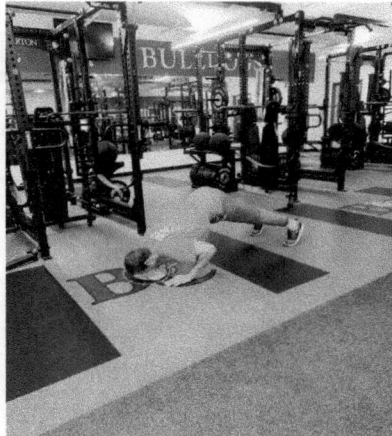

Body Weight Dive Bomber
Push Up Midrange Position

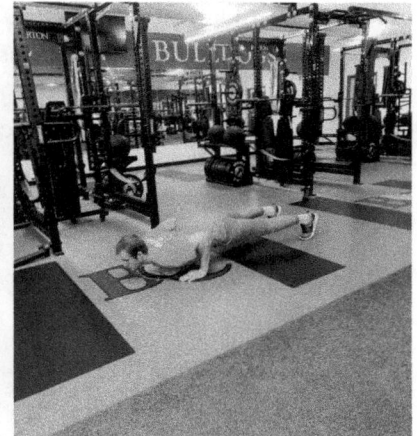

Body Weight Dive Bomber
Push Up Bottom Position

Pull Ups

- Using a bar that allows your body weight to hang with feet not touching the ground, grip the bar with an overhand grip (palms facing away), with hands outside the shoulders.
- Using your back and biceps muscles, pull your body up so that your chin is above the bar
  - Concentrating on squeezing your back helps to engage the back muscles
- Exhale as you pull yourself up and inhale as you lower yourself down to the starting position
- The torso should remain in an upright position as you control your body through the lifting and lowering movements

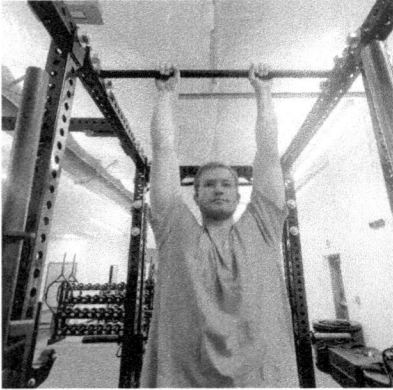

Pull Up Grip

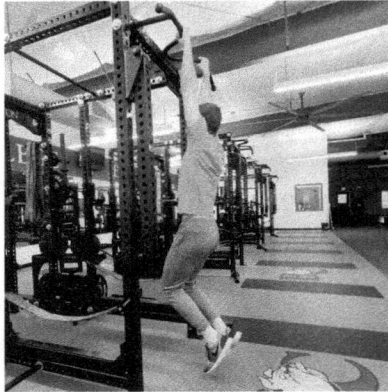

Pull Up Starting Position

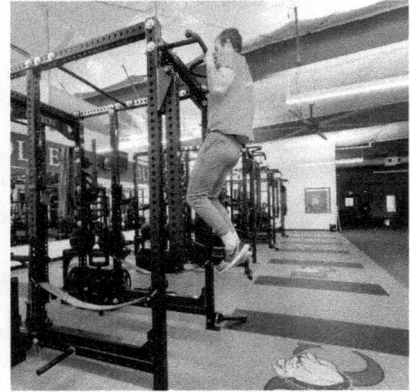

Pull Up Top Position

Pull Ups Variations

- Chin Up
  - Reversing the grip, using an underhand (palms facing the body) grip is often referred to as a chin up.
  - Using an underhanded grip utilizes the biceps to a greater extent.

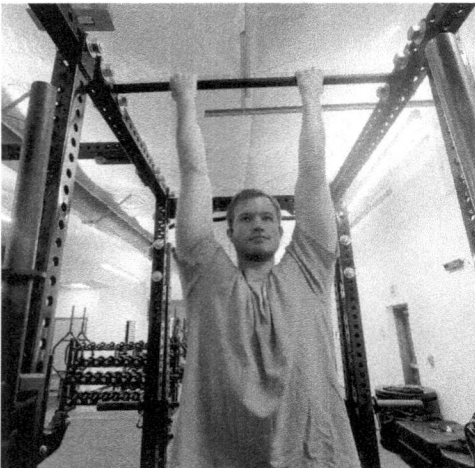

Chin Up Grip

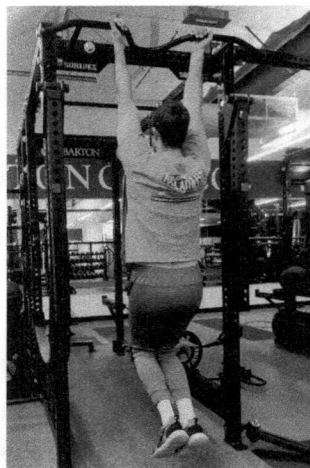

Chin Up Starting Position

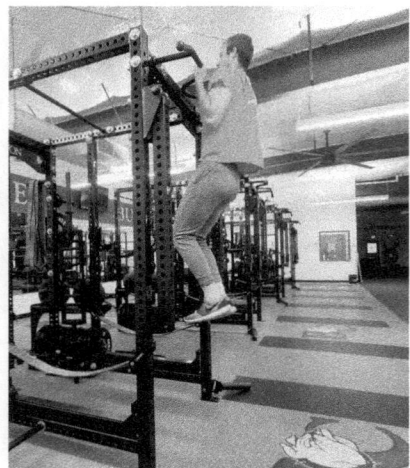

Chin Up Top Position

- Wide Grip
  - Using a grip that is wider than shoulder width, but with no greater than a 45-degree angle of the forearms, will utilize the rhomboids posterior deltoids and upper/outer area of the latissimus dorsi

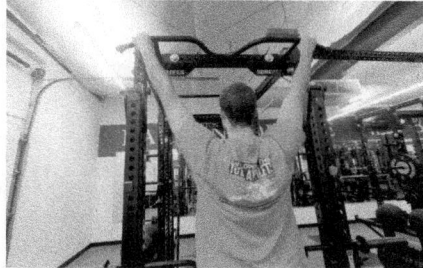

Wide Pull Up Grip

- Close Grip
  - Using a narrower than shoulder width grip will utilize the lower latissimus dorsi with more help from the chest and biceps

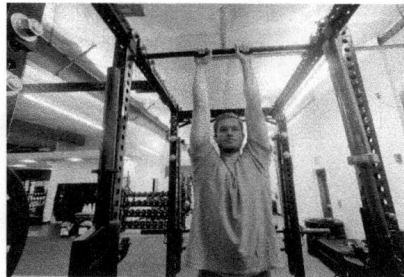

Close Pull Up Grip

- Towel Pull Up
  - Looping towels over the bar and grabbing the end using a neutral grip (palm facing in like you are shaking someone's hand) will utilize the forearms more and help increase grip strength to a greater degree

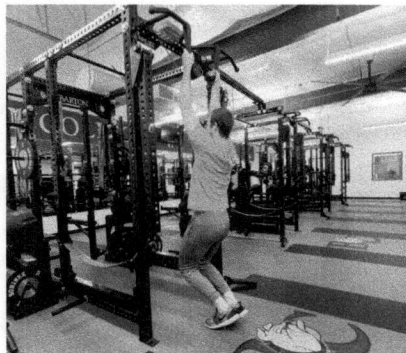

Towel Pull Up Bottom Position

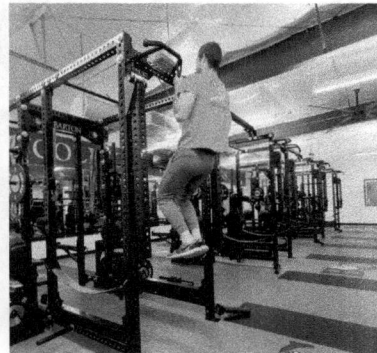

Towel Pull Up Top Position

- Assisted Pull Up
    - Using a counterbalance system, band or spotter assistant makes the exercise easier by decreasing the resistance being worked against to allow the exercise to be performed properly

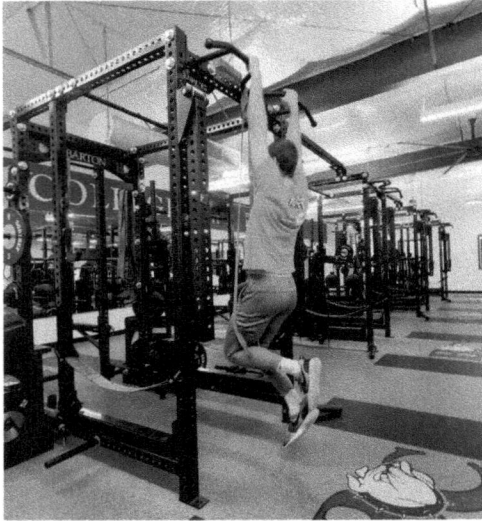

Assisted Pull Up Bottom Position

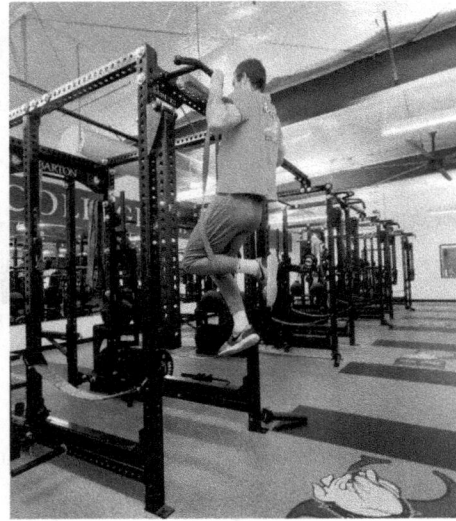

Assisted Pull Up Top Position

- Inverted Row
    - A bar at a lower height can be used to allow the feet to touch the ground
    - The steeper the incline of the body, the more resistance is utilized
    - Match the proper body angle based on the strength needs of the exerciser, allowing proper execution of the exercise and loading of the muscles

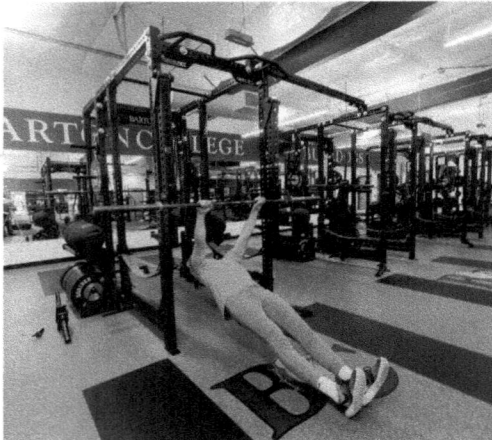

Inverted Row Bottom Position

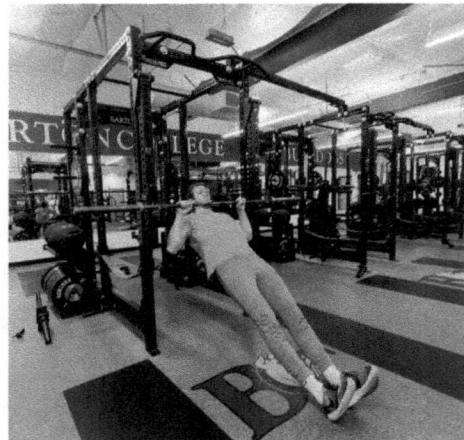

Inverted Row Top Position

Part 6 : Manual Resistance Exercises

Resisted Ankle Dorsiflexion

- Position the person performing the exercise with the leg outstretched, sitting on the ground or supported in some way.
- The person supplying the resistance places one hand above the ankle to stabilize the leg so that movement only occurs at the ankle joint.
- With the foot fully plantarflexed, place the other hand below the toes to provide resistance.
- Provide steady resistance as the person exercising pulls their toes back towards their shin into a fully dorsiflexed position.
- The person exercising and the person applying resistance must communicate properly to apply appropriate resistance.
  - Too much resistance and the foot cannot move; too little resistance and the muscle will not be overloaded.
  - Good communication is needed so that injury will not occur, movement should be slow and steady through the full range of motion.

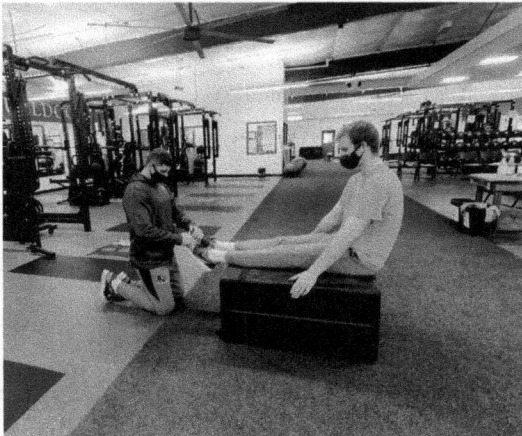

Resisted Ankle Dorsiflexion Starting Position

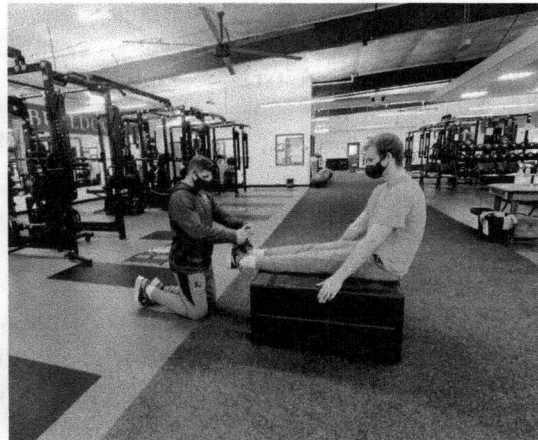

Resisted Ankle Dorsiflexion Finishing Position

Resisted Ankle Plantar Flexion

- Position the person performing the exercise with the leg outstretched, sitting on the ground or supported in some way.
- The person supplying the resistance places one hand above the ankle to stabilize the leg so that movement only occurs at the ankle joint.
- With the foot fully dorsiflexed, place the other hand on the ball of the foot to provide resistance.
- Provide steady resistance as the person exercising extends their foot, pointing their toes towards their shin into a fully plantarflexed position.
- The person exercising and the person applying resistance must communicate properly to apply appropriate resistance.

- o Too much resistance and the foot cannot move; too little resistance and the muscle will not be overloaded.
- o Good communication is needed so that injury will not occur. Movement should be slow and steady through the full range of motion.

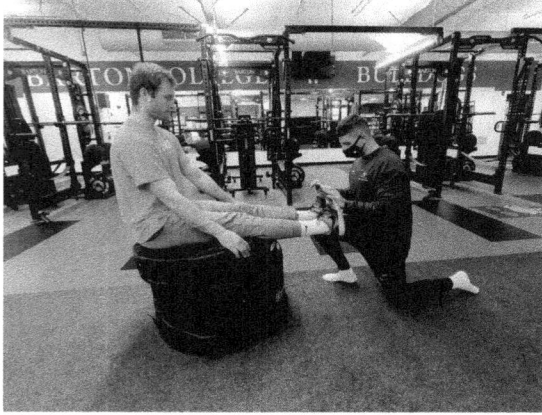

Resisted Ankle Plantar Starting Position

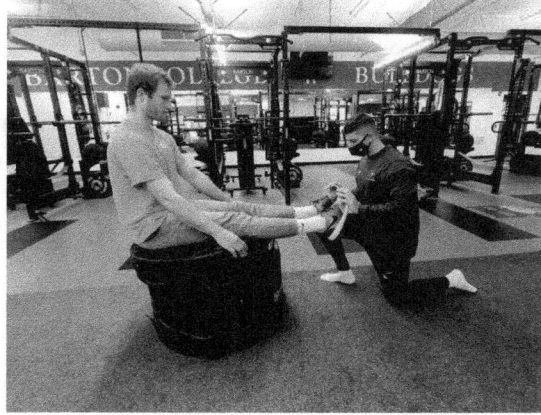

Resisted Ankle Plantar Finishing Position

Resisted Hamstring Curl

- Position the person performing the exercise on a chair with the bend of the knee against the end of the chair.
  - o Two chairs can be stacked or an object like a towel can be placed behind the knee so that the foot stays above the floor.
- The person supplying the resistance places one hand above the knee to stabilize the leg so that movement only occurs at the knee joint, with the person exercising extending the leg straight.
- Place the other hand above the ankle on the Achilles tendon to provide resistance.
  - o The hand is placed above the ankle to take pressure off the ankle joint while maximizing the axis of rotation.
- Provide steady resistance as the person exercising flexes at the knee, as they pull their foot towards the ground.
- The person exercising and the person applying resistance must communicate properly to apply appropriate resistance.
  - o Too much resistance and the foot cannot move; too little resistance and the muscle will not be overloaded.
  - o Good communication is needed so that injury will not occur. Movement should be slow and steady through the full range of motion.

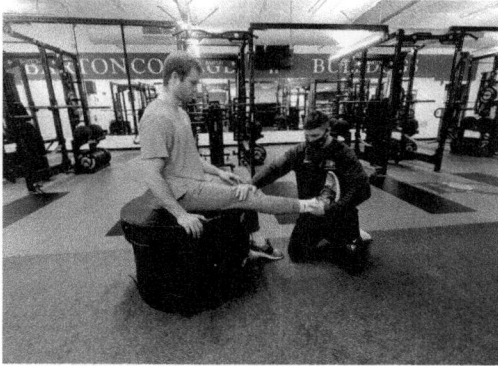

Resisted Hamstring Curl Starting Position

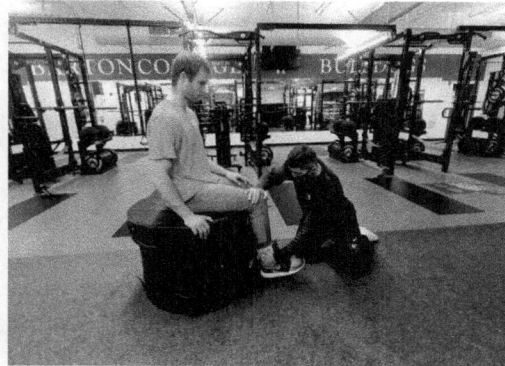

Resisted Hamstring Curl Finishing Position

Resisted Leg Extension

- Position the person performing the exercise on a chair with the bend of the knee against the end of the chair.
  - Two chairs can be stacked or an object like a towel can be placed behind the knee so that the foot stays above the floor.
- The person supplying the resistance places one hand above the knee to stabilize the leg so that movement only occurs at the knee joint, with the person exercising letting the other leg relax.
- Place the other hand above the ankle on bottom of the shin to provide resistance.
  - The hand is placed above the ankle to take pressure off the ankle joint while maximizing the axis of rotation.
- Provide steady resistance as the person exercising extends at the knee, as they extend their leg to straighten the leg.
- The person exercising and the person applying resistance must communicate properly to apply appropriate resistance.
  - Too much resistance and the foot cannot move; too little resistance and the muscle will not be overloaded.
  - Good communication is needed so that injury will not occur. Movement should be slow and steady through the full range of motion.

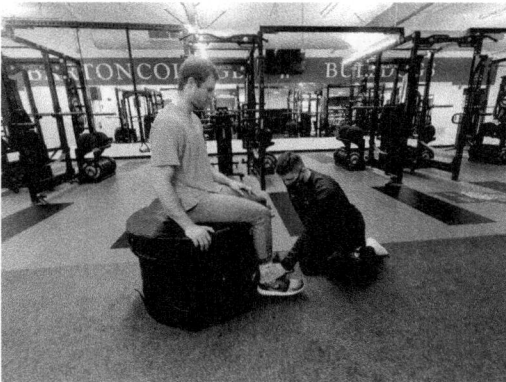

Resisted Leg Extension Starting Position

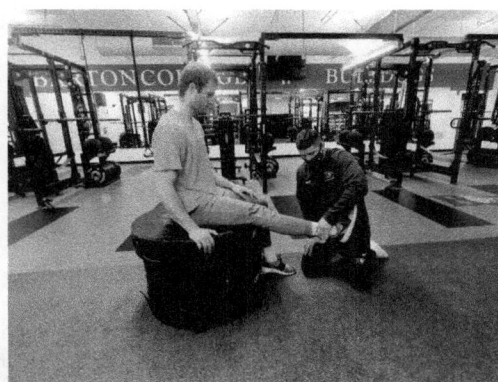

Resisted Leg Extension Finishing Position

Resisted Shoulder Press

- The person exercising can be sitting in a chair or sitting on the ground.
  - If the person exercising is stronger, having them sit lower with the person providing resistance higher helps provide leverage for the person providing resistance (this allows the needed resistance to be delivered).
- The person exercising should place their hands palm up, at shoulder height.
- The person providing resistance puts their palms on the other person's hands/palms and provides resistance as the exercises push up against resistance.
- Provide steady resistance as the person exercising extends their arms over head, to an almost straight position.
  - Leaving a little bend in the elbows, or any joint being exercised, takes pressure off the joint and keeps the resistance on the targeted muscle.
- The person exercising and the person applying resistance must communicate properly to apply appropriate resistance.
  - Too much resistance and the foot cannot move; too little resistance and the muscle will not be overloaded.
  - Good communication is needed so that injury will not occur. Movement should be slow and steady through the full range of motion.

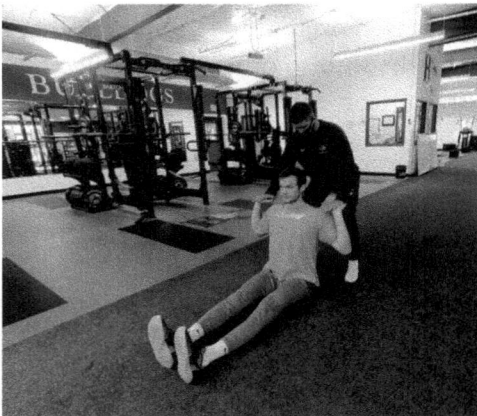

Resisted Shoulder Press Starting Position   Resisted Shoulder Press Finishing Position

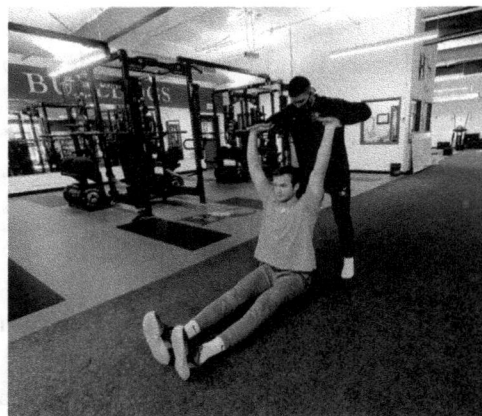

Resisted Lat Pulldown

- Start: Sitting with a natural arch in your back and slightly leaning back with your arms extended overhead.
- Movement: Pull your elbows downwards until your elbows come down to your sides. Pause momentarily and resist the negative to the starting position.
- Spotting: Position one leg against the lifter's back to add support. Grasp under the lifter's elbows and appropriately apply pressure.
- The person exercising and the person applying resistance must communicate properly to apply appropriate resistance.

- o Too much resistance and the foot cannot move; too little resistance and the muscle will not be overloaded.
- o Good communication is needed so that injury will not occur, movement should be slow and steady through the full range of motion.

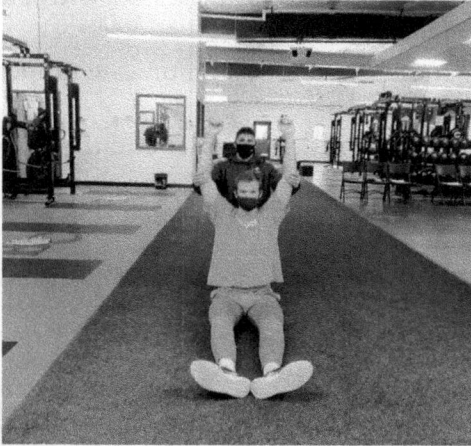

Resisted Lat Pulldown Starting Position

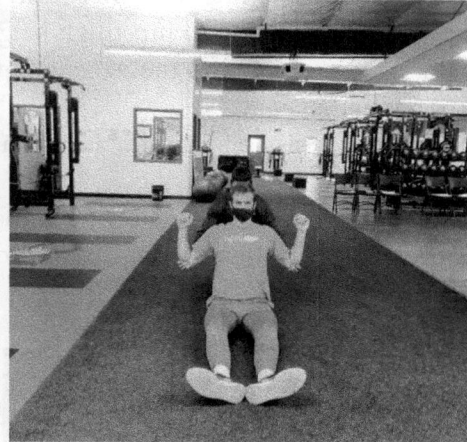

Resisted Lat Pulldown Finishing Position

Resisted Towel Biceps Curl

- Stand with feet shoulder width apart and knees slightly bent.
- With an end of a short towel in each hand (palms up), start with arms extended at thigh height.
- With a partner providing resistance from below, keep the elbows at the sides and flex biceps to pull the towel up to shoulder height.
- The person exercising and the person applying resistance must communicate properly to apply appropriate resistance.
  - o Too much resistance and the foot cannot move, too little resistance and the muscle will not be overloaded.
  - o Good communication is needed so that injury will not occur. Movement should be slow and steady through the full range of motion.

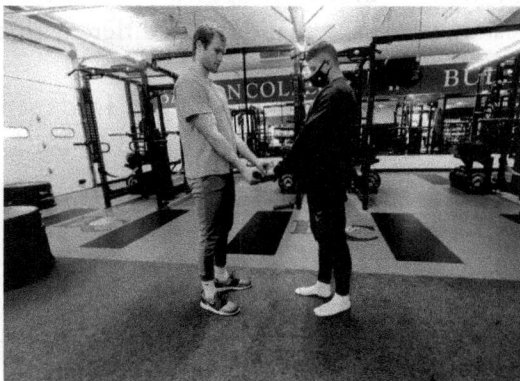

Resisted Towel Biceps Curl Starting Position

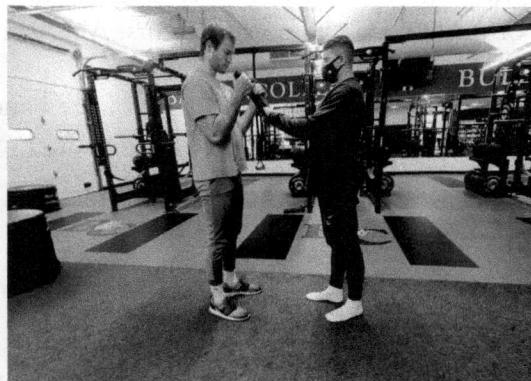

Resisted Towel Biceps Curl Finishing Position

Resisted Towel Triceps Extension

- Stand with feet shoulder width apart and knees slightly bent.
- With an end of a short towel in each hand (palms down), start with arms flexed and hands at chest height.
- With a partner providing resistance from above, keep the elbows at the sides and extend triceps, pushing the towel down to hip/thigh height.
- The person exercising and the person applying resistance must communicate properly to apply appropriate resistance.
  - Too much resistance and the foot cannot move; too little resistance and the muscle will not be overloaded.
  - Good communication is needed so that injury will not occur. Movement should be slow and steady through the full range of motion.

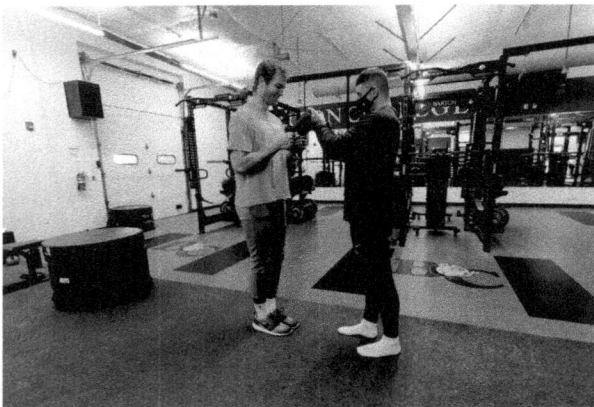

Resisted Towel Triceps Extension Starting Position

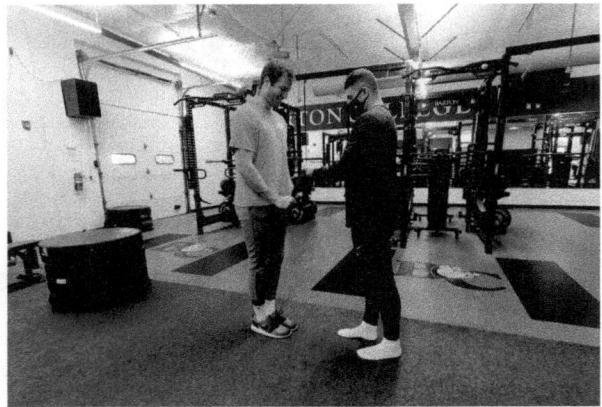

Resisted Towel Triceps Extension Finishing Position

Part 7: Resistance Band Exercises

Fitness bands provide a self-contained source of resistance, referred to as dynamic progressive resistance, which does not rely on gravity or other external forces for resistance. To the body, and specifically the muscle, the source of the resistance is not as important. What is important is that the muscle is overloaded or pushed past its normal limits. Alter band resistance by using bands with different thickness. Thinner bands will have less resistance.

You can also change the resistance of the band by anchoring it narrower or wider. In these images anchoring with two feet makes the band shorter, providing more resistance.

Less Resistance

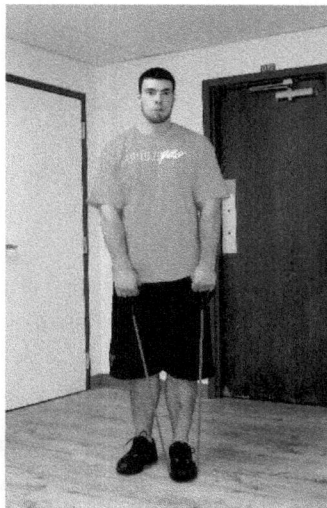

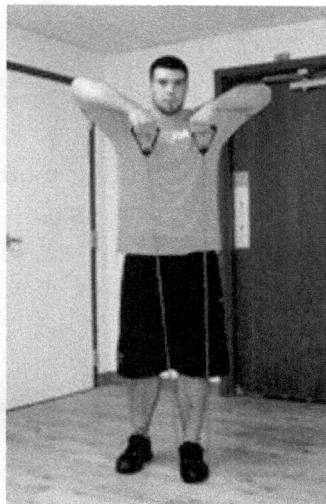

More Resistance

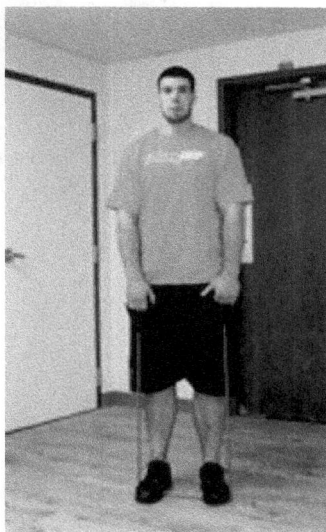

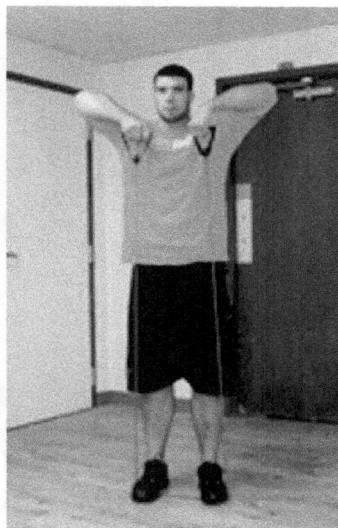

To maximize the workout and reduce the chance of injury when working with resistance bands:

- Keep the upper body stable with movement occurring only at the shoulder and elbow joints when doing upper body resistance band exercises.
- Maintain tension on tubing through a whole range of motion.
- Do not let the pull of the tubing cause the elbows to lock out and shoulders to raise up at top of movement.
- Exhale on exertion as you pull and inhale as you return to the starting position
- Always perform movements in a steady, controlled manner.
- Do not lock elbows

Narrow (Underhand) Grip Lat Pulldown

Anchor Point: High
Primary Muscle Group: Latissimus Dorsi (lateral fibers) (Back)

- Start in a kneeling position with arms extended, using an underhand close grip (hands about six inches apart).
- Torso should be flexed forward (but more upright than with wide grip variation) so that upper body is at the same angle as the stretched tubing (the line from the anchor point through the hands and shoulders down through the hips should be straight).
- Pull handles (maintaining width) to shoulder height leading with the elbows. Pause briefly, and then extend arms, keeping elbows slightly flexed, back to starting position.

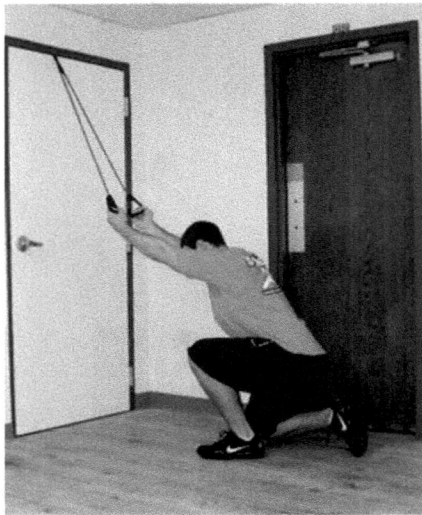

Starting Position

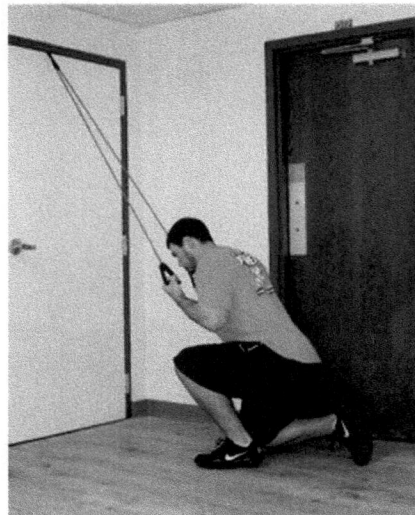

Pull Down Position

Wide (Overhand) Grip Lat Pulldown

Anchor Point: High
Primary Muscle Group: Latissimus Dorsi (lateral fibers) (Back)

- Start in a kneeling position with arms extended
- Use an overhand grip slightly wider than shoulder width.
- Torso should be flexed forward so that upper body is at the same angle as the stretched tubing (the line from the anchor point through the hands and shoulders down through the hips should be straight).
- Pull handles (maintaining width) to shoulder height leading with the elbows. Pause briefly, and then extend arms, keeping elbows slightly flexed, back to starting position.

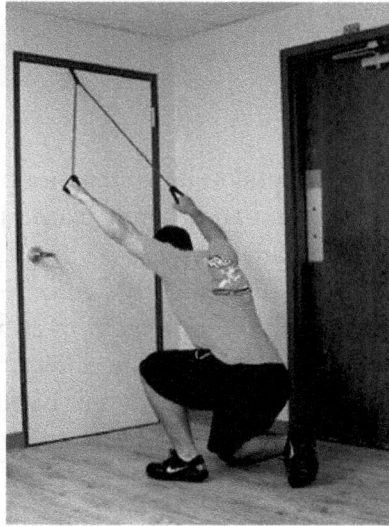

Starting Position   Pulldown Position

Standing Row

Anchor Point: Middle
Primary Muscle Group: Latissimus Dorsi (Back)

- Start with feet shoulder width apart and sit back into a high squat position (chest at anchor height) with arms extended using a shoulder-width, neutral grip.
- Torso should be upright and held stable throughout movement.
- Pull handles back to just outside the chest, leading with the elbows. Pause briefly and then extend arms, keeping elbows slightly flexed, back to starting position.

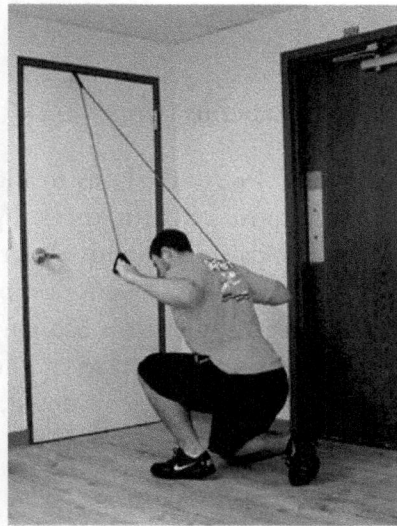

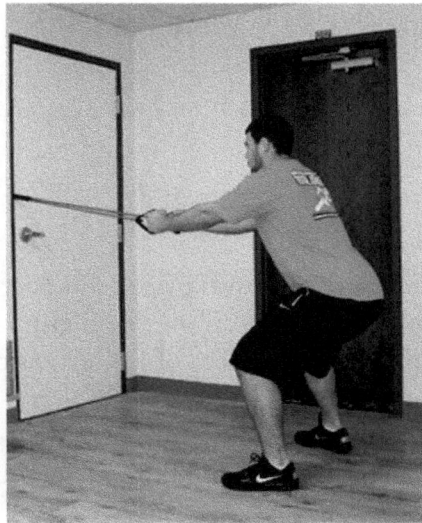

Standing Row Starting Position   Standing Row Finishing Position

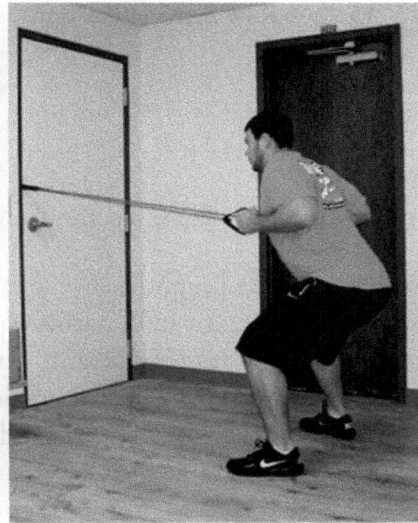

Upright Row

Anchor Point: Low
Primary Muscle Group: Trapezius (Upper Back)

- Stand with the tube close to the body to allow the line of pull to be as straight upwards as possible.
- Start in a standing position with knees slightly flexed and with hands placed in front of thighs using an overhand close grip (hands about six inches apart).
- Body should remain stable throughout movement with knees slightly flexed (to take pressure off the lower back). Common error is using upper body or knee movement to create momentum.
- Pull handles (maintaining width) to shoulder height, leading with the elbows.
- Pause briefly, and then extend arms down, keeping elbows slightly flexed, back to starting.

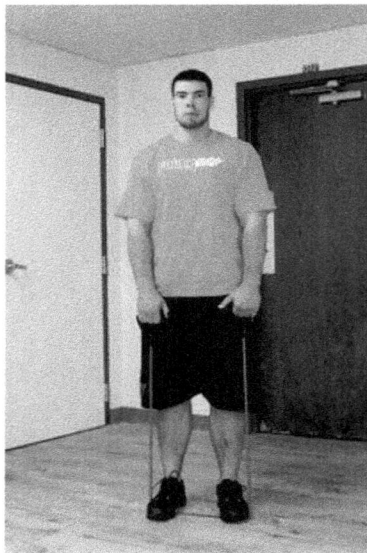

Upright Row Starting Position   Upright Row Finishing Position

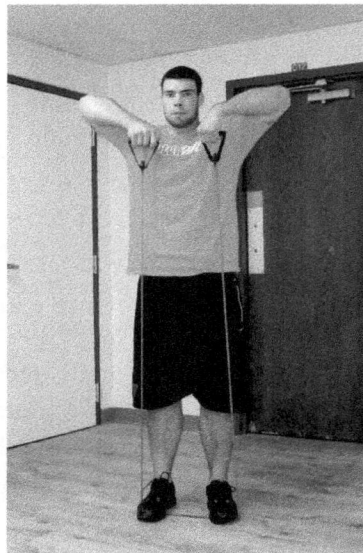

Chest Press

Anchor Point: Middle
Primary Muscle Group: Chest Press: Pectoralis Major (Chest)

- Start with feet staggered slightly, shoulder width apart and hands placed shoulder width apart at chest height. Let tubing sit under arms and grip handles with an overhand grip.
- Press straight forward at chest height, extending arms just short of full extension. Pause for a second and bring hands back to just outside the chest.
  - Do not lock out the elbows at the end of the press.
  - Keeping a slight bend in the elbows at the end of the pressing movement will take stress off the elbow joint and help prevent tendonitis.
- Push back off of front foot to return to starting position.
- Repeat, lunging forward with the opposite leg.

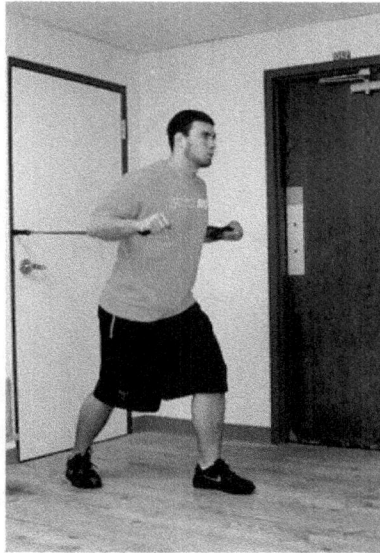

Chest Press Starting Position   Chest Press Finishing Position

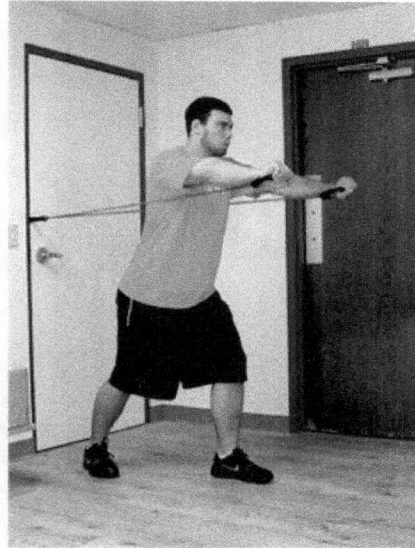

Chest Press/Lunge

Anchor Point: Middle
Primary Muscle Group: Lunge-Gluteus Maximus (Buttocks) and Quadriceps; Chest Press - Pectoralis Major (Chest)

- Start with feet shoulder width apart and hands placed shoulder width apart at chest height. Let tubing sit under arms and grip handles with an overhand grip.
- Take a large enough step forward with one leg so that the angles of the front and back leg are both 90 degrees.
  - When lunging, the optimal step places both knees at 90 degrees (front knee stays over mid foot to balls of feet).
  - Stepping too far will place the front knee over or behind the heel.
  - Stepping too short will allow the front knee to travel in front of toes.
- Keep hands at chest height, hold lunging position while keeping back knee a couple inches off the ground.
- Then press straight forward at chest height, extending arms just short of full extension. Pause for a second and bring hands back to just outside the chest.
  - Maintain tension on tubing through whole range of motion. Do not let your back knee touch or rest on the ground.
  - Upper body should remain upright during lunge and remain stable throughout movement.
- Push back off of the front foot to return to starting position.
- Repeat, lunging forward with the opposite leg.

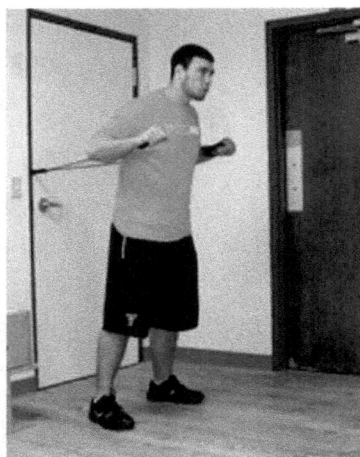

Chest Press/Lunge Position 1

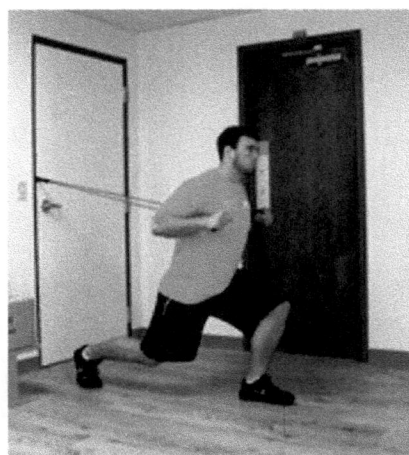

Chest Press/Lunge Position 2

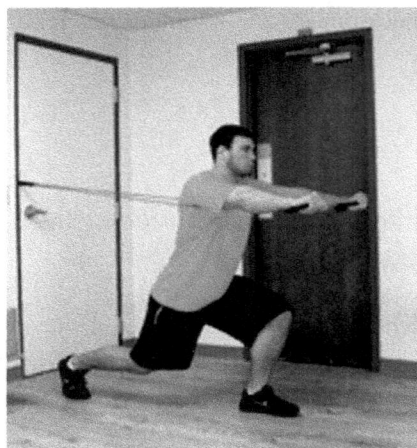

Chest Press/Lunge Position 3

Chest Fly

Anchor Point: High
Primary Muscle Group: Pectoralis Major (Chest)

- Stand with feet shoulder width apart in a staggered stance (one foot in front of the other).
- Flex at the hips, leaning chest forward and grip handles using an overhand grip with arms outstretched at chest height.
- Body should remain stable throughout movement with knees slightly flexed (to take pressure off the lower back).
- Pull handles together as you squeeze your chest and arms together, finishing with handles together out in front of your chest.
- Pause briefly, then abduct arms, keeping elbows slightly flexed, back to starting position.
- Due to tension, this can be a difficult movement; you may need to use lighter tubing or perform exercise one arm at a time.

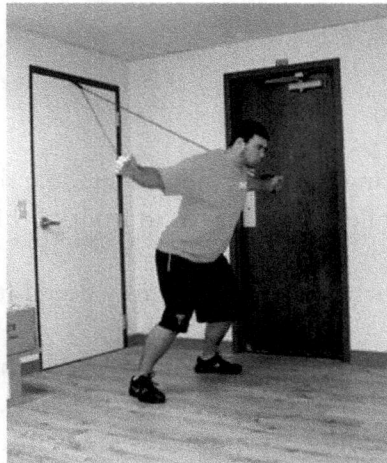

Chest Fly Starting Position

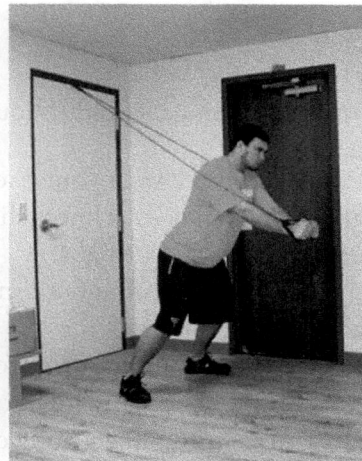

Chest Fly Finishing Position

Lateral Raise

Anchor Point: Low
Primary Muscle Group: Middle Deltoid (Shoulders)

- Stand with the tube close to the body to allow the line of pull to be as straight upwards as possible.
- Start in a standing position with knees slightly flexed and hands facing in on the side of thighs using an overhand close grip.
- Body should remain stable throughout movement with knees slightly flexed (to take pressure off the lower back).
- Pull handles vertically raising/abducting the arms to shoulder height leading with the hands/wrist.
  - Movement should not go any higher than hands slightly above shoulders.
  - Common error is using upper body or knee movement to gain momentum.
- Pause briefly, then lower arms down, keeping elbows slightly flexed, back to starting position.

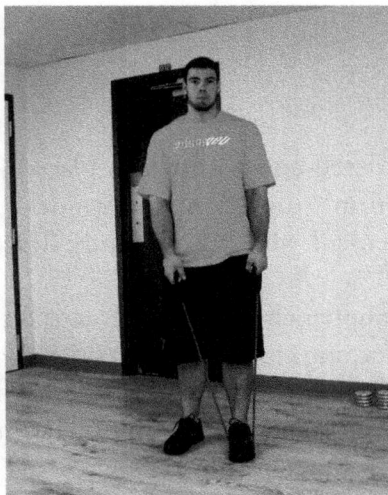

Lateral Raise Starting Position

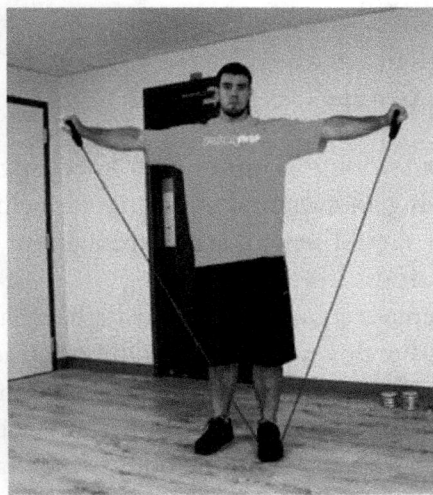

Lateral Raise Finishing Position

Front Raise

Anchor Point: Low
Primary Muscle Group: Anterior Deltoid (Shoulders)

- Stand close to the machine with your back facing the machine and straddle the tubing.
- Start in a standing position with knees slightly flexed and hands in front of thighs using an over-hand close grip (hands facing thighs).
- Body should remain stable throughout movement with knees slightly flexed (to take pressure off the lower back).
- Pull handles vertically, raising the arms to shoulder height, leading with the hands/wrists
  - Movement should not go any higher than hands slightly above shoulders.
  - Common error is using upper body or knee movement to gain momentum.
- Pause briefly, then lower arms down, keeping elbows slightly flexed, back to starting position.

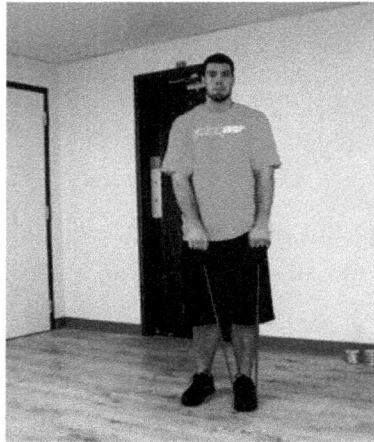

Front Raise Starting Position   Front Raise Finishing Position

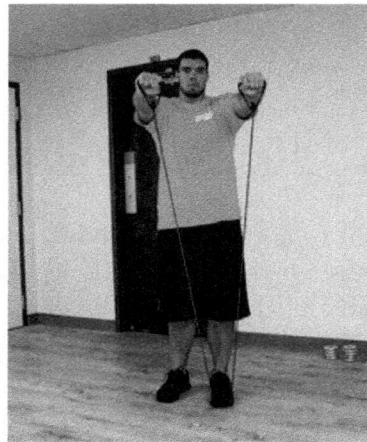

Triceps Pushdown

Anchor Point: High
Primary Muscle Group: Triceps

- Start in a standing position with knees slightly flexed and with hands placed just above chest height using an overhand close grip with elbows firmly tucked in against sides.
  - Body should remain stable throughout movement with knees slightly flexed (to take pressure off the lower back).
  - Movement should not go any higher than the upper chest, do not let tension pull elbows up.
- Push handles down just short of full extension, keeping elbows close to sides.
  - Keep elbows slightly flexed at the end of the movement to prevent elbow tendonitis.
  - Common errors are using upper body or knee movement to gain momentum and letting the elbows flare out from the body, which takes pressure off of triceps.
  - Do not lean forward and let the chest muscle be involved in the movement.
- Pause briefly, then raise hands back to starting position.

Variation:

- Same movement using an underhanded grip will place more emphasis on the lateral head of the triceps.

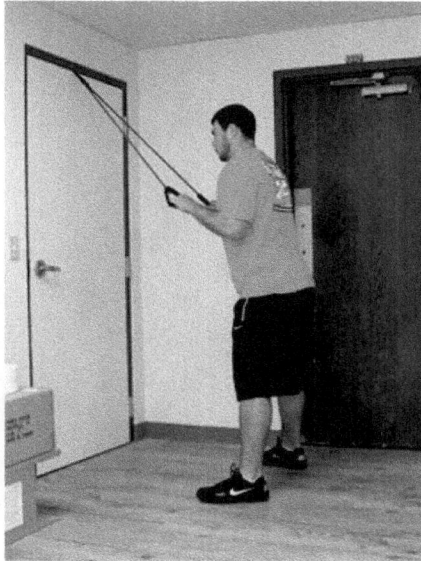

Triceps Pushdown Starting Position

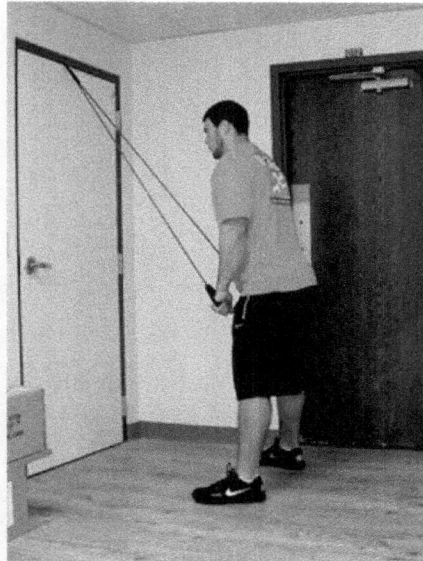

Triceps Pushdown Finishing Position

Rope Grip Triceps Pushdown

Anchor Point: High
Primary Muscle Group: Triceps (lateral head of triceps)

- Stand close to the machine facing the machine.
- Start in a standing position with knees slightly flexed, feet shoulder-width apart, with hands placed just above chest height using a neutral close grip (hands facing in like you are holding a rope) with elbows firmly tucked in against sides.
- Body should remain stable throughout movement with knees slightly flexed (to take pressure off the lower back).
- Push handles down just short of full extension, keeping elbows close to sides.
- To accentuate using the lateral head of the triceps, spread hands to the outside of legs at the end of movement.
- Keep elbows slightly flexed at the end of the movement to prevent elbow tendonitis.
- Pause briefly, then raise hands back to starting position.
- Movement should not go any higher than the upper chest, do not let tension pull elbows up.
- Common errors are using upper body or knee movement to gain momentum and letting the elbows flare out from the body which takes pressure off of triceps. Do not lean forward and let the chest muscle be involved in the movement.
- Exhale on exertion as you push down and inhale as you return to the starting position.
- Always perform movements in a steady, controlled manner.

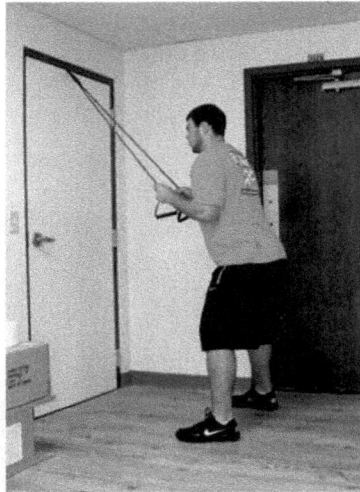

Rope Grip Triceps Pushdown
Starting Position

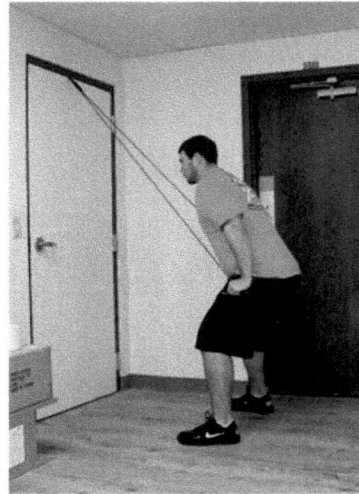

Rope Grip Triceps Pushdown
Finishing Position

Overhead Triceps Extension

Anchor Point: High
Primary Muscle Group: Triceps

Technique:

- Start in a standing position with knees slightly flexed, in a staggered stance—one foot in front of the other—with hands placed outside your ears using an overhand close grip, and with elbows in tight over shoulders.
- Upper body should lean forward slightly and the body should remain stable throughout movement with knees slightly flexed (to take pressure off the lower back).
- Push handles forward just short of full extension, keeping elbows in tight.
- Pause briefly, then return hands back to starting position

Training Tips:

- Upper body should remain stable with movement occurring only at the elbow joint. Maintain tension on tubing through the entire range of motion. Always keep elbows slightly flexed at the end of the movement to prevent elbow tendonitis. Do not let tension pull elbows up.
- Common error is letting the elbows flare out which takes pressure off of the triceps. Do not let the upper body be involved; isolate movement to the elbow joint only.
- Exhale on exertion as you press forward and inhale as you return to the starting position.
- Always perform movements in a steady, controlled manner.

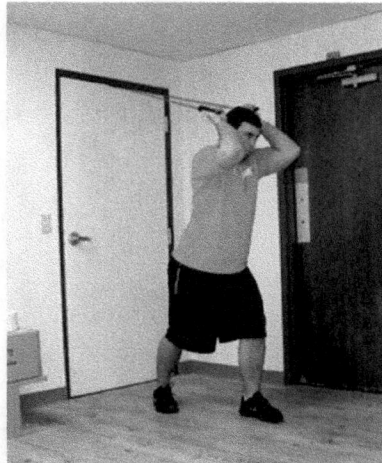

Overhead Triceps Extension
Starting Position

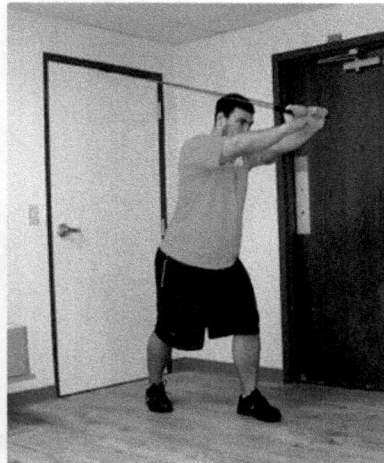

Overhead Triceps Extension
Finishing Position

Biceps Curl

Anchor Point: Low
Primary Muscle Group: Biceps

Technique:

- Start in a standing position with knees slightly flexed, with feet shoulder-width apart and arms extended with hands to the side of your thighs shoulder width apart using an underhand grip.
- Upper body should remain upright and stable throughout movement with knees slightly flexed (to take pressure off the lower back).
- Pull handles up to shoulder height, flexing only at the elbow joint (keeping elbows steady and in tight throughout movement).
- Pause briefly, then return hands back down to starting position.

Training Tips:

- Upper body should remain stable with movement occurring only at the elbow joint.
- Maintain tension on tubing through entire range of motion.
- Always keep elbows slightly flexed at the beginning of the movement to prevent elbow tendonitis.
- Do not let elbows pull up or outwards.
- Do not let the lower body be involved to create momentum; isolate movement to the elbow joint only.
- Exhale on exertion as you pull up and inhale as you return to the starting position.
- Always perform movements in a steady, controlled manner.

Variation:

- Same movement using overhand grip (reverse curl) will place more emphasis on the forearms.

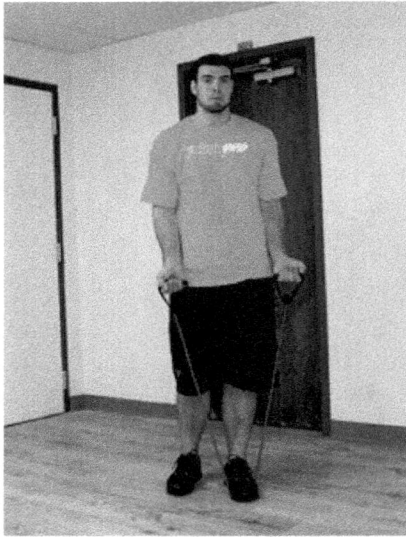

Biceps Curl Starting Position   Biceps Curl Finishing Position

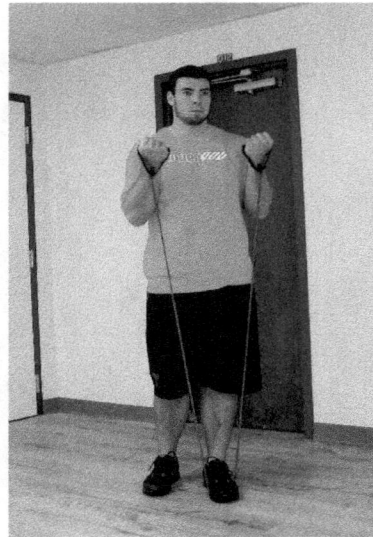

Biceps Curl/Resisted Squats

Anchor Point: Low
Primary Muscle Group: Biceps Curl: Biceps; Squats: Gluteus Maximus & Medius (Buttocks), Quadriceps

Technique:

- After completing the biceps curl with hands at shoulder height, sit back into a squatting position.
- To perform the squat, keep your chest up and head facing straight ahead, bend your knees and hips as if you are sitting back into a chair.
- Lower your hips until your upper thigh is parallel to the floor (knees should be at about 90 degrees).
- Keep your chest up, leaning forward slightly and stick your hips back as you squat in order to keep your balance and not fall back.
- Shifting hips back will also allow your knees to remain over your toes in a safe position.
- After squatting down to 90 degrees, pause and then extend knees and hips to return to a standing position.

Training Tips:

- Upper body should remain stable during the squat and not lean forward excessively.
- To keep the knees safe, don't let knees track out in front of toes.
- When performed properly, balls of feet, knees, and shoulders should be in alignment at bottom of the squat.
- Do not let knees drift inward while squatting.
- Maintain slight knee bend when squat is completed.
- Exhale on exertion as you stand up and inhale as you squat down.

- Always perform movements in a steady, controlled manner.
- Exhale on exertion as you stand up and inhale as you squat down.

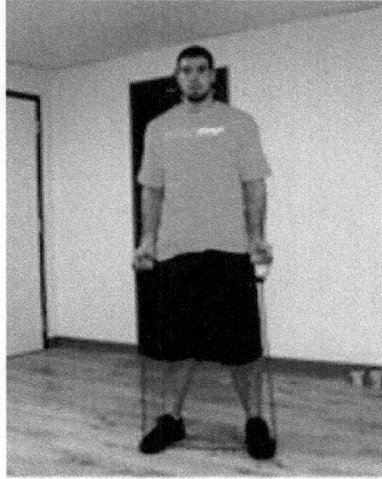

Biceps Curl / Resisted Squats
Position 1

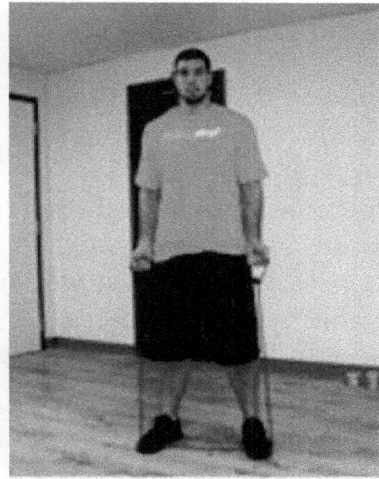

Biceps Curl / Resisted Squats
Position 2

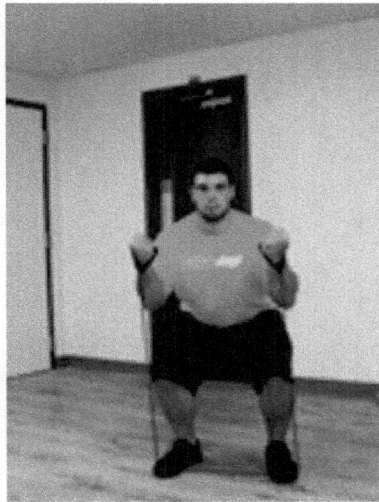

Biceps Curl / Resisted Squats
Position 3

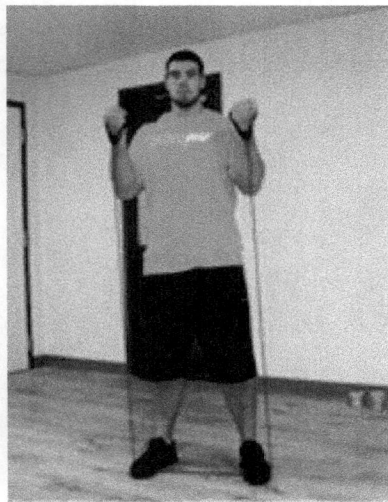

Biceps Curl / Resisted Squats
Position 4

Hammer Curl

Anchor Point: Low
Primary Muscle Group: Biceps with added emphasis on the Brachioradialis

Technique:

- Start in a standing position with knees slightly flexed, with feet shoulder width apart and arms extended with hands to the side of your thighs shoulder width apart using a neutral grip with palms facing in.
- Upper body should remain upright and stable throughout movement with knees slightly flexed (to take pressure off the lower back).
- Pull handles up to shoulder height, flexing only at the elbow joint (keeping elbows steady and in tight throughout movement).
- Pause briefly, then return hands back down to starting position.

Training Tips:

- Upper body should remain stable, with movement occurring only at the elbow joint. Maintain tension on tubing through the entire range of motion. Always keep elbows slightly flexed at the beginning of the movement to prevent elbow tendonitis. Do not let elbows pull up or outwards.
- Hammer curl hand grip places more emphasis on the forearm. Do not let the lower body be involved to create momentum, isolate movement to the elbow joint only.
- Exhale on exertion as you pull up and inhale as you return to the starting position.
- Always perform movements in a steady, controlled manner.

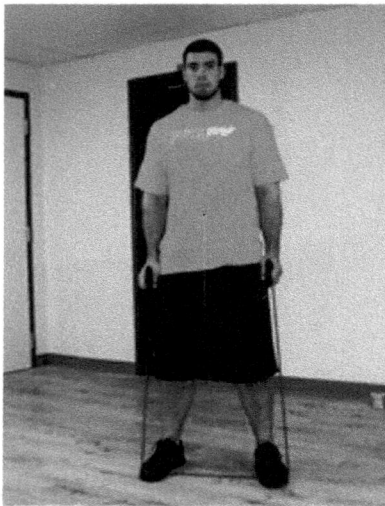

Hammer Curl Starting Position

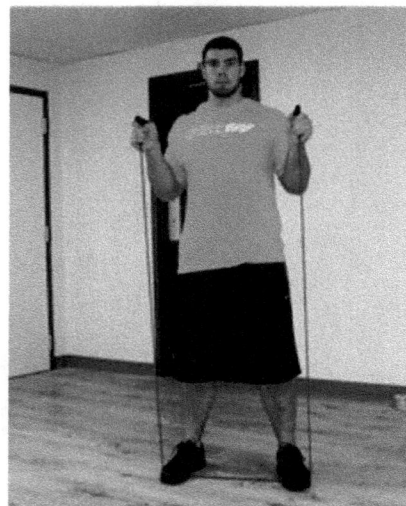

Hammer Curl Finishing Position

Hammer Curl/Resisted Squats

Anchor Point: Low
Primary Muscle Group: Biceps Curl: Biceps and Brachioradialis; Squats: Gluteus Maximus & Medius (Buttocks), Quadriceps

Technique:

- After completing the hammer curl with hands at shoulder height, sit back into a squatting position.
- To perform the squat, keep your chest up and head facing straight ahead, bend your knees and hips as if you are sitting back into a chair.
- Lower your hips until your upper thigh is parallel to the floor (knees should be at about 90 degrees).
- Keep your chest up, leaning forward slightly and stick your hips back as you squat in order to keep your balance and not fall back.
- Shifting hips back will also allow your knees to remain over your toes in a safe position.
- After squatting down to 90 degrees, pause and then extend knees and hips to return to a standing position.

Training Tips:

- Upper body should remain stable during the squat and not lean forward excessively.
- To keep the knee safe, don't let knees track out in front of toes.
- When performed properly, balls of feet, knees, and shoulders should be in alignment at the bottom of the squat.
- Do not let knees drift inward during squatting. Maintain slight knee bend when squat is completed.
- Exhale on exertion as you stand up and inhale as you squat down.
- Always perform movements in a steady, controlled manner.

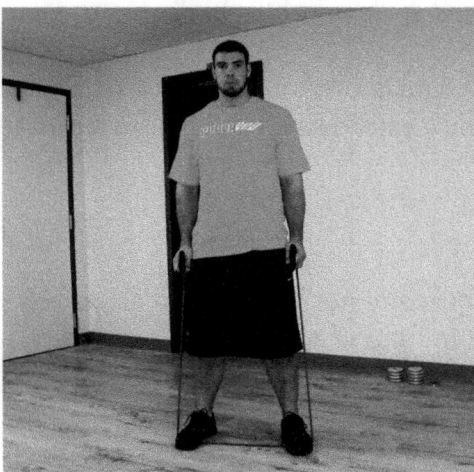

Hammer Curl / Resisted Squats Position 1   Hammer Curl / Resisted Squats Position 2

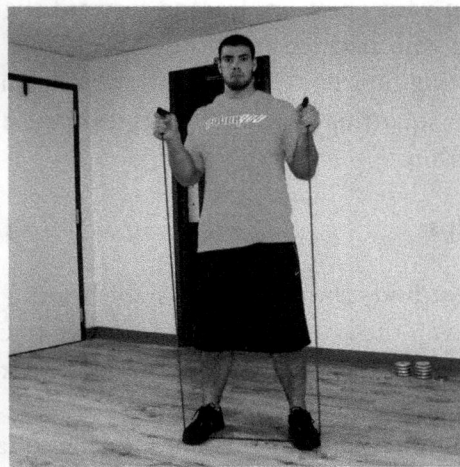

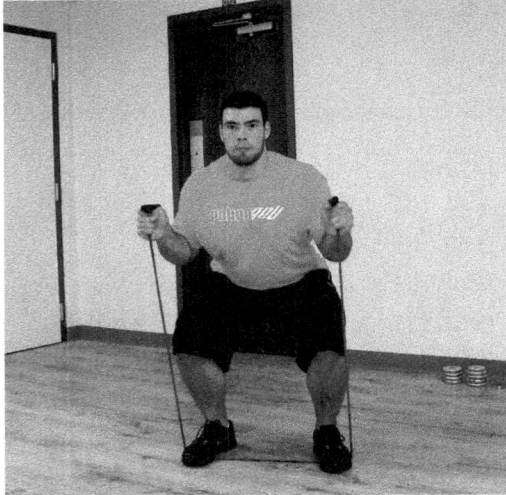

Hammer Curl / Resisted Squats Position 3

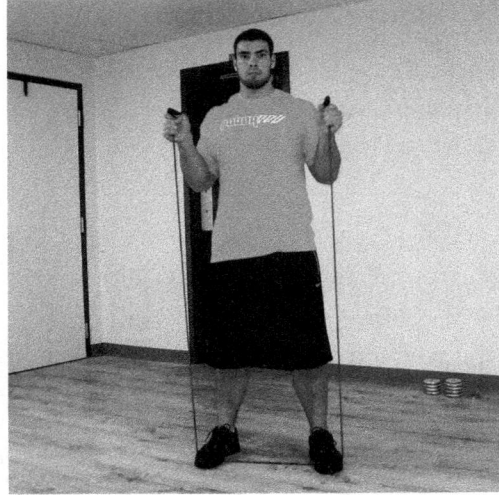

Hammer Curl / Resisted Squats Position 4

Resisted Squats

Anchor Point: Low
Primary Muscle Group: Squats: Gluteus Maximus & Medius (Buttocks), Quadriceps

Technique:

- With hands at shoulder height and tension on the tubing, sit back into a squatting position.
- To perform the squat, keep your chest up and head facing straight ahead, bend your knees and hips as if you are sitting back into a chair.
- Lower your hips until your upper thigh is parallel to the floor (knees should be at about 90 degrees).
- Keep your chest up, leaning forward slightly and stick your hips back as you squat in order to keep your balance and not fall back.
- Shifting hips back will also allow your knees to remain over your toes in a safe position.
- After squatting down to 90 degrees pause and then extend knees and hips to return to a standing position.

Training Tips:

- Upper body should remain stable during the squat and not lean forward excessively.
- To keep the knee safe, don't let knees track out in front of toes.
- When performed properly, balls of feet, knees, and shoulders should be in alignment at the bottom of the squat.
- Do not let knees drift inward during squatting.
- Maintain slight knee bend when squat is completed.
- Exhale on exertion as you stand up and inhale as you squat down.
- Always perform movements in a steady, controlled manner.

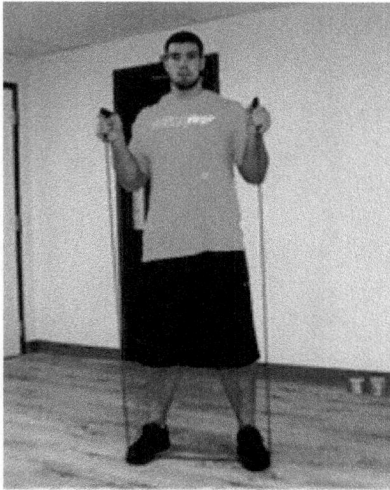

Resisted Squats Position 1

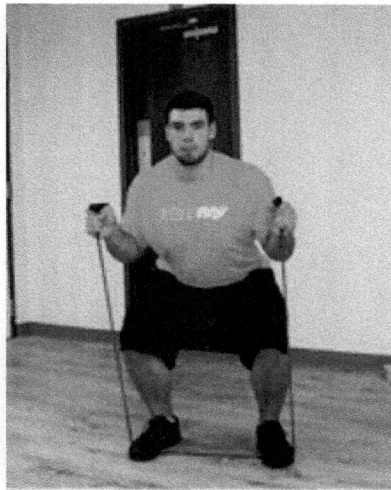

Resisted Squats Position 2

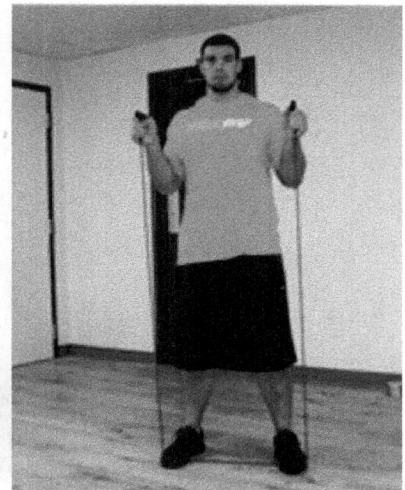

Resisted Squats Position 3

Resisted Crunch

Anchor Point: Middle / High
Primary Muscle Group: Rectus Abdominis (Abdomen)

Technique:

- Start in a kneeling position, holding handles slightly in front of shoulders.
- Begin with the upper body in a straight position with shoulders, hips and knees in line.
- Roll or curl your spine, pulling your chest towards your hips as you flex your abdominal muscles.
- This "crunch" movement does not require a large movement. You just want to move far enough to feel the abdominal muscles fully engage as they flex.
- Then extend back up to your starting position.

Training Tips:

- Hips and knees should remain relatively stable, with movement occurring only from the contraction of the abdominal muscles. Slight movement may occur at the hips due to the abdominals' relationship to the hip flexors.
- Maintain tension on tubing through the entire movement.
- Common error is having too much movement at the knees and hips, which takes the emphasis off the abdominals. If too much movement is happening with the knees and hips, then shift hips back slightly (sitting back on heels a little) to take the hip flexors out of the movement.
- Exhale on exertion as you curl/crunch forward and inhale as you return to the starting position.
- Always perform movements in a steady, controlled manner.

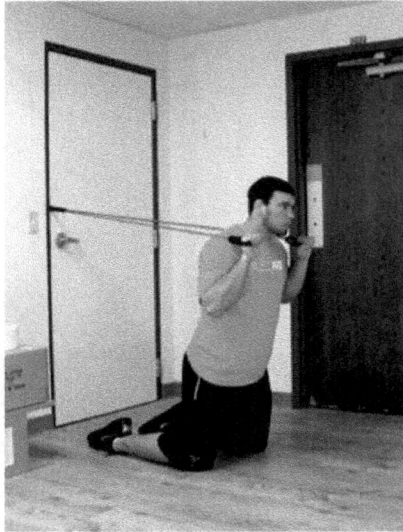

Resisted Crunch Starting Position   Resisted Crunch Finishing Position

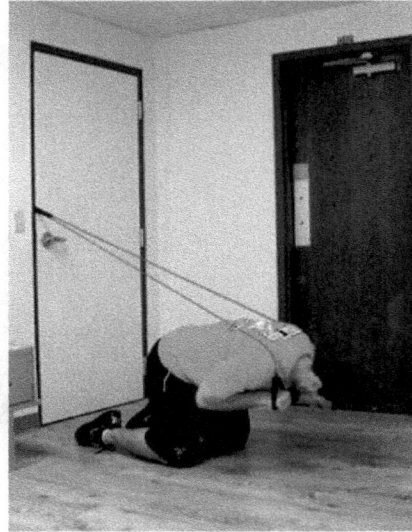

One Arm Rotational Row

Anchor Point: Middle
Primary Muscle Group: Torso & Hip Rotators, Abdominals, Latissimus Dorsi

Technique:

- Start standing perpendicular to the attachment with knees slightly bent and reach across body with your arm farthest away, grabbing the handle at chest height.
- Pull the band handle across your body to where your hand is outside the hip of the arm you are pulling with, then rotate your feet and hips 90 degrees.
- Then rotate back to the starting position.
- Repeat movement with the other side.

Training Tips:

- Upper body should remain stable, with initial pull using the back and arms and the rest of the movement should come from the rotating of the hips and feet.
- Maintain tension on tubing through the entire movement.
- Inside arm can be used to generate force by swinging the arm over the tube as you rotate.
- Be sure to allow the feet to naturally rotate on the balls of your feet with the hips.
- Keeping the feet stationary while twisting with the hip will place too much strain on the knees.
- Starting position should be perpendicular to the attachment and in the finishing position, you should be facing away from the attachment site.
- Exhale on exertion as you pull and rotate, and inhale as you return to the starting position.
- Always perform movements in a steady, controlled manner.

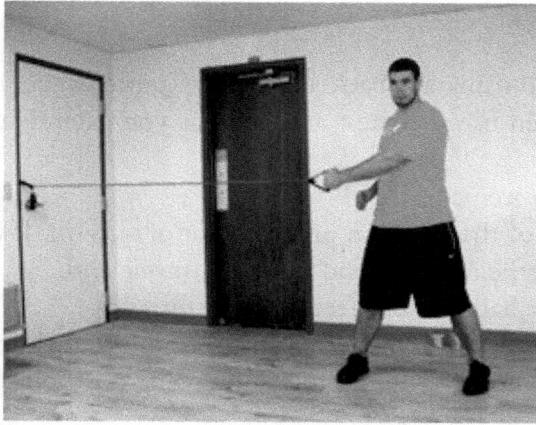

One Arm Rotational Rows Position 1

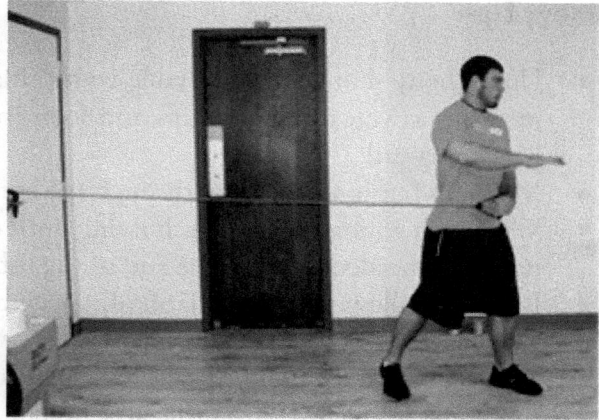

One Arm Rotational Rows Position 2

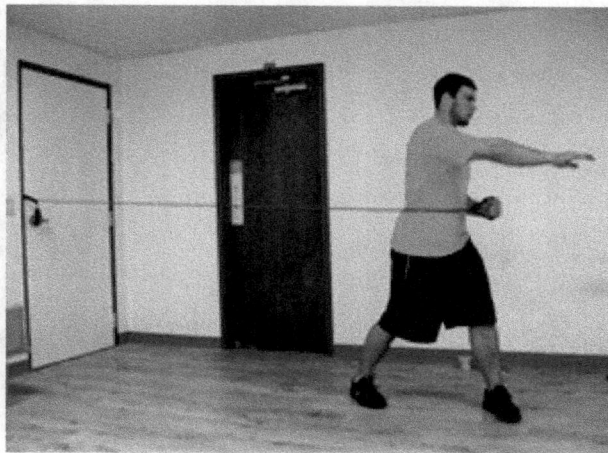

One Arm Rotational Rows Position 3

Lateral Chop

Anchor Point: Middle
Primary Muscle Group: Torso & Hip Rotators, Abdominals, Latissimus Dorsi, Chest & Triceps

Technique:

- Start standing perpendicular to the attachment with knees slightly bent and reach across the body with both hands grabbing the handle at chest height.
- Pull the band as you rotate your hips and feet 90 degrees. As you finish rotating your hips and feet, extend your arms out in front like you are chopping wood with an ax.
- Then rotate back to the starting position.
- Repeat movement with the other side.

Training Tips:

- Upper body should remain stable with initial pull using the back and arms. Continue the momentum as you rotate the hips and feet, and then use the chest and arms as you extend your hands forward.
- Maintain tension on tubing through the entire movement.
- With such a long movement, holding both ends of the tube can provide a lot of tension. If less tension is needed, anchor one end of the tube on the machine and pull on just one end.
- Be sure to allow the feet to naturally rotate on the balls of your feet with the hips.
- Keeping the feet stationary while twisting with the hip will place too much strain on the knees.
- Starting position should be perpendicular to the attachment and in the finishing position, you should be facing away from the attachment site.
- Exhale on exertion as you pull and rotate, and inhale as you return to the starting position.
- Always perform movements in a steady, controlled manner.

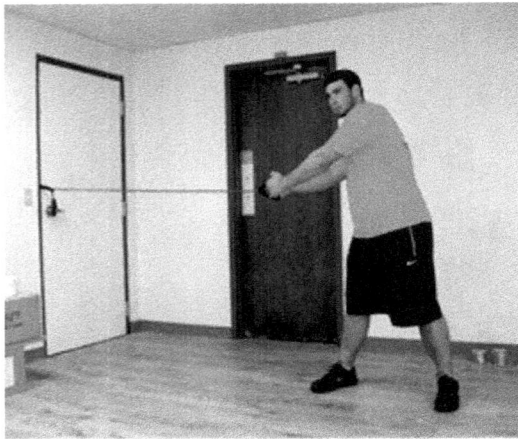

Lateral Chop Starting Position   Lateral Chop Finishing Position

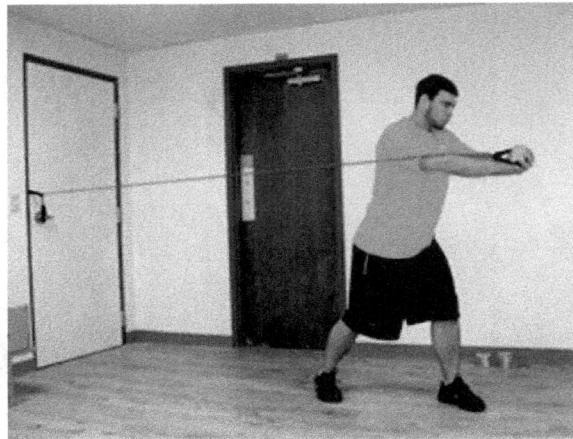

High/Low Chop

Anchor Point: Top
Primary Muscle Group: Torso & Hip Rotators, Abdominals, Latissimus Dorsi, Chest & Triceps

Technique:

- Start standing perpendicular to the attachment with knees slightly bent and reach up and across your body with both hands grabbing the handle slightly higher than your head.
- Pull the band down on an angle as you rotate your hips and feet 90 degrees. As you finish rotating your hips and feet, extend your arms out in front maintaining the same angle as the initial pull down, like you are chopping wood with an ax.
- Then rotate back up to the starting position.
- Repeat movement with the other side.

Training Tips:

- Upper body should remain stable with initial pull down using the back and arms. Continue the momentum as you rotate the hips and feet and then use the chest and arms as you extend your hands down and forward.
- Maintain tension on tubing through the entire movement.
- With such a long movement, holding both ends of the tube can provide a lot of tension. If less tension is needed, anchor one end of the tube on the machine and pull on just one end.
- Be sure to allow the feet to naturally rotate on the balls of your feet with the hips. Keeping the feet stationary while twisting with the hip will place too much strain on the knees.
- Starting position should be perpendicular to the attachment and in the finishing position you should be facing away from the attachment site.
- Exhale on exertion as you pull and rotate, and inhale as you return to the starting position.
- Always perform movements in a steady, controlled manner.

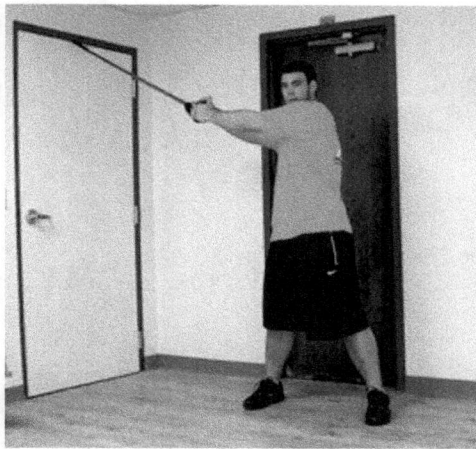

High Low Chop Starting Position   High Low Chop Finishing Position

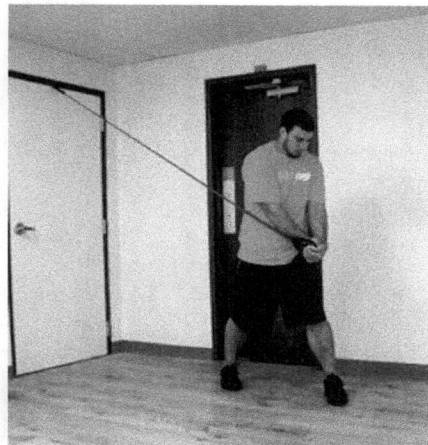

Low/High Chop

Anchor Point: Bottom
Primary Muscle Group: Torso & Hip Rotators, Abdominals, Latissimus Dorsi, Chest & Triceps

Technique:

- Start standing perpendicular to the attachment with knees slightly bent and reach up and across the body with both hands grabbing the handle below hip height.
- Pull the band up on an angle as you rotate your hips and feet 90 degrees. As you finish rotating your hips and feet, extend your arms out in front maintaining the same angle as the initial pull up, like you are chopping wood with an ax.
- Then rotate back up to the starting position.
- Repeat movement with the other side.

Training Tips:

- Upper body should remain stable with initial pull up using the back and arms. Continue the momentum as you rotate the hips and feet and then use the chest and arms as you extend your hands up and forward.
- Maintain tension on tubing through the entire movement.
- With such a long movement, holding both ends of the tube can provide a lot of tension. If less tension is needed, anchor one end of the tube on the machine and pull on just one end.
- Be sure to allow the feet to naturally rotate on the balls of your feet with the hips.
- Keeping the feet stationary while twisting with the hip will place too much strain on the knees.
- Starting position should be perpendicular to the attachment and in the finishing position you should be facing away from the attachment site.
- Exhale on exertion as you pull and rotate and inhale as you return to the starting position.
- Always perform movements in a steady, controlled manner.

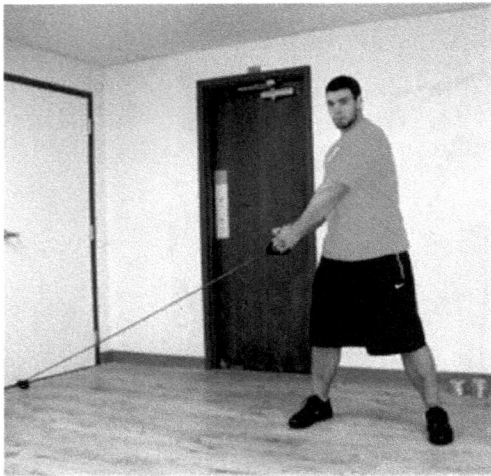

Low High Chop Starting Position   Low High Chop Finishing Position

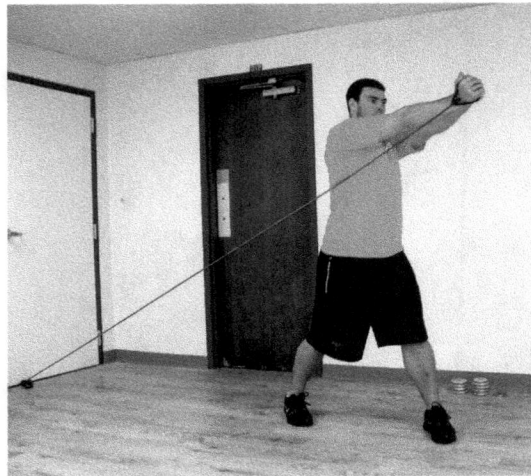

Internal Rotation

- Tubing should be placed at elbow height.
- Using an adequate resistance, step far enough from the anchor so that tube is tight without slack.
- Holding elbow steady at your side, start with your hand reaching out while your elbow is bent at 90 degrees.
- Keeping elbow stationary, internally rotate your shoulder to pull the cable or tube across your body.
- Externally rotate your shoulder to return to starting position.

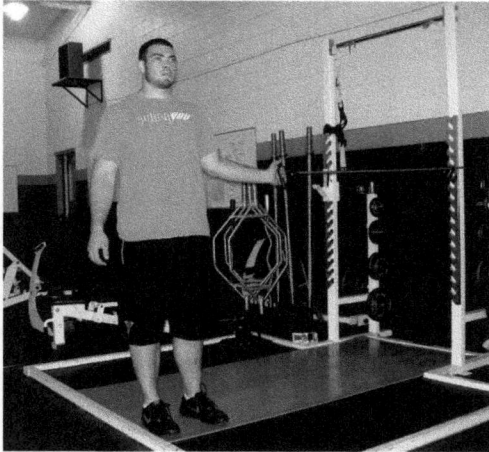

Internal Rotation Starting Position

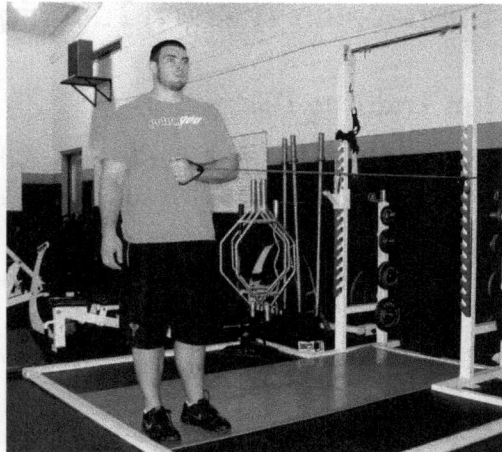

Internal Rotation Finishing Position

External Rotation

- Tubing should be placed at elbow height.
- Using an adequate resistance, step far enough from the anchor so that the tube is tight without slack.
- Holding elbow steady at your side, start with your hand across your body while your elbow is bent at 90 degrees.
- Keeping elbow stationary, externally rotate your shoulder to pull the cable or tube across your body until your hand is extended away from your body.
- Internally rotate your shoulder to return to starting position.

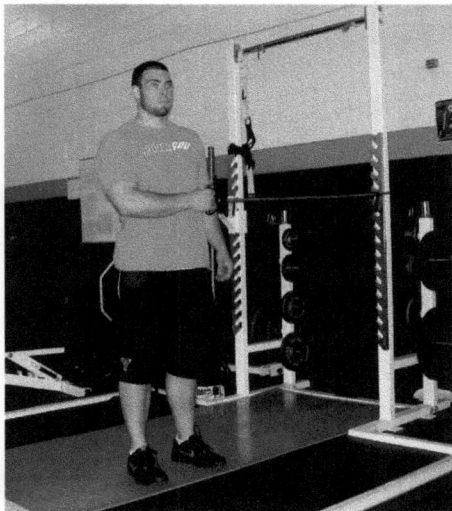

External Rotation Starting Position

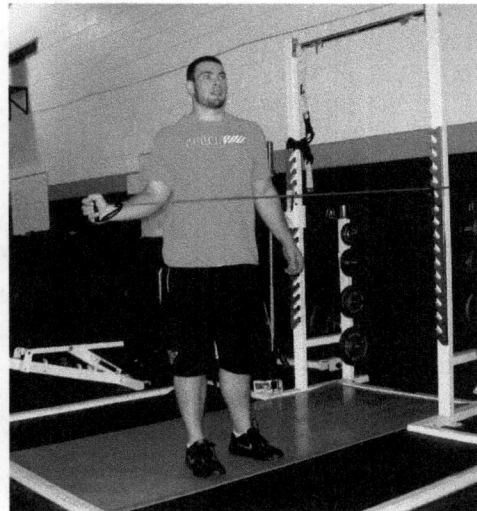

External Rotation Finishing Position

Part 8: Suspension Training Techniques

Suspension Training Basics

Body position and the base used can influence the difficulty of the exercise. Changing positioning is a great way to vary the intensity of suspension exercises and allows individuals at different strength and fitness levels to modify exercises to suit their needs and abilities. When combining vibration with suspension training, making the exercise more difficult intensifies the vibration effect on the targeted muscles.

Body Angle

When standing, changing the angle of your body changes the amount of body weight (resistance) that is used in the exercise. For pulling exercises, standing with feet farther away from the point where the suspension ropes are anchored (standing up straighter) lessens the resistance used, making the exercise easier. Placing the feet closer in line with the anchor point and leaning farther back increases the resistance used, making the exercise harder.

For pressing exercises, placing your feet closer to the anchor point and using a shorter strap/rope length (standing up straighter) will lessen the resistance used, making the exercise easier. By extending the strap/rope length and placing your feet farther away from the anchor point, you increase your body angle, increasing the resistance used and making the exercise harder.

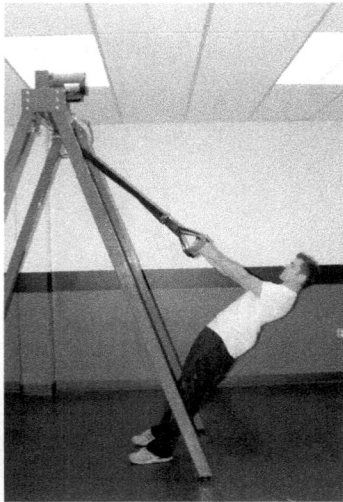

Pulling movement with feet closer (less body lean)

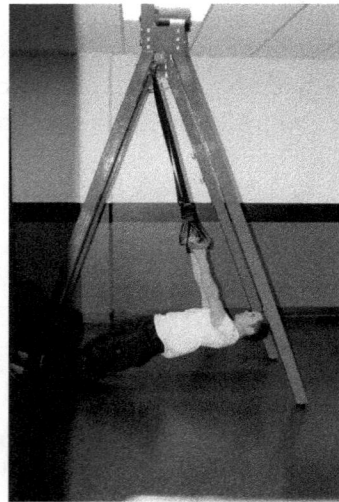

Pulling movement with feet farther away (more body lean)

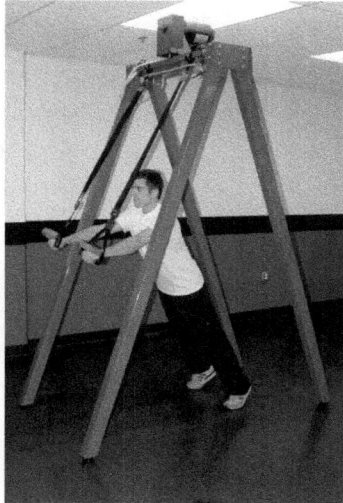

Pressing movement with feet closer (less body lean)

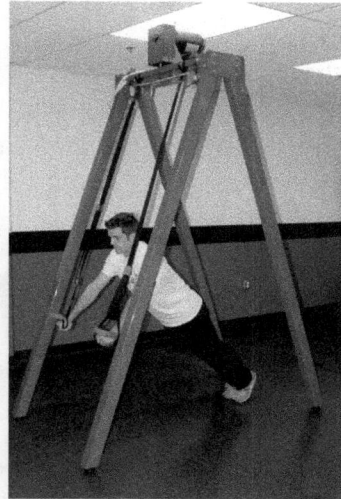

Pressing movement with feet farther away (more body lean)

Changing the Base of Support

Base Width

A second way to modify the difficulty of a suspension exercise is changing your base of support. Placing your feet apart and widening your base makes you more stable and lessens the difficulty of the exercise. To make the exercise more difficult, you can lessen your stability by bringing your feet together. The exercise can be progressed even further by balancing on one foot instead of two. This increases the instability, making the exercise much harder to perform. The less stable you are, the more muscles and balance you need to use in performing the exercise.

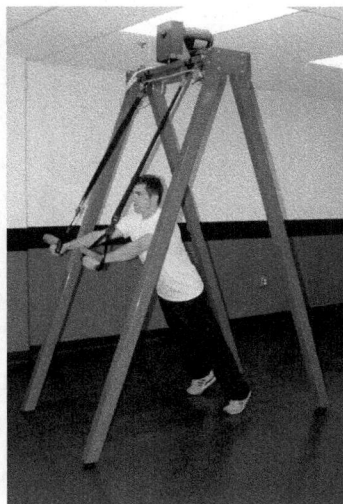

Wider, more stable base

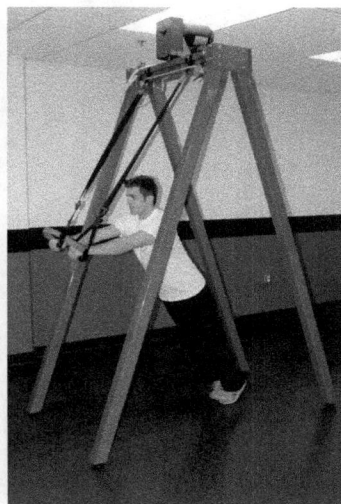

Narrower, less stable base

Length of Stance

Similar to changing the width of your stance, changing the length of your stance also changes your stability. Performing exercises with a stagger-stance provides more stability, making the exercise less difficult. As you shorten the distance your feet are staggered, you become less stable, increasing the difficulty of the exercise. Having feet together is the most difficult form of this modification.

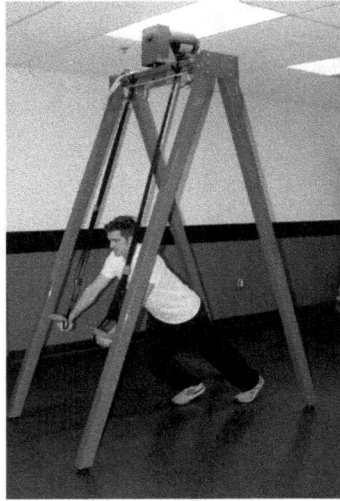

Staggered, more stable base

Changing Starting Position (Floor Exercises)

Lining up your feet directly under the anchor point lessens the amount of body weight resistance you use, making the exercise easier to perform. The farther away your feet are positioned from the anchor point, the more body weight resistance you use, which makes the exercise more difficult.

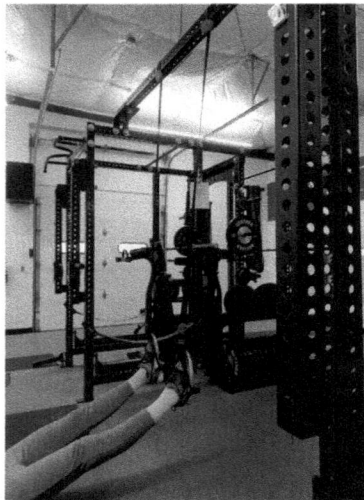

Feet under the anchor point   Feet farther away from the anchor point

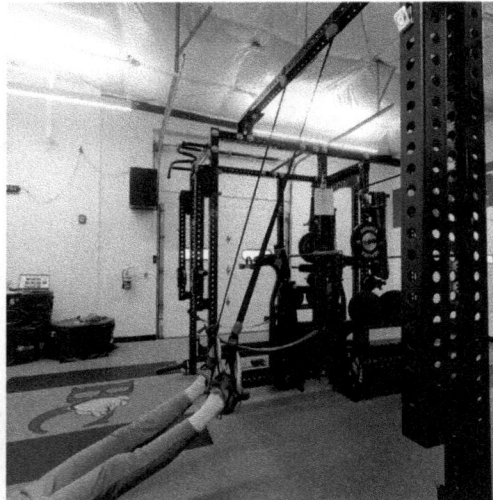

Changing Your Center of Gravity (Floor Exercises)

Floor exercises, such as planks, can be made easier or harder depending on your center of gravity. Exercises are easier to perform when you support your body with your forearms. When you support the weight of your body on your hands, you are less stable, which increases the difficulty of the exercise.

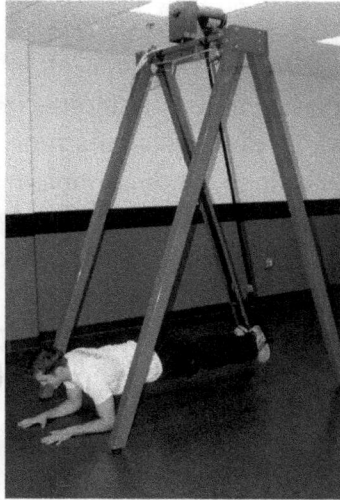

Supporting your body weight on your forearms (easier)

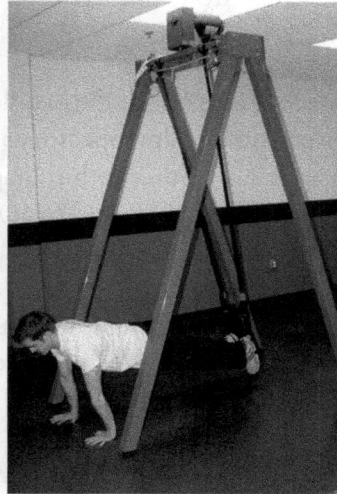

Supporting your body weight on your hands (harder)

Single Handle Configuration

You can change the two handles into one handle by aligning the two handles—with one hand above the other. Feed the bottom handle through the triangle of the top handle and then take the handle that is now on the bottom and feed it through the triangle on the top handle. Tug on the handles to tighten the two together and to make sure the handles are adjusted correctly.

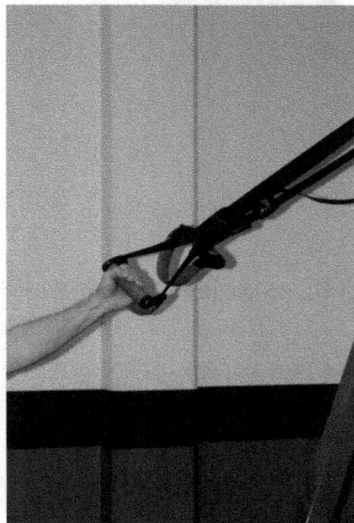

Suspension Stretching Exercises

Static passive exercises place a muscle in an extended static stretching position.

Quad Stretch

Targeted Muscle: Quadriceps (front of thigh)
Attachment: Foot/ankle

- Put the toe of one foot into one of the handles so the handle rests against the front of your ankle joint.
- Shorten the suspension strap/rope so your foot is elevated—with your flexed knee pointing downward and your heel closer to hip height (or as high as comfortable).
  - You may want to hold the other strap/rope or the machine to balance yourself.
- Bend the knee of your standing leg to lower your hips, feeling a stretch in your quadriceps (front of thigh).
- The more you bend the standing knee, the more you will feel the stretch.
- Do not stretch to the point of feeling discomfort or pain. If you feel any pain, immediately release the stretch. Hold a comfortable stretch for 20 to 30 seconds.

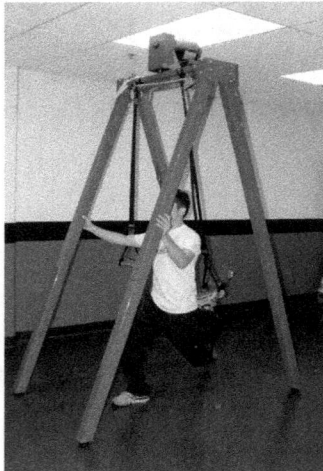

Chest Stretch

Targeted Muscle: Pectoralis major (chest)
Secondary Muscle: Deltoids (shoulder)
Attachment: Handles

- Stand with the suspension anchor point behind you and lift your arms to shoulder height with your palms facing forward.
- Step forward and stop when you feel a stretch through your chest.
- To accentuate the stretch, lean your weight forward more.
- Do not stretch to the point of feeling discomfort or pain.
- If you feel any pain, immediately release the stretch. Hold a comfortable stretch for 20 to 30 seconds.

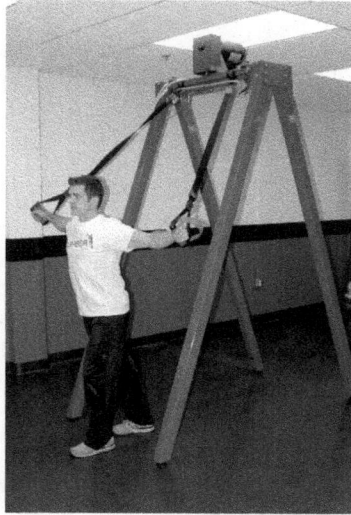

Shoulder Stretch

Targeted Muscle: Deltoids (shoulder)
Attachment: Handles

- Stand with the suspension anchor point behind you and lift your arms to shoulder height, reaching straight ahead.
- Raise your arms straight up as you step forward with one leg.
- With your hands directly over your head and your palms facing forward, lean your body forward to initiate a stretch in your shoulders.
- Do not stretch to the point of feeling discomfort or pain. If you feel any pain, immediately release the stretch.
- Hold a comfortable stretch for 20 to 30 seconds.

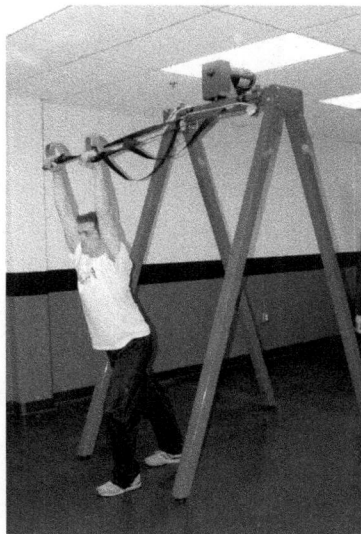

Lat Stretch

Targeted Muscle: Latissimus dorsi (back)
Attachment: Handles

- Stand facing toward the anchor point and step back until your arms are fully extended in front of your chest and the straps/ropes have no slack.
- With your feet shoulder-width apart, bend your knees as you shift your weight back like you are sitting in a chair.
- Let the straps/ropes pull at your arms as you feel the muscles stretching across your back.
- Do not stretch to the point of feeling discomfort or pain.
- If you feel any pain, immediately release the stretch. Hold a comfortable stretch for 20 to 30 seconds.

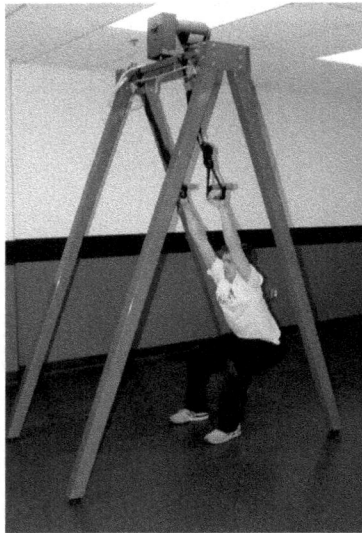

Suspension Resistance Exercises

Suspension Push Up

- Facing away from the anchor point, lean your body forward with a staggered stance and lower your chest toward your hands—like you are doing a push up.
- Perform a push-up but lower your chest to the height of your hands and press up to just short of fully extending the arms.
- Having the hands slightly higher than during a standard push up (more toward the shoulders) will help direct the straps/ropes out of your way.
- Perform the exercise in a slow, controlled manner.
- Increasing the body angle, narrowing the stance or using a one-foot stance will make the exercise more difficult.

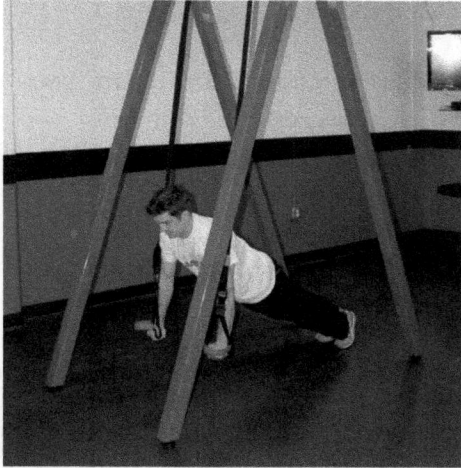

Top position for the suspension push up

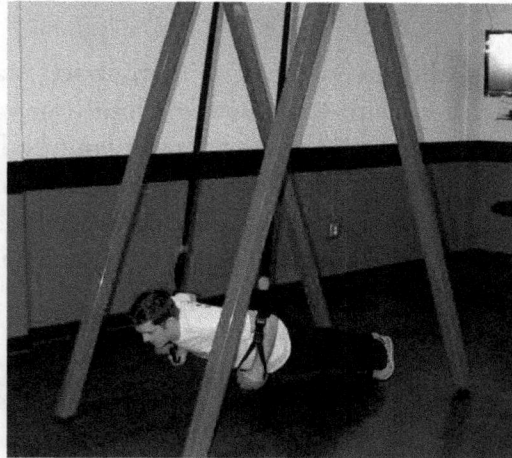

Bottom position for the suspension push up

Chest Fly

- Facing away from the anchor point, lean your body forward.
- Starting with your hands extended straight in front of you with your palms facing together, lower your body as you horizontally abduct (widen out) your arms at shoulder height, keeping your elbows almost completely straight.
- Perform a chest fly by lowering yourself by fully abducting your arms to be even with your shoulders and then horizontally adduct the arms together back to the starting point.
- Try to maintain the same arm angle (slight elbow bend) throughout the whole exercise.
- Perform the exercise in a slow, controlled manner.
- Increasing the body angle, narrowing the stance or using a one-foot stance will make the exercise more difficult.

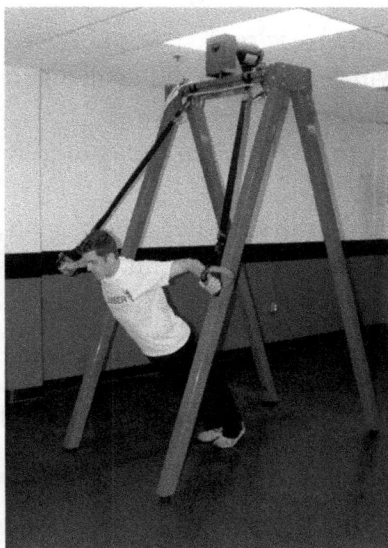

Starting position for the chest fly

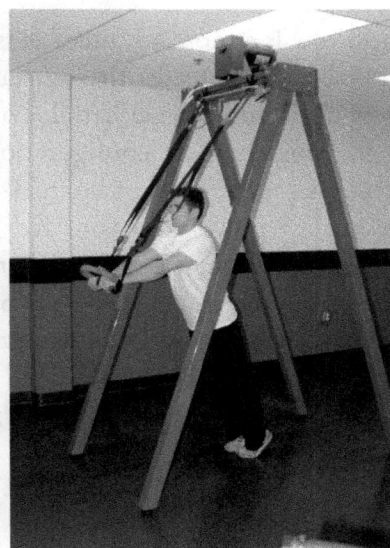

Finishing position for the chest fly

Row

- Facing the anchor point with your feet staggered and shoulder width apart, start with your hands even with your chest and lean your weight back as you extend your arms.
- When performing the row, lower your body by extending your arms fully and then pull your body up until your hands are even with your chest.
- Perform the exercise in a slow, controlled manner.
- Increasing the body angle, narrowing the stance or using a one-foot stance will make the exercise more difficult.

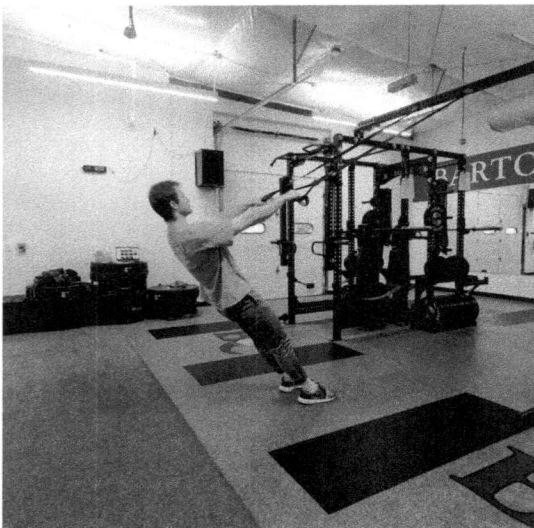

Starting position for the row

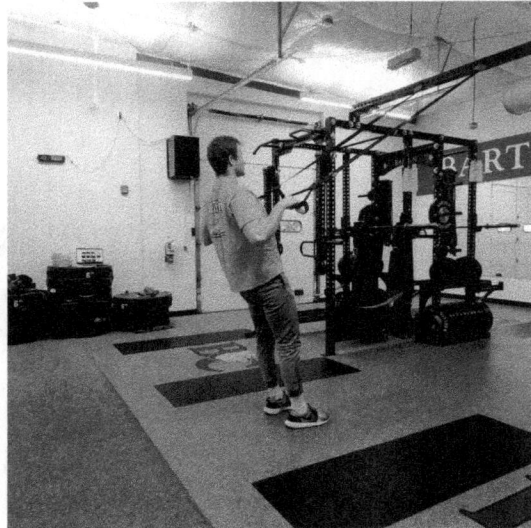

Finishing position for the row

One-Arm Row

- The one-arm row is a more advanced version of the basic row.
- Using just one arm increases the resistance, which increases the challenge to the body. The one-arm row utilizes the single-handle configuration.
- To set up the single-handle configuration, refer to the one handle configuration instructions earlier in this chapter (see Insert figure 3-12).
- Facing the anchor point with your feet staggered and shoulder width apart, start with your hands even with your chest and lean your weight back as you extend your arms.
- When performing the row, lower your body by extending your arms fully and then pull your body up until your hands are even with your chest.
- Perform the exercise in a slow, controlled manner.
- Increasing the body angle, narrowing the stance or using a one-foot stance will make the exercise more difficult.

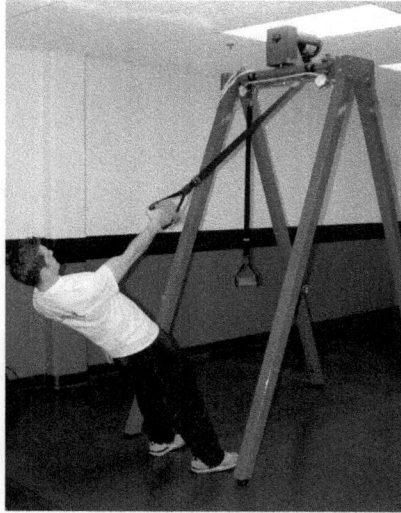

Starting position for the one-arm row

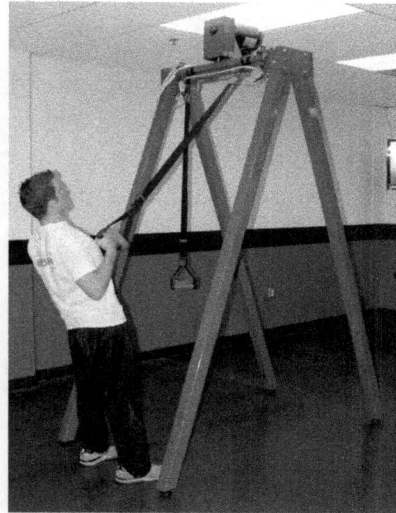

Finishing position for the one-arm row

Dip

- Standing under the anchor point with your arms at your side and your palms facing in, hold the handles just outside your shoulders (adjust the strap/rope so the handles are below your hips).
- Walk your feet slightly forward or back (placing your feet behind you may be more comfortable for your shoulders), shifting the remainder of your body weight on the handles.
- Dips are performed by lowering your hips as you bend your elbows to a 90 degree angle and then pressing your body back up to the starting position.
- To keep pressure on the triceps, keep the elbows in tight. Do not let the elbows flare out to the sides.
- Perform the exercise in a slow, controlled manner.
- The farther you place your feet in front or behind your hips, the more body weight resistance you will use.

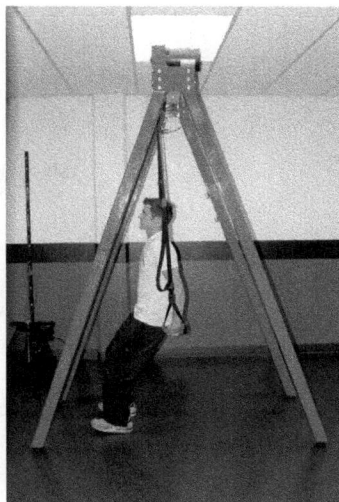

Starting position for the dip

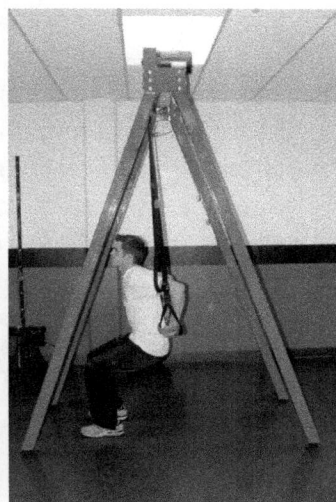

Bottom position for the dip

Triceps Extension

- Standing under the anchor point, extend your arms out at head height.
- Lean your body forward so the straps/ropes are taut.
- To perform the full triceps extension, keep your hand position stable and lower your body as you bend your elbows, so your hands are even with your forehead and then push your body back to the starting position by extending your arms. To keep pressure on the triceps, keep the elbows in tight.
- Do not let the elbows flare out to the sides.
- Perform the exercise in a slow, controlled manner.
- Increasing the body angle, narrowing the stance or using a one-foot stance will make the exercise more difficult.

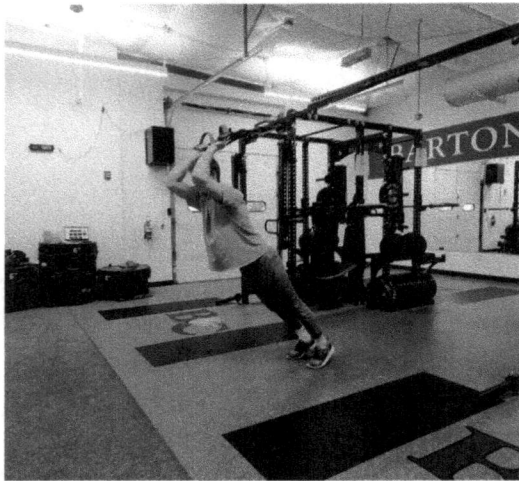

Starting position for the triceps extension

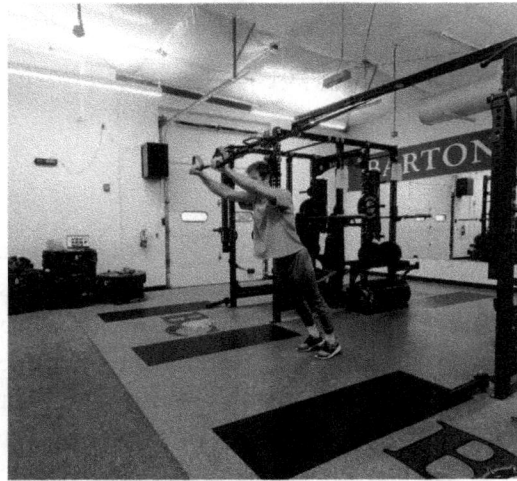

Bottom position for the triceps extension

Biceps Curl

- Facing the anchor point with your feet staggered and shoulder-width apart, start with your hands even with your chest and lean your weight back as you extend your arms. With your palms facing up, flex your elbows, bringing your hands to your chin as you pull your body up.
- Then, extend your arms as you lower your body back to the starting position.
- To keep pressure on the biceps, keep the elbows in tight.
- Do not let the elbows flare out to the sides.
- Perform the exercise in a slow, controlled manner.
- Increasing the body angle, narrowing the stance or using a one-foot stance will make the exercise more difficult.

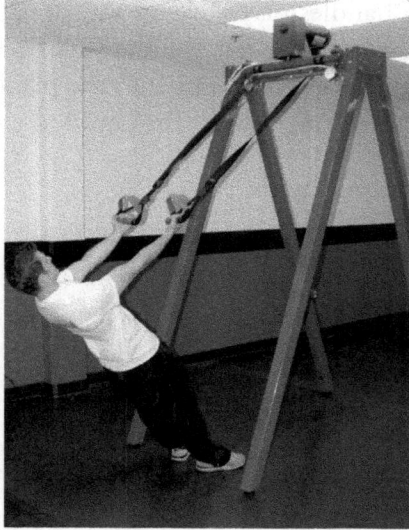

Starting position for the biceps curl   Finishing position for the biceps curl

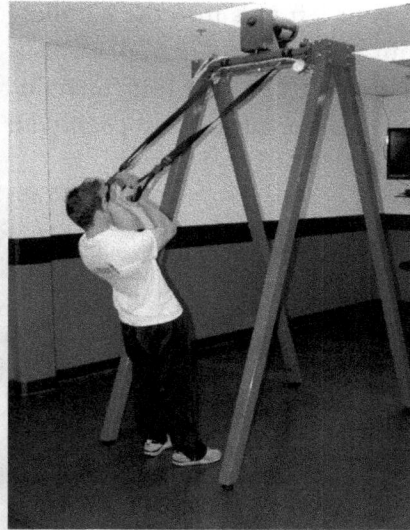

Utilizing the Handles for Core and Lower-Body Movements

Heels in the Handles (Exercises Facing Upward)

Extend the straps/ropes to about 8 inches off the ground. Sitting close to the handles and facing the straps/ropes, steady the handles with your hands and then roll back slightly, bringing your knees to your chest, and place your heels into the handles. (Some handles may have an additional loop below the hand grips for your heels.) As you lay back, push your heels down into the handles and extend your legs.

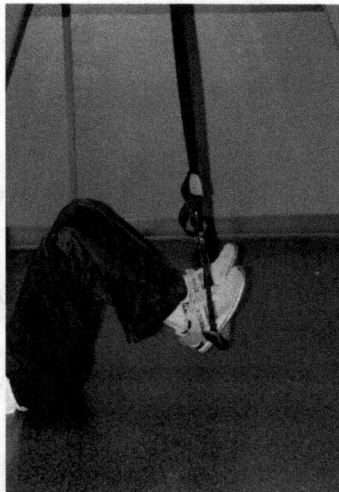

Toes in the Handles (Exercises Facing Downward)

Extend the straps/ropes to about 8 inches off the ground. Sitting close to the handles and facing the straps/ropes, grab the right handle with your right hand and cross your left foot over the top of your right leg, putting your left toes into the handle. (Some handles may have an additional loop below the hand grips for your toes/heels). Then, place your right toes in the left handle. Roll over, bringing your left shoulder over the top. Let your feet rotate in the handles as you rotate into the plank position. Your feet should now be positioned so the tops of your feet are resting against the handles.

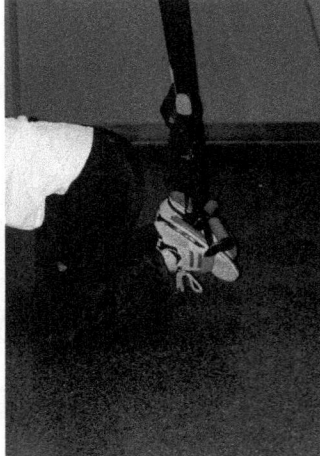

Front Plank

Targeted Muscle: Abdominals
Attachment: Foot/ankle

- Extend the straps/ropes to about 8 inches off the ground.
- Position your toes in the handles as described at the beginning of the core/lower-body section.
- Start out in the resting position—with your knees and forearms resting on the ground.
- Consciously think about keeping your abdominal muscles tight while keeping good posture, maintaining a straight line from your ankles through your hips to your shoulders.
- To make the exercise more difficult, perform the exercise on your hands—with your arms extended—instead of on your forearms.

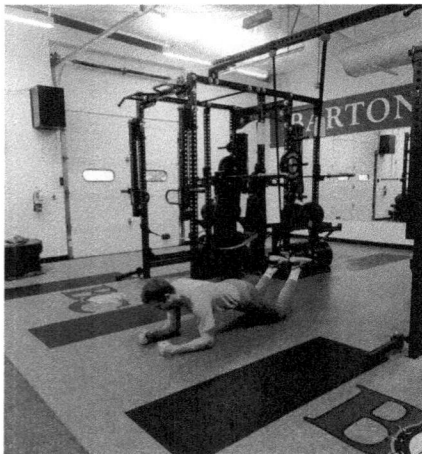

Front plank resting position (forearm base)

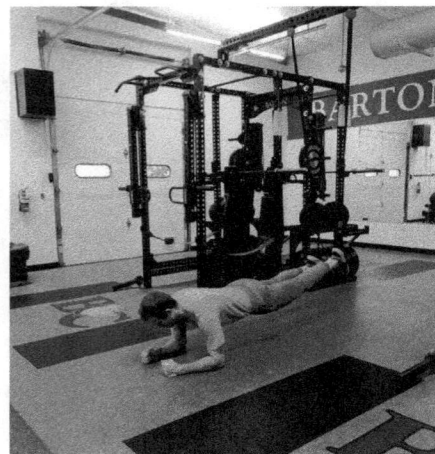

Front plank (forearm base)

160

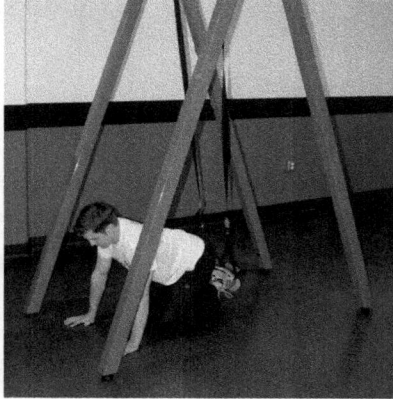

Front plank resting position
(from knees, arms extended base)

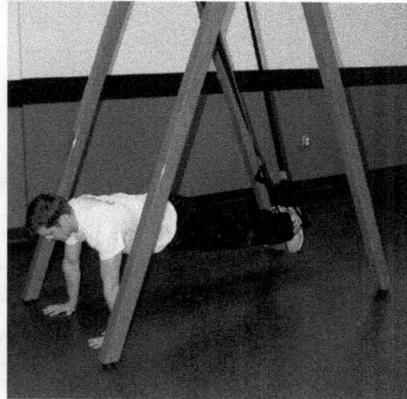

Front plank (arms extended base)

Side Plank

Targeted Muscle: Obliques (side abdominals)
Attachment: Foot/ankle

- Extend the straps/ropes to about 8 inches off the ground. Position your toes in the handles as described at the beginning of the core/lower-body section.
- Start in the resting position turned to one side—with your hip resting on the ground—and with your feet offset (top leg forward) and your body resting on your forearms.
- Engage your oblique muscles by lifting your hip up in the air, maintaining a straight line through the center of your body. Keep your body stable, resting your top hand on your hip.
- To make the exercise tougher, raise your top arm straight in the air.
- To further increase the intensity of the exercise, balance on one hand with an arm extended instead of resting your weight on your forearms.
- The most difficult variation involves balancing on your straight arm and extending your top arm straight up in the air.
- Perform this exercise equally on both sides.

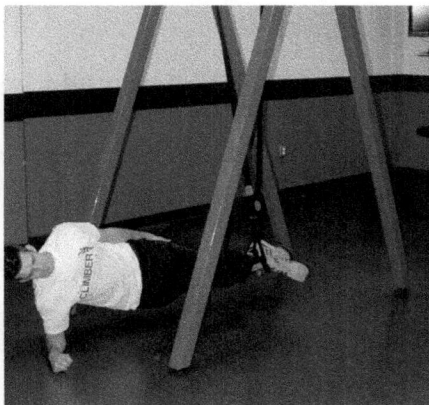

Side plank (forearm base)

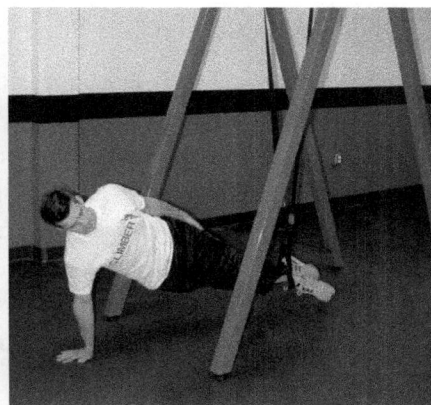

Side plank (arm extended base)

Glute Bridge

Targeted Muscle: Gluteus maximus
Attachment: Foot/ankle

- Extend the straps/ropes to about 8 inches off the ground.
- Position your heels in the handles as described at the beginning of the core/lower-body section.
- Start in the resting position—with your knees bent at 90 degrees and lying with your hips and back on the ground.
- With feet suspended and knees bent, lift your hips off the ground.
- Think about tightening your abdominals and gluteus maximus as you maintain a straight line from your shoulders through your hips to your knees.

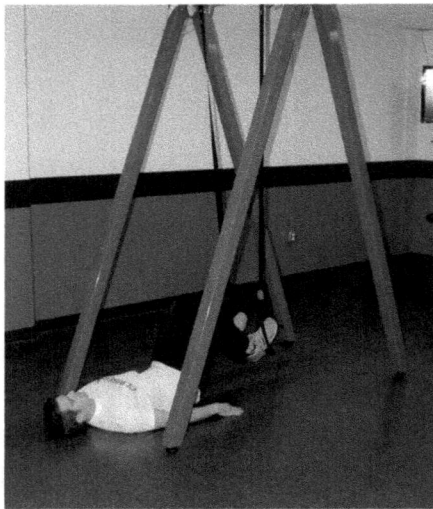

Starting position for the glute bridge   Finishing position for the glute bridge

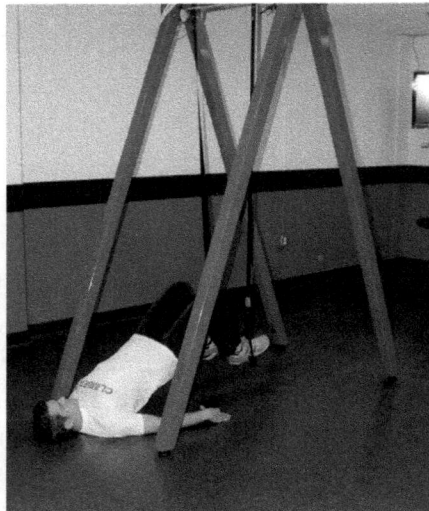

Pike-Ups

Targeted Muscle: Abdominals
Attachment: Foot/ankle

- To perform the pike-up, start in the front plank resting position on your knees with your arms extended and your hands on the ground.
- Lift your knees up into the extended arm front plank position and execute the pike by raising your hips up while keeping your legs straight.
- Your hips will rise up higher as your feet move closer toward your hands.
- Pause for a second or two at the top of the pike (where your hips are at their highest point) and then slowly—in a controlled manner—lower your hips while keeping your legs straight to the arms extended front plank starting position.

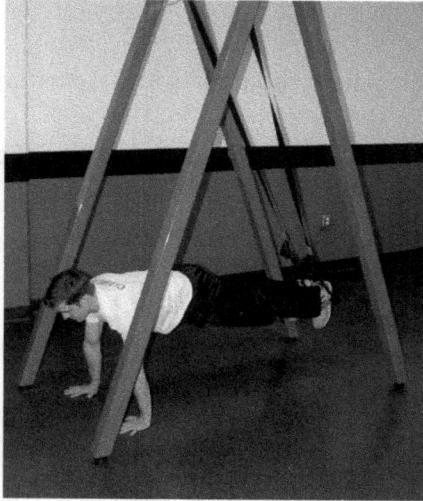

Starting position for the pike-up
(extended arms front plank position)

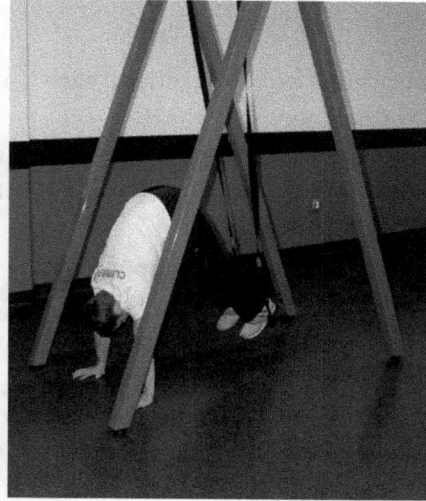

Top position for the pike-up
(high hip position)

Squat

- Stand with your arms extended, with your feet placed shoulder width apart and holding the handles for balance.
- To perform the squat, keep your chest up and your head facing straight ahead.
- Bend your knees and hips as if you are sitting back into a chair.
- Lower your hips until your upper thigh is parallel to the floor (knees should be at about 90 degrees).
- Keep your chest up, leaning forward slightly, and stick your hips back as you squat to keep your balance and not fall back.
- Shifting your hips back will also allow your knees to remain over your toes in a safe position.
- After squatting down to 90 degrees, pause and then extend your knees and hips to return to a standing position.

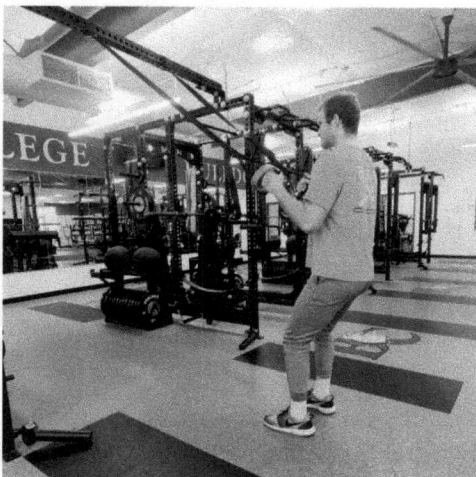

Suspension squat top position

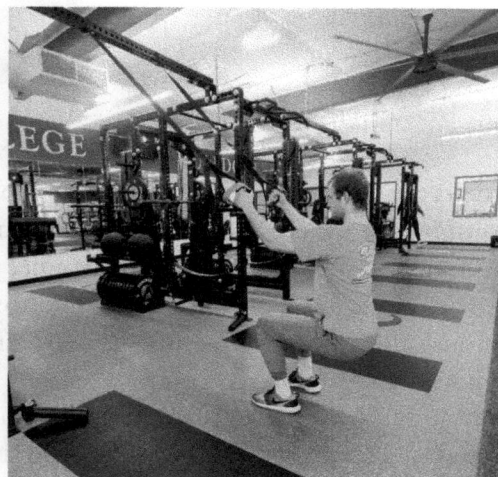

Suspension squat bottom position

Single-leg Squat

- Stand with your arms extended, with your feet placed shoulder-width apart and holding the handles for balance.
- To perform the single-leg squat, keep your chest up and your head facing straight ahead.
- Straighten one leg out in front and bend the knee and hip of the stance leg as if you are sitting back into a chair.
- Lower your hip until your upper thigh is parallel to the floor (knee should be at about 90- degrees).
- Keep your chest up, leaning forward slightly, and stick your hips back as you squat to keep your balance and not fall back.
- Shifting your hips back will also allow your knees to remain over your toes in a safe position.
- After squatting down to 90 degrees, pause and then extend your knee and hip to return to a standing position.

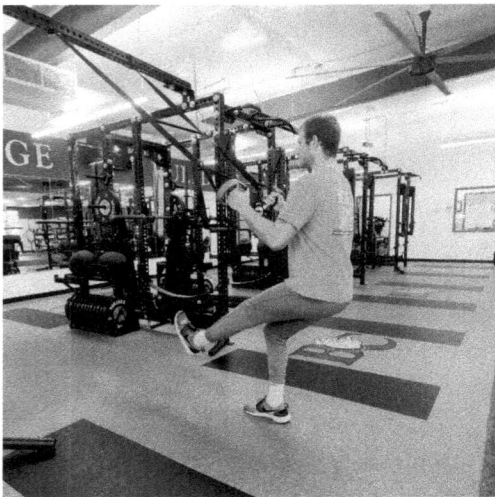

Suspension single-leg squat top position

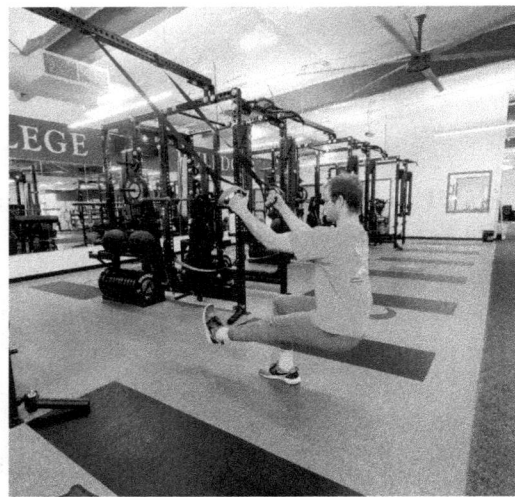

Suspension single-leg squat bottom position

Rear Elevated Split Squat

Attachment: Foot/ankle

- Extend the straps/ropes to a comfortable position off the ground for the rear leg.
- Position your toes in the handles as described at the beginning of the core/lower-body section.
- With the rear leg supported in the handle, position the front foot far enough forward that, when the back leg is lowered to the floor, the front knee does not extend out in front of the toes.
- Bending the front knee, drop the hips straight down into 90-degree bend of both front and back legs.
- Push up on the front leg, extending the knees and hips back to the starting position.
- If needed, something like a wooden dowel can be used for balance, just be sure to keep the emphasis on the leg muscle.

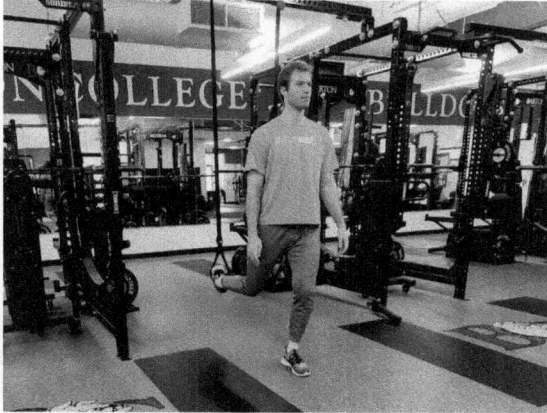

Suspension rear elevated split squat top position

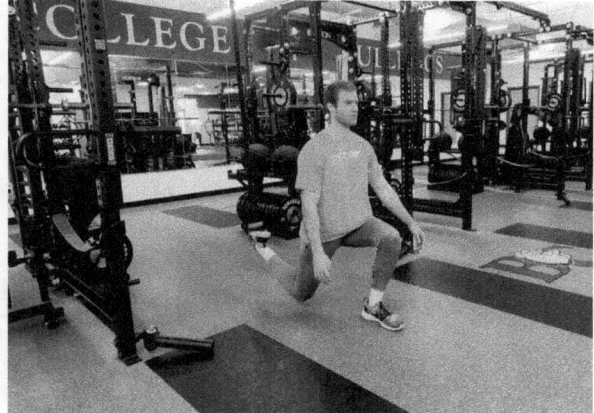

Suspension rear elevated split squat bottom position

Knees to Elbows

Targeted Muscle: Hip flexors/abdominals
Attachment: Foot/ankle

- Extend the straps/ropes to about 8 inches off the ground.
- Position your toes in the handles as described at the beginning of the core/lower-body section.
- Start out in the resting position similar to the front plank, with your knees and your forearms on the ground.
- Lift your knees off the ground and then bend your knees, bringing your knees forward toward your elbows, tucking your knees to your chest.
- Then, extend your legs out straight into the front plank position.
- Keep your abdominals tight as you tuck your knees forward and then extend your legs out straight in a slow, controlled manner.
- To make the exercise more difficult, start from your hands with your arms extended instead of from your forearms.

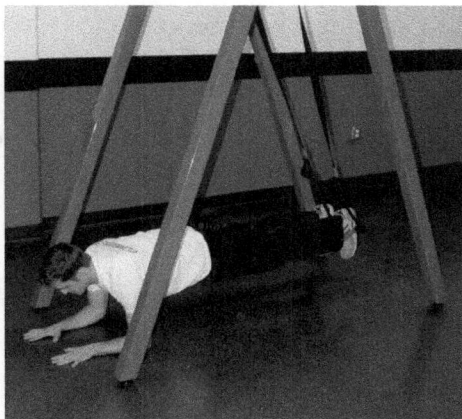

Starting position for the knees to
elbows (forearms front plank position)

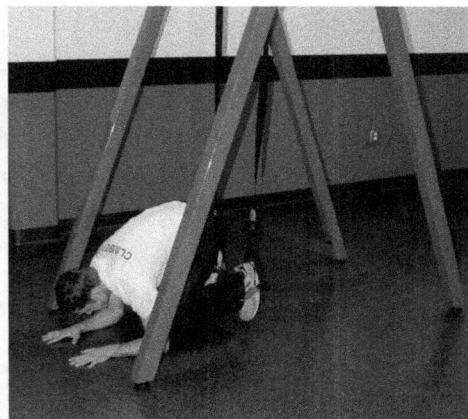

Finishing position for the knees
to elbows (knee tuck position)

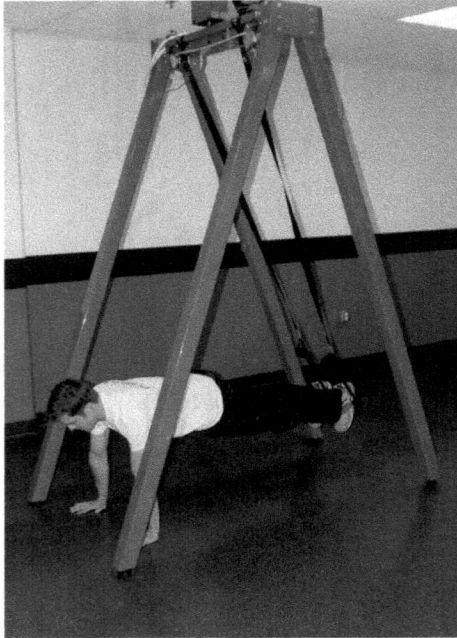

Starting position for the extended knees
to elbows (extended arms front plank position)

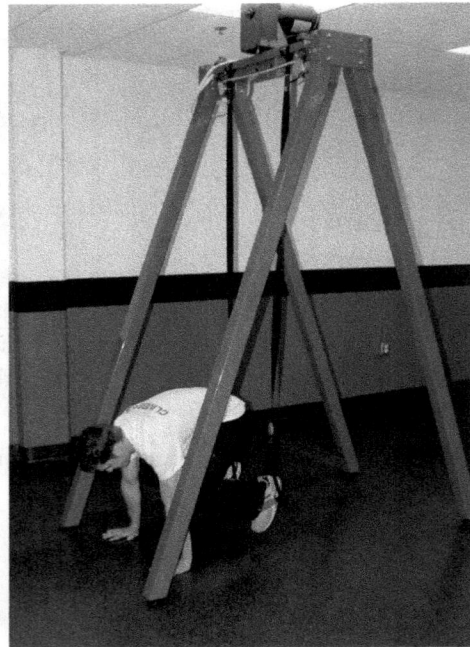

Finishing position for the extended
knees to elbows (knee tuck position)

Twisting Knees to Elbows

Targeted Muscle: Hip flexors/abdominals and obliques
Attachment: Foot/ankle

- Extend the straps/ropes to about 8 inches off the ground.
- Position your toes in the handles as described at the beginning of the core/lower-body section.
- Start out in the resting position similar to the front plank, with your knees and your forearms on the ground.
- To involve the oblique muscles, add in a twist by bringing your knees to one side.
- Lift your knees off the ground and then bend them, bringing your knees forward toward your elbow on one side, tucking your knees into the outside of your elbow.
- Then, extend your legs out straight into the front plank position.
- Keep your abdominals tight as you twist and tuck your knees forward and then extend your legs out straight in a slow, controlled manner.
- Perform the exercise by alternating repetitions to each side.
- To make the exercise more difficult, start from your hands with your arms extended instead of from your forearms.

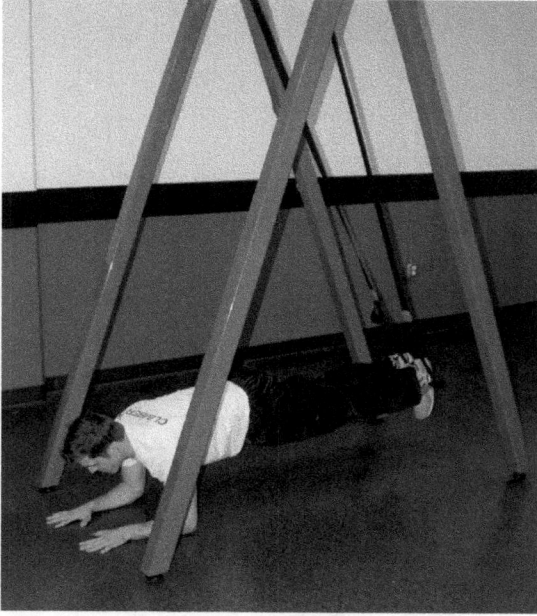

Starting position for the twisting knees
to elbows (forearms front plank position)

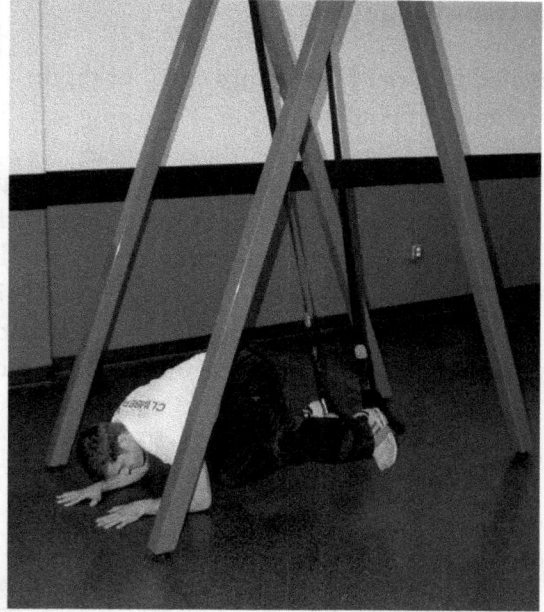

Finishing position for the twisting knees
to elbows (twisting knee tuck position)

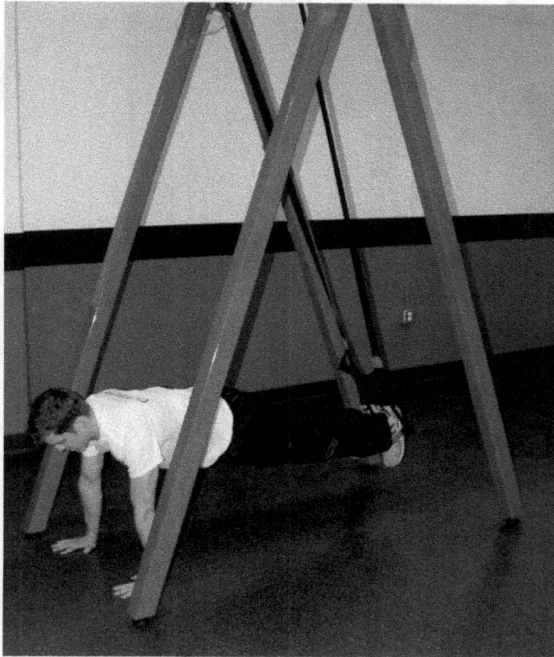

Starting position for the extended twisting knees
to elbows (extended arms front plank position)

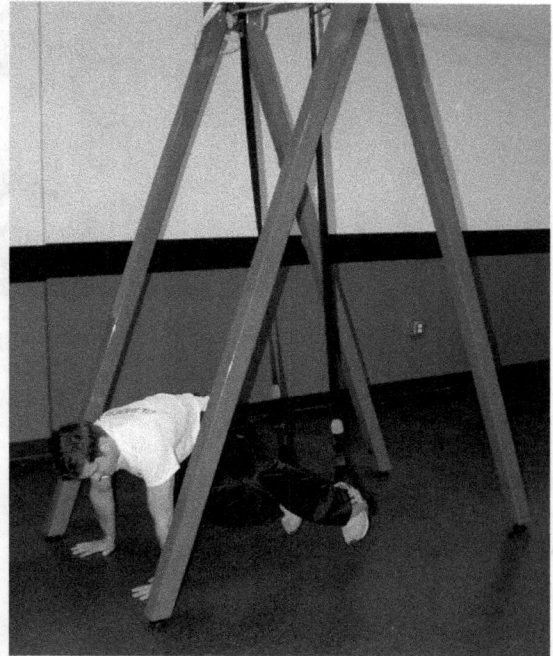

Finishing position for the extended knees
to elbows (knee tuck position)

Leg/Hamstring Curl

Targeted Muscle: Hamstrings (back of thigh)
Attachment: Foot/ankle

- The leg/hamstring curl movement is opposite to the knees-to-elbows movement.
- Extend the straps/ropes to about 8 inches off the ground. Position your heels in the handles as described at the beginning of the core/lower-body section.
- The resting position is like the glute bridge resting position—with knees bent at 90 degrees and your body lying with your hips and back on the ground.
- Lift your hips off the ground like in the glute bridge exercise.
- Keeping your abdominal and gluteus maximus muscles tight, extend your legs out straight in a slow and controlled manner.
- As you keep the hips elevated, engage the hamstring muscles to bend your knees as you return to the resting bridge position.

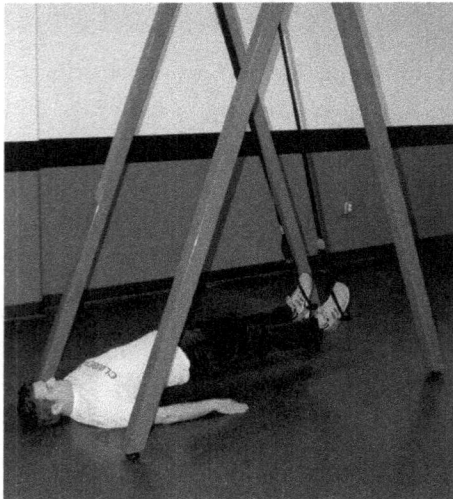

Starting position for the leg/hamstring (legs straight position)

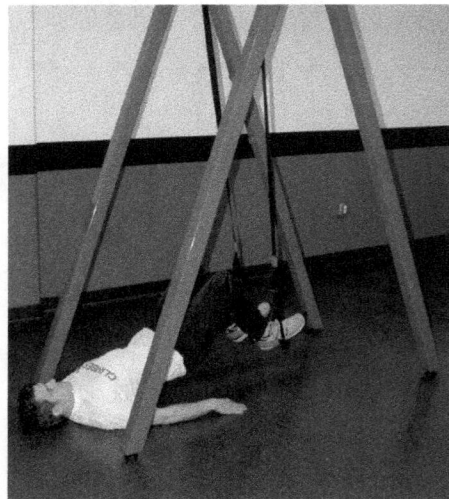

Finishing position for the leg/hamstring

Runners (Face Down)

Targeted Muscle: Hip flexors/abdominals
Attachment: Foot/ankle

- Facedown runners are similar to the knees-to-elbows exercise, except the emphasis is placed on one leg instead of both legs.
- Start facing down—with your knees resting on the ground—and then lift your knees up and extend your legs into the front plank position.
- Keeping your toes flexed toward your shin, bend one knee, bringing your knee forward toward your chest as far as you can.

- To perform the exercise, keep your hips elevated and alternate legs in a running-type motion. Try to keep your upper body stable on the ground and concentrate on not rotating from side to side.
- To add more emphasis on hip flexors/abdominals, the movement can be slowed down with pauses between alternating the positions of the leg.

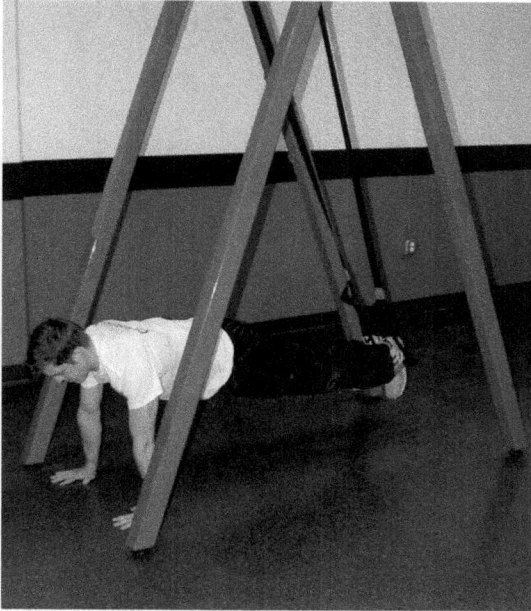

Starting position for the runners (face down) (front plank/legs straight position)

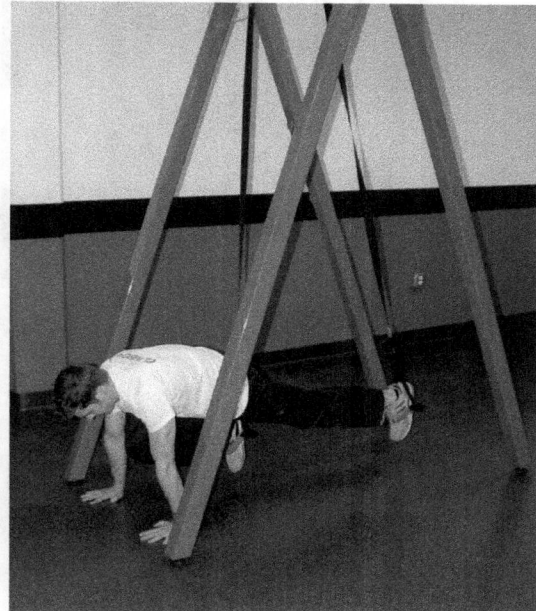

Finishing position for the runners (face down)

Runners (Face Up)

Targeted Muscle: Hamstrings (back of thigh)
Attachment: Foot/ankle

- Face up runners are similar to the leg/hamstring curl exercise, except the emphasis is placed on one leg instead of both legs.
- Start facing up, with your legs extended, and elevate your hips off the ground to help engage the muscles.
- Keeping your toes flexed toward your shin, bend one knee, bringing your heel back toward your glutes as far as you can.
- To perform the exercise, keep your hips elevated and alternate legs in a running-type motion.
- Try to keep your upper body stable on the ground and concentrate on not rotating from side to side.
- To make the exercise easier if needed, you can actually rest your hips lightly on the ground to lessen the load placed on the hamstrings.
- To add more emphasis on hamstrings, the movement can be slowed down with pauses between alternating the positions of the leg.

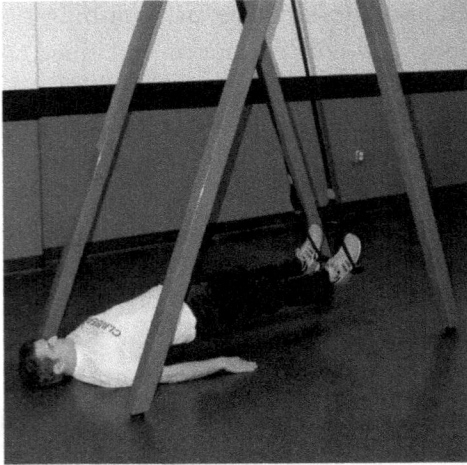

Starting position for the runners (face up)
(legs straight position)

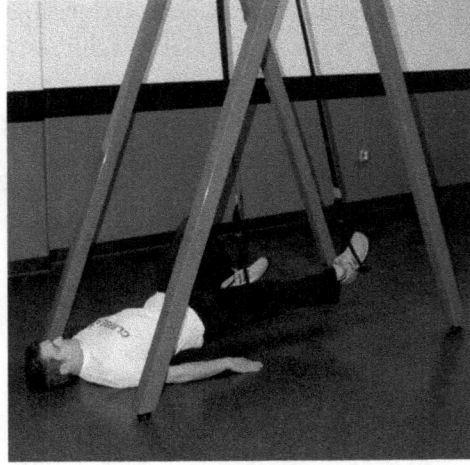

Finishing position for the runners (face up)

Fall Out

Targeted Muscle: Abdominals
Secondary Muscles: Deltoids (shoulders) and triceps brachii (back of upper arm)
Attachment: Handles

- Stand with your feet shoulder-width apart. Facing away from the anchor point, grab the handles with your arms at your side.
- Leaning your body-weight forward slowly, raise your arms to make a straight line from your hands to your ankles.
- Keeping your arms straight and abdominals tight, pull your arms down to the starting position.
- To make the exercise harder, start from your knees as you face away from the anchor point.
- To further increase the exercise intensity, perform the exercise from your knees while facing the anchor point.

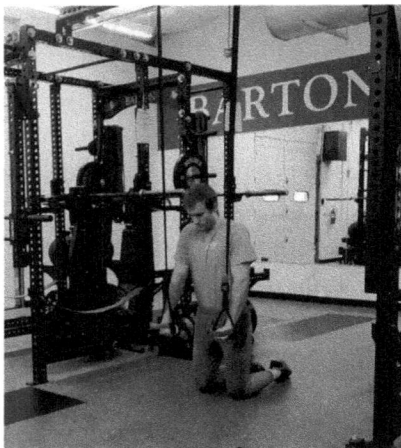

Starting position for the fall out

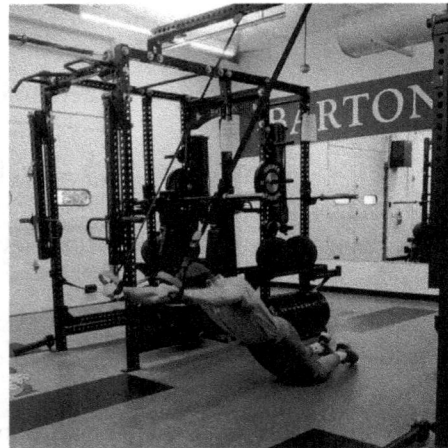

Finishing position for the fall out

References: Chapter 6

Sections in this chapter are adapted from my previously published books:

1. Dornemann, T. M. *POWERREV Youth Athletic Development Program: Building Champions in Sports and in Life*. Ronkonkoma, NY: Linus, 2015.

2. Dornemann, T. M. and A. Mikheev. *Russian Vibration Training: The Mikheev Method*. Monterey, CA: Healthy Learning, 2013.

7

POWER DEVELOPMENT: TRIPLE EXTENSION EXPLOSIVE LIFTING

By: Dave Kemble

Teaching Instructor East Carolina University
Program Coordinator for Health Fitness Specialist East Carolina University
USA Weightlifting National Coach and Instructor

IN THE PHYSICAL development of athletes, power output is king. While being strong is important, if an athlete cannot produce high force over a short amount of time, he/she will not perform on the field or court at a high level. This is due to the fact that in most sports there is a limited amount of time an athlete can produce force into the ground or other implement during competition. For example, let's compare the bench press lift to the shot put event in track and field. During a 1-RM bench press, barbell velocity in advanced lifters is approximately 0.17 ± 0.04 m/s (1), while the average shot put release maximal velocity in elite males is 13.69 ± 0.26 m/s (IAAF World Championships 2017–Men's Shot Put). From this data, it is clear to see the velocities between these two maximal effort activities are vastly different. Therefore, athletes must train for power when doing training activities outside of their sport.

Terms and Definitions

Before we dive deeper into how to influence power production in athletes, we must first define certain variables related to power production:

- *Force (F)* is the push or pull impacted on an object and is the product of mass multiplied by acceleration. In the weight room, body weight and external resistance (barbells, resistance bands, medicine balls, etc.) are often used as resistance forces in order to bring about positive adaptations of the musculature, skeletal, and connective tissues. Force is typically measured in Newtons (N). $N = 1\text{kg} \cdot 1 \text{ m/s}^2$

- *Velocity (V)* is the change in position of an object in reference to time. Velocity is typically measured in m/s. In the weight room, training can involve a variety of velocities ranging from 0 m/s (isometric exercise) to maximal (jumping, throwing and sprinting).
- *Force-Velocity Curve (FV)* is a display of how force and velocity interact with one another. In this curve one can clearly see there is a negative relationship between the two variables. For an athlete to create maximal force, velocity of movement must be low. In contrast, for an athlete to reach high velocities there is not enough time to produce high forces, therefore forces are quite low. Terms such as *maximal strength, strength-speed, power, speed strength and speed* are often used in conjunction with the FV curve.

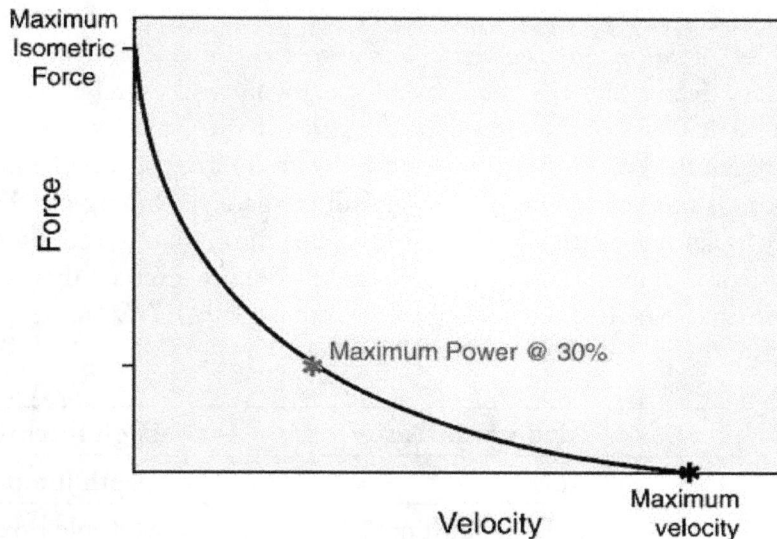

- *Strength* is an ability to produce force at a given velocity. Strength can be directly evaluated using a 1-repetition maximum (1-RM) test or estimated using data from a repetition maximum test (RM). Maximal strength or low-speed strength is typically measured using a 1-repetition maximum (1-RM) test for lifts such as the back squat, bench press or deadlift. Utilizing these lifts during training typically results in athletes gaining strength because the velocities displayed during maximal efforts are quite low. These lifts have mean velocities of 0.30 ± 0.05 m/s, 0.17 ± 0.04 m/s and 0.15 ± 0.15 m/s respectively (1). Thus, allowing more time for force development. Dynamic or high-speed strength can be evaluated using 1-RM testing for explosive lifts such as the snatch, clean or jerk. These explosive lifts are recognized as producing the highest power output amongst all forms of resistance training, as they have both high force and high velocity requirements. For example, maximal barbell velocities for these lifts are as follows: snatch = 1.65 m/s to 2.0 m/s, clean = 1.2 – 1.6 m/s, and jerk = 2.0 – 2.5 m/s (3). *NOTE: maximal velocity ranges for each lift are due to height differences amongst athletes.*
- *Power (P)* is a product of force and velocity (P = F · V). Power is best produced at moderate forces and moderate velocities. Looking at the FV curve again, one can clearly see this interaction once power output is displayed too.

Power Development for Athletes

Now that you understand the rationale for developing power in athletes and the basic background in how force, velocity and power interact, you can train for power output.

Plyometrics

Hopping, skipping, jumping, running, throwing and tossing are all forms of plyometric activities. Plyometric exercises rely on the concept of rate of force development (RFD). Simply put, muscles reach high forces over short time periods. This high RFD is possible due to the stretch-shortening cycle (SSC) all plyometric exercises have in common. The SSC uses stored energy and reflexive properties of the specialized muscle fibers to create high force output over short time periods. Phases of the SSC include: *eccentric (muscle stretches), amortization (isometric) and concentric (muscle shortens).*

The eccentric phase determines the intensity of the plyometric exercise. The more loading that occurs during the eccentric phase of the movement, the greater the intensity of the plyometric exercise. For example, let's compare the box jump (a jump from the ground to the top of a box) to a depth jump (jumping from the top of the box to the ground and immediately jumping off the ground). There is more potential energy in landing on the ground during a box jump than the countermovement of a box jump. Therefore, the depth jump is a much more intense plyometric exercise than a box jump. Below is a table of various plyometric exercises and their absolute intensities (4). *NOTE:* Relative intensity should be established for each individual athlete.

Low Intensity	Medium Intensity	High Intensity
Skip	Tuck Jump	Depth Jump
Vertical Jump	Split Squat Jump	Multiple Box Jump
Broad Jump	Hurdle Hop	Bounding
Box Jump	Jump from Box	Multiple Hurdle Hop
MB Chest Pass	Clap Push-ups	
MB Scoop Toss	Depth Push-ups	
MB Slams		
MB Rotational Pass		

Before you implement plyometrics into a program, your athletes should have a base level of strength supported by several months of resistance training (4). Other prerequisites include appropriate levels of speed, flexibility, balance and landing mechanics (for lower-body drills).

Weightlifting Movements

The sport of weightlifting has been described as the sport for all sports (5). That's because all three movements in the sport of weightlifting involve triple extension, which is extension of the hips, knees and ankles. Athletes in various sports display triple extension during competition. Activities such as sprinting, jumping and even throwing a baseball involve triple extension of the lower body. During explosive phases of the competition lifts in the sport of weightlifting (second pulls of snatch and clean and the drive phase of the jerk) is where peak power output occurs, as the barbell is still being accelerated and will not reach its maximal velocity until after the athlete has ceased to apply upward force to it. Compare this barbell acceleration to the actions seen in the back squat, bench press and deadlift. The barbell will decelerate as the athlete completes upward force. It is easy to see how the lifts involved in the sport of weightlifting are superior in the development of power output in athletes.

Readiness to Perform Weightlifting Movements

Before adding weightlifting movements into an athlete's training, one first must establish basic strength and flexibility minimums for each athlete. If athletes cannot properly perform the assessments, extra strength and flexibility training may be necessary before progressing. USA Weightlifting recommends the following assessments before beginning snatch, clean and jerk-related training:

Overhead Squat (OHS): is used to ensure your athletes possess appropriate levels of strength and flexibility to perform snatch-related lifts overhead and in the deep squat position. Before beginning the OHS assessment, the snatch-grip must be determined.

There are a number of ways to determine the appropriate grip to use. One recommended way to find this grip is to place the bar in the hip crease while hinging at the hips (pushing the hips back). With the barbell still in the hip crease, slide the hands out until the elbows are fully extended. This should be just about right for most athletes. *NOTE: Taller athletes may find their hands are in contact with the sleeves of the barbell. This is fine and appropriate due to their arm lengths.*

To perform the OHS, the barbell will be overhead above the shoulders with elbows extended while shoulders are externally rotated and the scapula retracted and in upward rotation. Feet should be shoulder width apart. Begin the movement by flexing the knees and hips until your hip crease is below the superior border of the patella. In the bottom position of the OHS, the torso ideally will be held vertical. Some forward incline in the torso will probably occur, but the torso should not incline more than the tibias. The spine is held rigid with no observable flexion and the barbell is balanced over the middle of the foot (between the heel and ball of the foot). Knees are in line with the feet while the feet are flat on the ground. After pausing in the bottom position for 2-3 seconds, stand and recover.

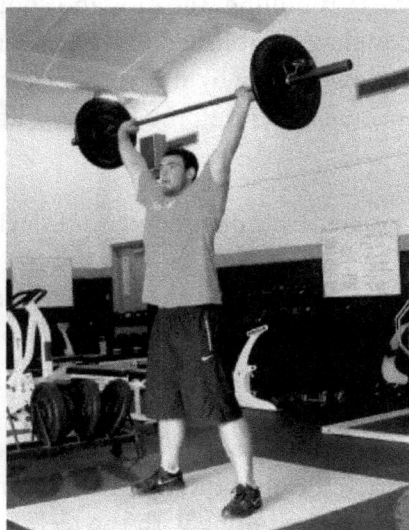

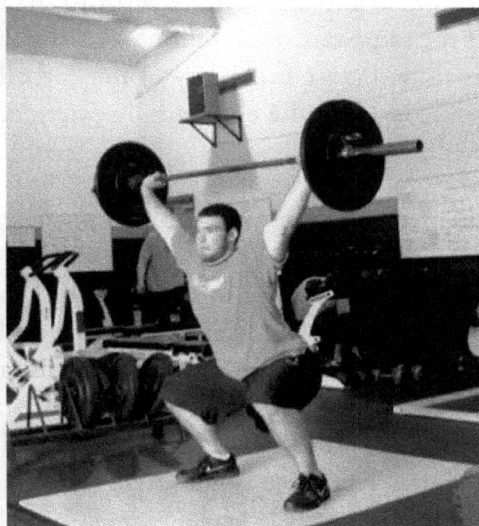

Snatch-grip Pull: is used to ensure your athletes possess appropriate levels of strength and flexibility to perform snatch-related lifts when pulling from the floor.

The stance will be hip to shoulder width with the feet in contact with the floor through the entire movement. The barbell should be over the widest part of the foot (the first metatarsal). The grip width will be the same as the one used in the OHS. *NOTE: The use of a hookgrip is strongly recommended to get your athletes used to pulling the snatch and clean with this style of grip.*

A hookgrip is a version of an overhand, closed grip (closed referring to the thumb being wrapped around the bar). In the hookgrip the thumb is tucked under the fingers to provide a stronger grip.

a. overhand
b. underhand
c. alternating
d. hook

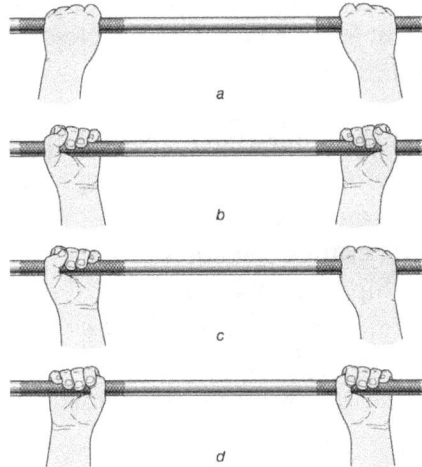

*Essentials of Strength Training and Conditioning – NSCA (4th ed.)

The get-set position is established by lowering the hips, pushing the knees forward (tibia more horizontal touching or almost touching the barbell) and raising the torso until the shoulders are stacked directly over or slightly in advance of the barbell. The shoulders should never be behind the barbell. Using the musculature of the legs and hips, drive the feet into the platform, allowing the knees to displace rearward (tibia will become more vertical). As the athlete is pulling, the hips and shoulders should rise together at the same rate, maintaining a constant back angle as established in the get-set position. As the bar rises, maintain close proximity of the barbell to the lower body by utilizing the latissimus dorsi musculature while keeping the elbows fully extended. Continue extending the hips and knees until the torso is fully erect.

Front Squat: is used to ensure your athletes possess appropriate levels of strength and flexibility to perform clean-related lifts.

To begin, the barbell will be in the front rack position. Stand behind the bar with the bar resting high on your chest. Keep your deltoids with the elbows high (humerus approximately parallel to the ground). Feet are shoulder width apart. Begin the movement by flexing the knees and hips until your hip crease is below the superior border of the patella. In the bottom position, the torso ideally will be held vertical. Some forward incline in the torso will probably occur, but the torso should not incline more than the tibias. The spine is held rigid with no observable flexion, the barbell is balanced over the middle of the foot (between the heel and ball of the foot), knees are in line with the feet, feet flat on the ground. After pausing in the bottom position for 2-3 seconds, stand and recover.

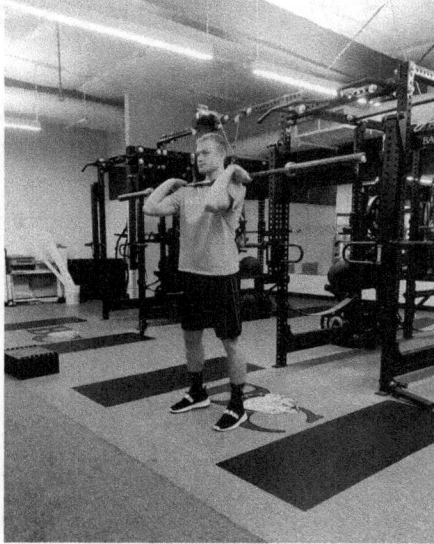

Front squat top position

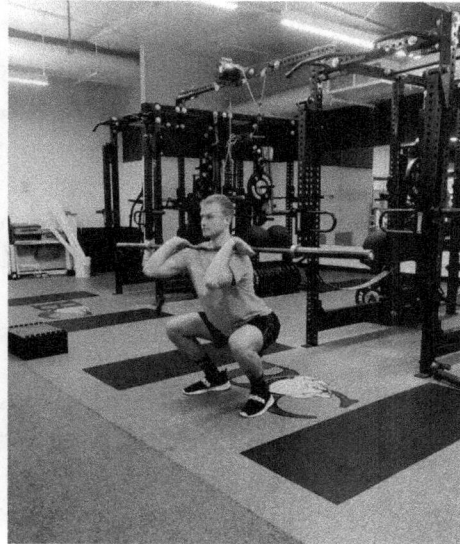

Front squat bottom position

Press: is used to ensure your athletes possess appropriate levels of strength and flexibility to perform jerk-related lifts.

The barbell should sit high on the deltoids using a closed grip just outside shoulder-width. The elbows spread down and out (just ahead of the barbell). Stand with feet approximately hip width apart. The movement is executed by using only the musculature of the upper body (deltoids and triceps). Press the barbell from the shoulders into the overhead position, which will cause the barbell to travel both up and slightly back behind the ears. In the overhead position, the barbell should be directly above the shoulders, hips, knees and ankles. After pausing in the overhead position for 2-3 seconds, lower the barbell back to the shoulders.

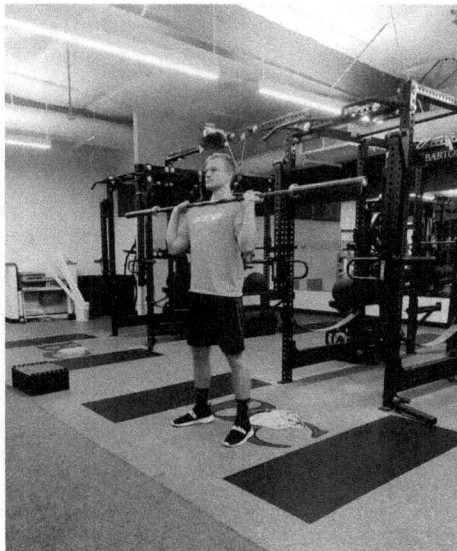

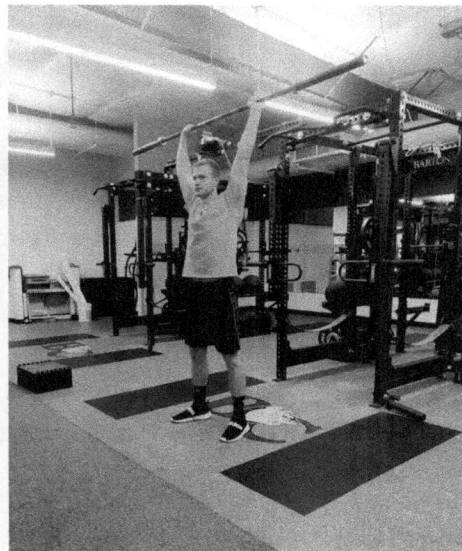

Training with the Snatch, Clean and Jerk and Weightlifting Nomenclature

USA Weightlifting endorses the use of a top-down and partial movements approach when teaching the lifts. What this means is that athletes should perform hang or block variations for the snatch and clean before starting lifts from the platform. It is also generally recommended that athletes perform power variations before attempting to execute the deep squats used in the snatch and clean or split technique of the jerk. Below is a description of the nomenclature–or common words used in the discipline of weight-lifting–needed to fully understand all of the variations of the snatch, clean and jerk.

Hang: this term is used to describe a starting position in which the barbell and discs (bumper plates) are "hanging" above the platform.

There are an infinite number of hanging positions that could be used. Here are some common positions: *high hang (sometimes referred to the power position), above the knee, middle of the knee and below the knee.* By performing hanging variations, coaches are removing portions of the pull in the snatch or clean, thus removing some of the technical work, especially when performed in the high hang or above the knee positions. Hanging variations are great for developing positional strength, as the athlete must hold the barbell as he/she assumes the correct position to hang from. Hanging variations can also be used when trying to remove additional stress from executing the full pull from the platform. Again, this is especially true when hanging from the high hand and above the knee positions, as pulling from below the knee increases fatigue to the lower back.

Block: this term is used to describe a starting position in which the discs (bumper plates) are resting on an object (i.e., pulling blocks) elevated above the platform.

Block work is an excellent option when working on technique, as the coach can focus on positional work by getting his/her athletes in the correct starting position each rep. Additionally, block variations can also remove stress from training, as the athlete does not have to hold positions as is required during hanging variations. Finally, when coaches want to work on RFD, block variations are ideal as the athlete will begin with very little force since the weight of the barbell is resting on the blocks and there is a shorter time frame to develop force in the pull compared to pulling from the platform. When pulling blocks are not available, coaches may choose to rest the barbell on safety arms of racks. However, athletes should be encouraged to slowly return the barbell to the arms to avoid damaging the barbells.

Power: this term is used to describe the squatting depth in the receiving positions of the snatch, clean and jerk. During training when these lifts are received in an above parallel squat, power variations are being implemented. Additionally, power variations are lighter than full squat variations due to the greater barbell displacement. So, when programming calls for greater barbell velocity, power variations can be used with great success.

Teaching the Snatch and Clean

Each phase of the lift is equally important and thus must be fully understood by the coach in order to effectively teach the full lift.

Get-set: To execute a technically sound snatch or clean from the platform, the get-set position must be well established. In this position you will want to see the following:

- Feet flat and approximately shoulder width apart: toes may be turned out slightly in order to accommodate hip mobility and/or torso to limb ratios.
- Shoulders in internal rotation: elbows should point to bar ends.
- Appropriate grip width: snatch-grip vs. clean grip. The use of a hookgrip should be encouraged.
- Knees: as your athlete lowers his/her body down, the knees will push forward, inclining the tibias in the process. This will place a little more pressure towards the balls of the feet, but heels should stay down.
- Hips and shoulders: these joints are dependent upon one another. The hips are low but not too low. Hip starting position will have an impact on the shoulder starting position. The hips should be lowered to a position in which the shoulders are stacked directly over the barbell or slightly in front of it. Lowering the hips should never cause the shoulders to travel behind the barbell.
- Back angle: the angle of the torso relative to the platform. This back angle is created in the get-set position and should not significantly change during the first pull.
- Spine: set in complete extension with no observable flexion.

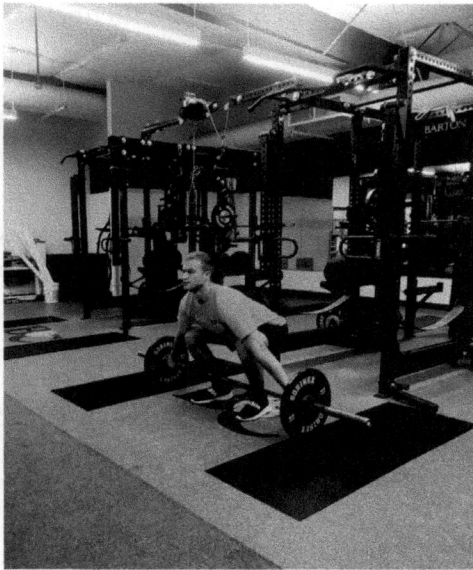

Snatch Get Set   Clean Get Set

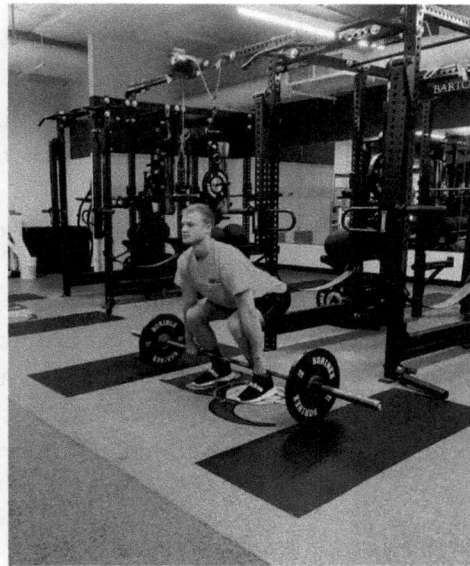

1ˢᵗ Pull: The first pull is described as the displacement of the barbell to just beyond the knee. This portion of the pull lasts until the knee has reached its greatest extension.

During the first pull, the musculature of the legs (quadriceps) should be the primary driving force. As the athlete performs the first pull, his/her knees should displace rearward and begin shifting his/her weight from the ball of the foot towards the heel gradually. This rearward shifting of the athlete's weight should not cause a significant change in the back angle created in the get-set position. This will cause the athlete's tibia to become more vertical. Along with the use of the latissimus dorsi, this should facilitate an upward and rearward displacement of the barbell. At the end of the first pull, as the barbell has moved up and back, the athlete's shoulders should be in advance of the barbell.

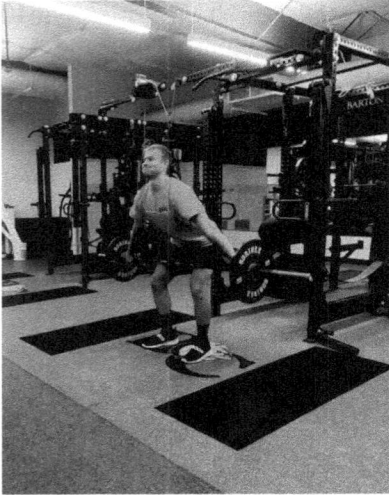

Snatch 1st Pull

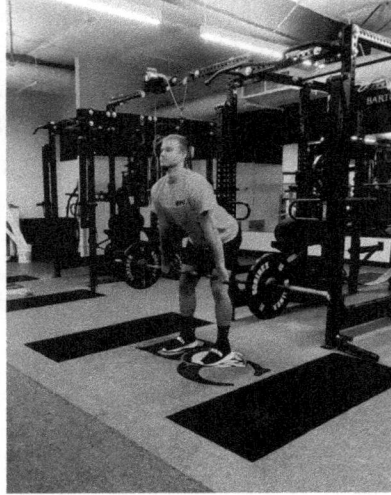

Clean 1st Pull

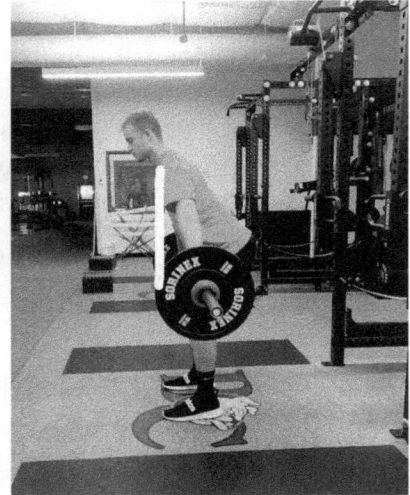

Line indicates how shoulders stay
in advance (in front) of the bar

Reposition: This phase has been called by many different names such as the *transition, scoop or double-knee bend*. Whatever you choose to call it, this is how the athlete gets into a strong power position in order to execute a powerful second pull.

At the completion of the first pull, the torso will rapidly move upright while the knees flex and shift forward of the barbell. The distribution of weight should once again move forward on the foot (just behind the ball of the foot), but the heels should remain down. As the athlete is performing the reposition, coaches should observe barbell contact with the athlete. In the snatch, this point of contact should be on the hip and during the clean it should be on the middle to upper thigh. In advanced lifters, coaches may also hear an audible sound that occurs with this contact. It is important to note that during the reposition the athlete should attempt to keep his/her shoulders in front of the barbell as long as possible.

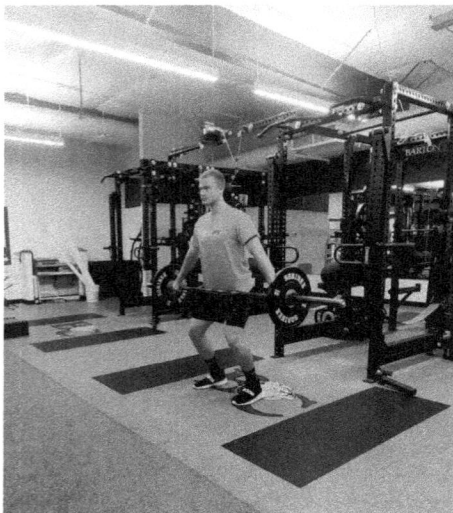

Snatch Reposition

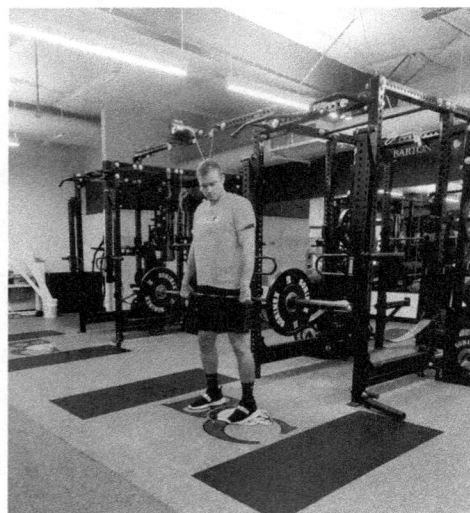

Clean Reposition

2nd Pull: In the power position the athlete will be in a very strong position to exert maximal force into the platform. Here the musculature of the legs and hips will drive into the platform and the athlete will reach a point of triple extension as the heels elevate from the platform. The final event that should occur in the second pull is an aggressive shoulder shrug. With a properly executed second pull, the barbell will continue to accelerate beyond this point of triple extension.

The musculature of the arms should be relaxed with no elbow flexion. Only the legs, hips and back musculature is involved in the pull. Coaches should work hard to correct any elbow flexion that occurs before the second pull.

Pull-under: Now it is time for the musculature of the arms and shoulders to take over. As the barbell is still accelerating upward, the athlete should aggressively pull him/herself under the barbell using the arms and shoulders. As the athlete does so, his/her feet shift quickly and outward into the receiving position (approximately shoulder width).

Snatch: The athlete should focus on pulling his/her elbows up and out when pulling under the barbell. As the barbell travels past the chest, the elbows will rotate behind the barbell and the athlete will then push him/herself down under the barbell to prepare to receive the barbell overhead.

Clean: The athlete should focus on pulling his/her elbows up and back when pulling under the barbell. As the barbell travels past the waist, the elbows will rotate forward and up as the athlete prepares to receive the barbell high on the deltoids.

Receive: This can also be called the catch phase. Receiving the barbell should always occur at its greatest height.

Snatch: As the athlete pulls under the bar, he/she will then begin pushing the body under the bar as arms fully extend to position the bar over the shoulders/upper-back and over the base of support. The depth at which the athlete receives the bar partially determines how we name the lift.

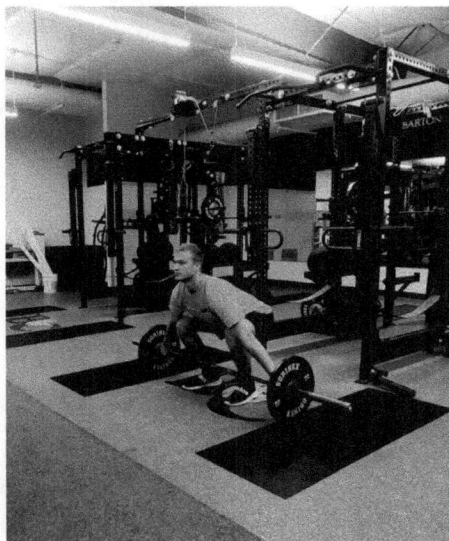

Snatch Get Set

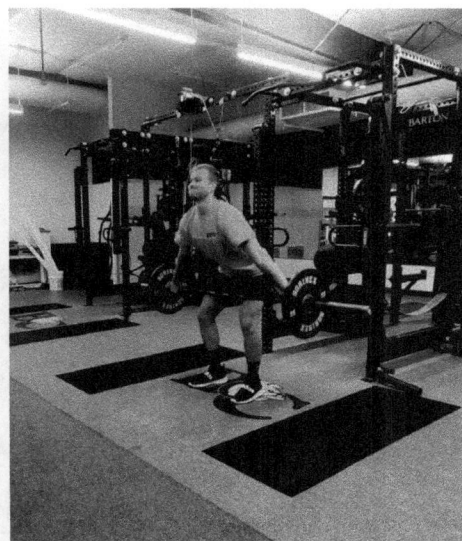

Snatch First Pull

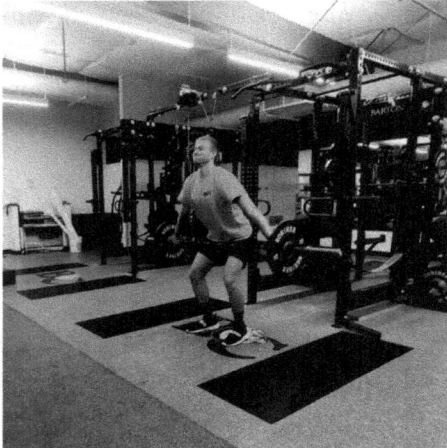

Snatch Power Position

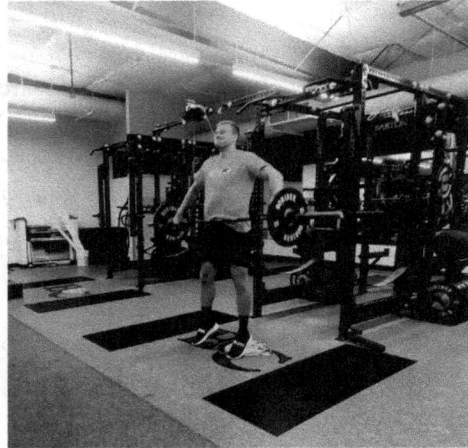

Snatch Triple Extension

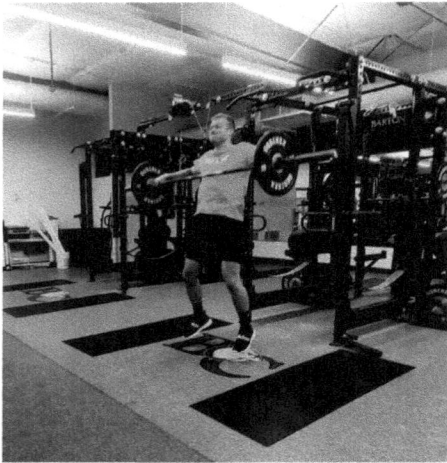

Snatch Pull Under

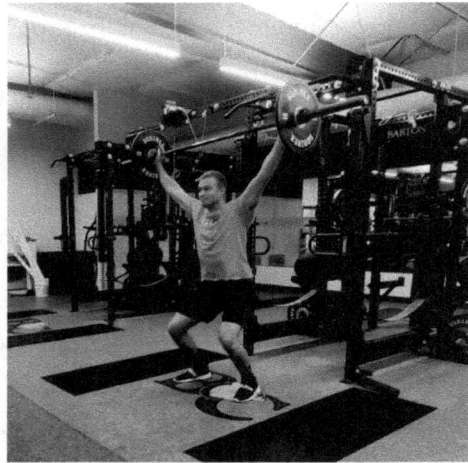

Snatch Catch

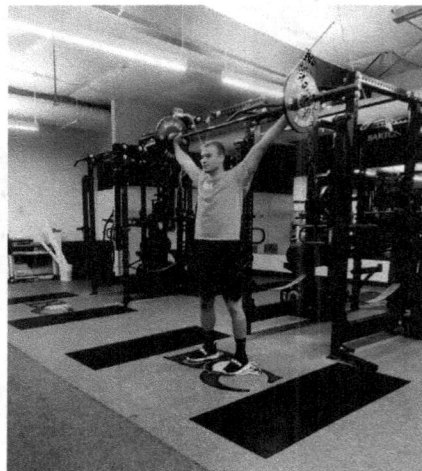

Snatch Recover

Clean: As the athlete pulls under the bar, he/she will then push the elbows up and in front of the barbell, receiving the barbell high on the deltoids and over the base of support. The depth at which the athlete receives the bar partially determines how we name the lift.

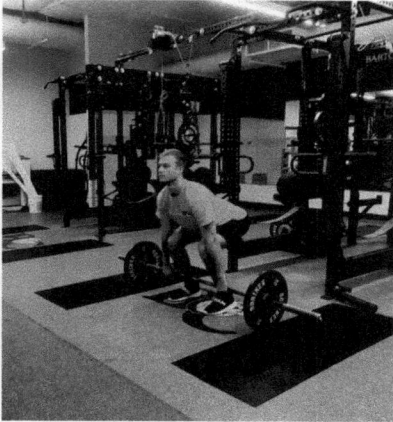

Clean Get Set

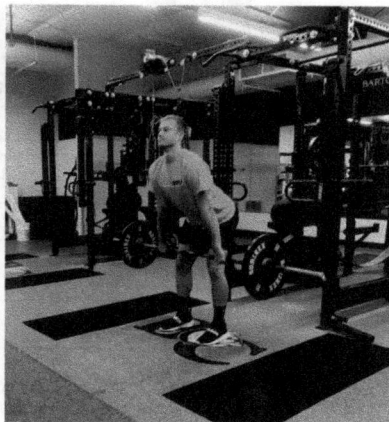

Clean First Pull

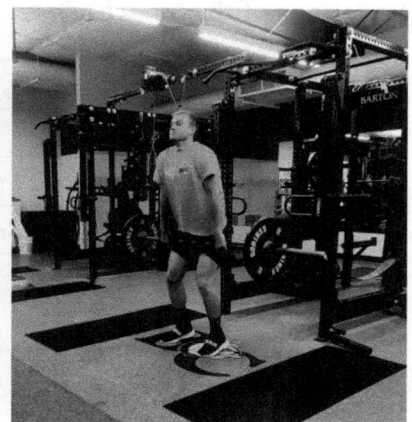

Clean Power Position

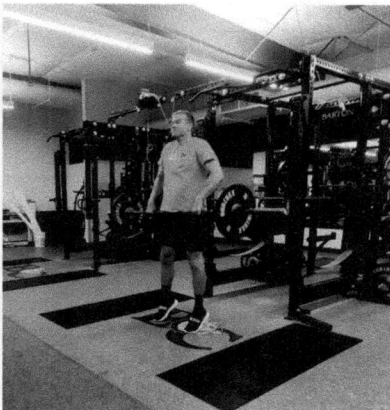

Clean Triple Extension

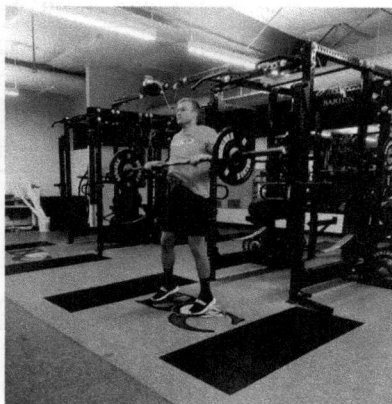

Clean Pull Under

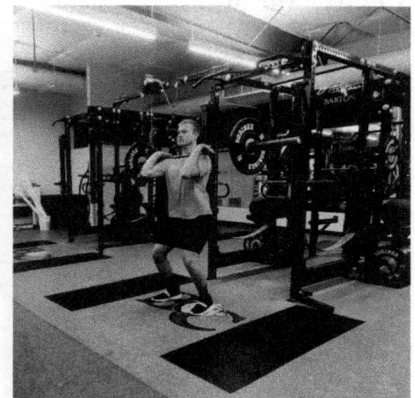

Clean Catch

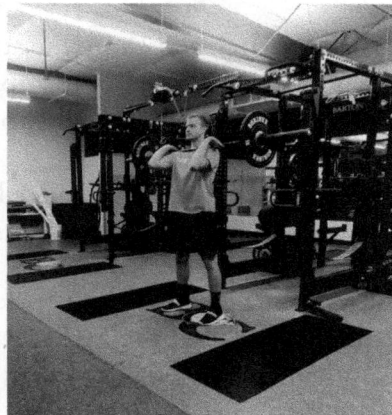

Clean Recover

Recover: After receiving the barbell overhead or on the deltoids in a balanced state, the athlete should once again use the musculature of the legs and hips to stand tall before lowering the barbell back down to the platform.

Variations of the Snatch

Power Variations	Deep Squat Variations
High-hang Power Snatch	High-hang Snatch
Hang Above the Knee Power Snatch	Hang Above the Knee Snatch
Hang Below the Knee Power Snatch	Hang Below the Knee Snatch
Power Snatch	Snatch
Power Snatch + OHS*	

* Example complex to get athletes ready for the full deep squat snatch

Variations of the Clean

Power Variations	Deep Squat Variations
High-hang Power Clean	High-hang Clean
Hang Above the Knee Power Clean	Hang Above the Knee Clean
Hang Below the Knee Power Clean	Hang Below the Knee Clean
Power Clean	Clean
Power Clean + FS*	

* Example complex to get athletes ready for the full deep squat clean

Teaching the Jerk

As we described in the section above when teaching the snatch and clean lifts, there are also phases of the jerk.

Get-set: Similar to the pulling stances of the snatch and clean, the athlete's feet should be approximately hip width. The barbell should rest high on the deltoids with the scapula protracted and slightly elevated. The elbows should be spread out and point down slightly. A full grip (barbell in palm of hand) is recommended but not required. The athlete's hands should be relaxed.

Behind the neck variations exist too. Basically all that is changed is that the barbell will rest on high on the trapezius muscles and the elbows should be directly under the barbell.

Dip: The dip involves the athlete sitting down (and slightly back) in ~¼ squat with feet flat. Your athlete should have a preference for the front edge of the heel when dipping. A dip depth is approximately 8-12% of the athlete's height. When teaching the dip, first start by encouraging a deep breath and bracing of the core musculature. Keep the torso vertical during the dip to ensure the bar path stays vertical. The dip should be short and quick (think SSC as described in the plyometric section above) but controlled–positions and change of direction (COD) are most important. Upper-body angles remain constant during the dip phase.

Athletes will generally want to dip deeper than necessary. This will more than likely cause problems in either their upright posture or ability to change directions quickly.

Drive: The musculature of the legs and hips drive the barbell off of the shoulders through rapid triple extension (max power output). The drive phase too must be vertical. Encourage the athlete to stay back during the drive phase. Athletes that tend to dip too far back on the heels will then drift forward in their drive phase. Make sure their dip is more balanced in the middle of the foot.

Push-under: After a full extension of legs and hips, the athlete quickly begins to push his/her body down under the bar with arms and shoulders. The athlete receives the bar behind head at arm's length with torso vertical (although in power jerk variations a slight incline of the torso is necessary as the hips sit back and down).

Footwork: As the arms and shoulders are pushing the athlete down, the feet will either shift outward to shoulder width in a power jerk or shift to the split position in a split jerk. Split stance is typically more comfortable for most athletes, especially those with thoracic spine and overhead mobility limitations. In the split position the main points of emphasis are:

- Front foot flat
- Front tibia vertical, knee stacked over heel
- Back knee flexed
- Back heel up with ball of the foot down
- Hips under the barbell
- Feet move in sagittal plane (do not let move inward)

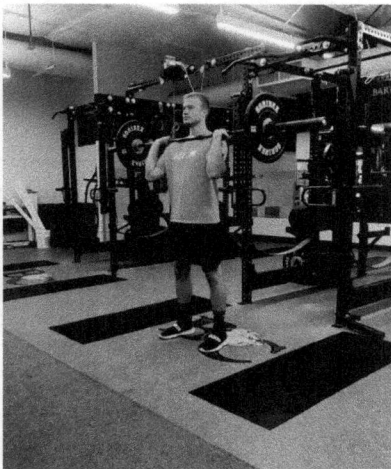 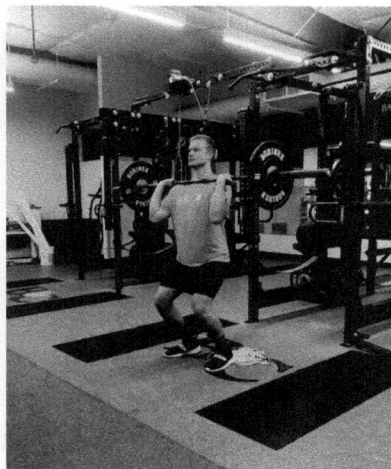 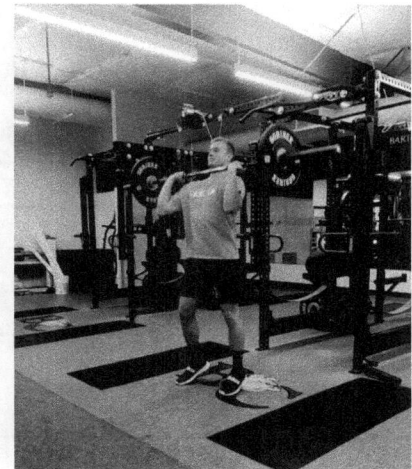

Get Set   Dip   Drive

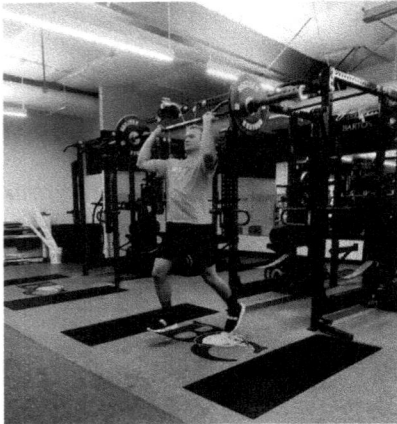

Push-under

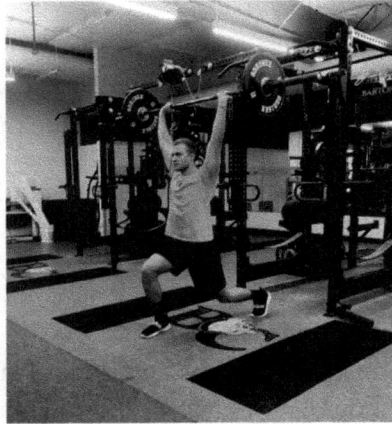

Footwork (Split Jerk Position)

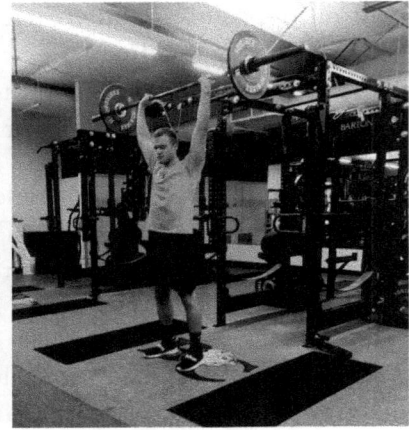

Power Jerk Position

Variations of the Jerk

Behind the Neck Variations	Front Rack Variations
Push Press	Push Press
Power Jerk	Power Jerk
Split Jerk	Split Jerk

Below are some example workouts with progressions when teaching the snatch, clean and jerk. There are no definitive time frames for these progressions to occur. Some athletes may advance weekly, while others may take more time before they have mastered the skills needed to advance. Please use your best judgment for your particular circumstance.

Example Snatch-related Workouts with Progressions

Start of Snatch Training:

High-hang Snatch Extension	3 x 5
Snatch-grip Push Press	3 x 5
Snatch Pull	3 x 5
Back Squat	3 x 5

Progression 1:

High-hang Snatch High Pull*	3 x 5
Snatch-grip Push Press + Overhead Squat#	3 x 3 + 3 (3 push press + 3 OHS)
Snatch Pull	3 x 5
Back Squat	3 x 5

* If athlete is using legs and hips well in extension, then progression can be made to snatch high pull.
# If overhead position has been established, then progression can be made to OHS.

Progression 2:

High-hang Muscle Snatch + Overhead Squat*	3 x 3 + 1 (3 muscle snatch + 1 OHS)
Overhead Squat	3 x 3
Snatch Extension+	3 x 5
Back Squat	3 x 5

* If timing of extension to high pull is occurring well, then progression can be made to muscle snatch.
+ If athlete is pulling well, then progression can be made to snatch extension.

Progression 3:

High-hang Power Snatch + Overhead Squat*	3 x 3 + 1 (3 power snatch + OHS)
Snatch Balance+	3 x 3
Snatch Extension	3 x 5
Back Squat	3 x 5

* If arm action is proper in muscle snatch, then progression can be made to power snatch.
+ If OHS training has gone well, the progression can be made to snatch balance.

Progression 4:

High-hang Snatch*	3 x 3
Snatch Balance	3 x 3
Snatch Extension	3 x 5
Back Squat	3 x 5

* If power snatch + OHS has been established, then progression can be made to full snatch.

Example Clean & Jerk-related Workouts with Progressions

Start of Clean & Jerk Training:

High-hang Clean Extension	3 x 5
Press	3 x 5
Clean Pull	3 x 5
Front Squat	3 x 5

Progression 1:

High-hang Clean High Pull	3 x 5
Push Press+	3 x 5

Clean Pull	3 x 5
Front Squat	3 x 5

* If athlete is using legs and hips well in extension, then progression can be made to clean high pull.
+ If the overhead position has been established, then progression can be made to push press.

Progression 2:

High-hang Muscle Clean + Front Squat*	3 x 3 + 1
Push Press	3 x 5
Clean Extension+	3 x 5
Front Squat	3 x 5

* If timing of extension to high pull is occurring well, then progression can be made to muscle clean.
+ If athlete is pulling well, then progression can be made to clean extension.

Progression 3:

High-hang Power Clean + Front Squat*	3 x 3 + 1
Power Jerk+	3 x 3
Clean Extension	3 x 5
Front Squat	3 x 5

* If arm action is proper in muscle snatch, then progression can be made to power snatch.
+ If dip and drive are good in push press, then progression can be made to power jerk.

Progression 4:

High-hang Clean + Power Jerk*^	3 x 3 + 3
Split Footwork	3 x 5
Clean Extension	3 x 5
Front Squat	3 x 5

* If power clean + FS has been established, then progression can be made to full clean.
^ Here we have put clean and power jerk together.

Progression 5:

High-hang Clean + Split Jerk*	3 x 3 + 3
Clean Extension	3 x 5
Front Squat	3 x 5

* If footwork has been established for split position, then progression can be made to split jerk.

References: Chapter 7

1. Weightlifting: sport for all sports https://www.abebooks.com/9788860282705/Weightlifting-Sport-sports-Urso-Antonio-8860282705/plp

2. NSCA's Essentials

3. VBT Paper

4. Soviet Manual

5. Hamill, Knutzen, and Derrick. *Biomechanical Basis of Human Movement* (5th edition). Philadelphia, Pennsylvania: Wolters & Kluwer, 2022.

8
AGILITY TRAINING

By: Tim Dornemann, Ed. D., CES, PES, CSCS, OS Pro

Exercise Science Program & Kinesiology Director, Barton College
Associate Professor of Exercise Science, Barton College
&
Scott O'Dell
Director of Strength & Conditioning, East Central University

"AGILITY GENERALLY REFERS to two sorts of motor functions. On the one hand, it is integral to the ability to explosively start, decelerate, change direction, and accelerate again quickly while maintaining body control and minimizing loss of speed (Costello and Kreis 1993). Agility, in this respect, is important in sport because movements are often initiated from various body positions. So athletes need to be able to react with strength, explosiveness, and quickness from these different positions in short bursts of 10 yards (9 meters) or less before a change of direction is required. On the other hand, agility refers to the ability to coordinate several sport-specific tasks simultaneously, such as when a player dribbles a basketball around a full-court press while looking for an open teammate to whom he or she can pass the ball (Barnes & Cissick 2004). Studies show that agility in these tasks is the primary determining factor to predict success in a sport (Halberg 2001)." Definition of agility taken from *Training for Speed, Agility, and Quickness* (2005).

In *High-Performance Sports Conditioning* (2001), the importance of balance in agility training is emphasized with the following definition: "Balance—The ability to maintain the center of body mass over a base of support—has long been classified as an important aspect of motor development. It is the underlying component of all movement skills, especially agility."

By the previous points of emphasis and definitions with agility, agility is much more than creative drills performed in short distances around a bunch of cones. As you see in the definition above, there are words such as "explosively start," "strength," "quickness," "balance" and "body control," among many others used to describe exactly what it is. Agility consists of everything we have done in this book and will consist of factors covered in the rest of this book as well. As was covered in linear speed training and to be covered in plyometrics, there is a systematic, progressional approach to take with developing agility properly for injury prevention and sports performance.

190

Every area of sports performance can be agility, just as agility can be in every area of sports performance. All areas of sports performance are relative to each other. In this chapter, we will cover the "norm" in thinking when we use the word agility. During the training plan, when looking at a change of direction, or agility, day of emphasis in the field/court work, there is a process to take in progressing the drills and using them for maximum performance and injury prevention. As suggested in the acceleration start, the center of gravity should always be out in front of the direction the body is moving, creating movement and good acceleration angles.

Lateral Movement

Initiating the lateral movement from a previous movement is taught in two different ways by various coaches. There is the crossover step, which seems to be more popular—this consists of the athlete immediately turning their hips and committing their body as soon as they make the decision to move in the given direction. The crossover step will typically have a faster time compared to the open/shuffle step during the initial phase of training.

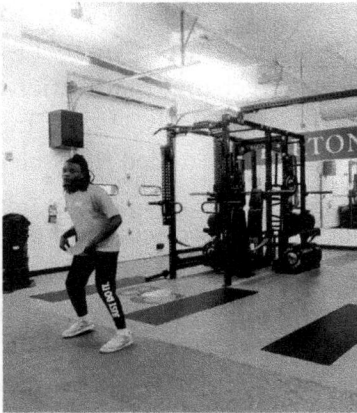

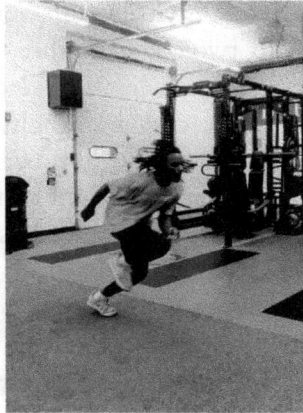

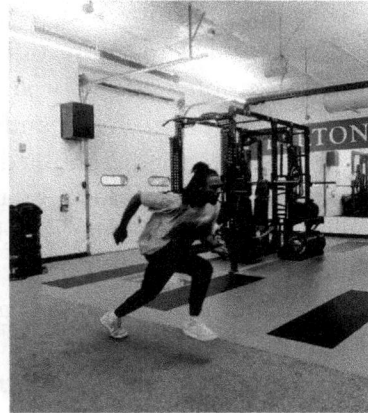

Then there is the open step. This is where the athlete pushes off of both feet and opens up the knee and toe of the nearest leg in the direction they are planning to move. The open step allows the body to commit in the direction of movement with more time to still be in a better position to unexpectedly cut back the other direction.

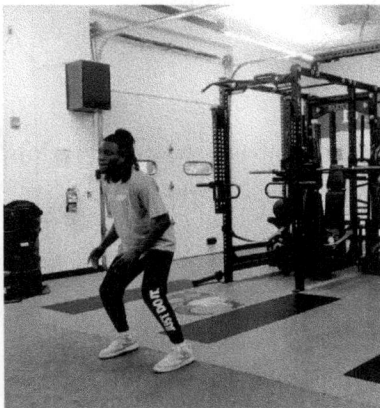

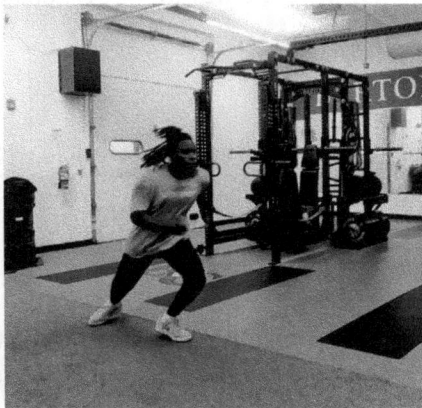

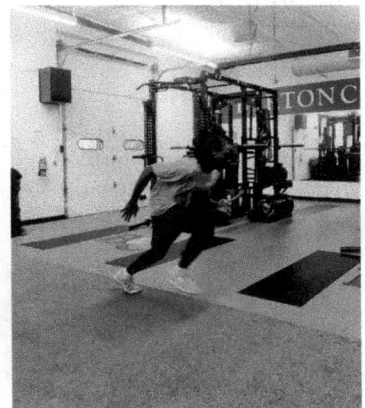

University of Oregon Head Strength and Conditioning Coach James Radcliffe reveals some good research and analyses to this debate over which lateral step is better to train in his book *Functional Training For Athletes At All Levels* (2007):

> In much of the University of Oregon Strength & Conditioning Program and Exercise and Movement Science's experience and data collection, we have found simple answers to the debate on whether a crossover is better than an open step, or vice versa. In novice performers, the cross-over step has shown faster initial get-off. Video analysis reveals that without practice they push off with both feet and project the hips better than unpracticed open steps. The hips are often held higher as with higher-velocity running and speed cuts. In many sports, however, the crossover step can lead to improper positions on the field or court. Crossover technique may also lead to step sequences that are not as efficient as open technique due to other change-of-direction needs. Once trained in the art of projecting the hips from the open technique, the get-off times become more comparable, and may be more useful in certain positions and patterns on the field or court.

The purpose of the agility program is to teach body control, acceleration, deceleration and change direction skills. The agility program progressively utilizes cutting, change of direction and quick feet drills, using multiple movement patterns to teach participants how to better control their bodies, accelerate, decelerate and change direction. Initially two cone and three cone drills, like the pro-agility (5-10-5) drill using three cones, are incorporated to teach acceleration, deceleration and change of direction using the outside foot. Next, inside and outside foot cuts are taught using five-cone drills. As the training progresses, shuffling and combined forward and backward movement patterns are added into the drills. Speed cuts introduce inside foot cuts with a series of straight cones.

Use of drills like the figure-eight drill, can be introduced as an advanced power cut, and different variations of the pro-agility drill can be added using shuffling and combined forward and backward movement patterns. Transitional agility drills are incorporated by combining different drills and movements. Square drills can be designed in a vast variety of ways to challenge athletes by using unlimited combinations of movement patterns and cutting techniques. Transitional agility drills are designed to prepare athletes to be able to transition quickly in preparation for the demand of their sport. During upper level progressions, reaction agilities, like shadowing drills and coach response drills, are added to help improve reaction time.

Rope and ladder drills are used throughout the levels to help improve footwork and foot speed. Rest periods are held constant at 45 seconds between repetitions to allow adequate recovery. These drills are designed for teaching movement skills and the conditioning aspect is secondary. However, as conditioning improves over the the course of training, the number of repetitions per drill is increased.

Agility Basics

Agility is an expression of an athlete's coordinative abilities, which are the basis of acceleration, maximum-velocity and multidirectional skills.

Agility Progression

As with any aspect of training, proper progression is key. While the ultimate goal is to be able to change direction based on reading and reacting to an opponent's movements like in competition, training cannot start there.

A good coach systematically progresses an athlete through exercises, having athletes master each level of the progression before moving on. Agility technique drills, featuring the use of two or three cones, create an environment to repeatedly practice basic change of direction technique. Once basic change of direction skills have been established, five-cone drills in a zig zag or "W" pattern can be used to develop inside and outside foot cutting technique. When an athlete has the ability to properly execute 90-degree cuts, then use transitional agility drills with a four cone "square" configuration to teach how to transition from one movement pattern to another. Sports commonly require athletes to be able to transition from moving forward to moving laterally or backwards. The four cone pattern provides an opportunity for athletes to practice and perfect transitional change of direction skills. Line and agility ladder drills provide a structured way of developing footwork and foot speed that are important to many sports. After athletes are proficient in basic technique, cutting skills, transitioning between movement patterns, and footwork, then reaction agility drills can be introduced. Coach reaction and mirror drills allow athletes to use the agility skills that have been developed in a read-and-react situation, similar to how they would play their sport.

- Agility Technique (2 or 3 cone drills)
- Cutting Skills (5 cone drills)
- Transitional Agilities (4 cone drills)
- Quick Feet Work (ladder drills)
- Reaction Agilities

Basic Change of Direction Technique & Cues

Drop: As you decelerate prior to changing direction, lower the body (hips) down. This puts you in a strong position to stop quickly.

Stop: From this strong and low position, stop your forward momentum.

Drive: Drive your body explosively in the new direction. From your lowered body position, drive out (not up) in as close to the optimal 45-degree body angle as possible and re-accelerate in the new direction.

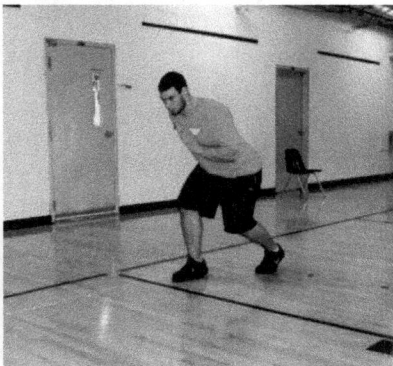

Drop low to decelerate

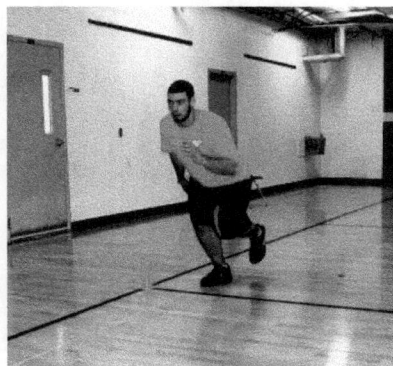

Load plant leg to stop

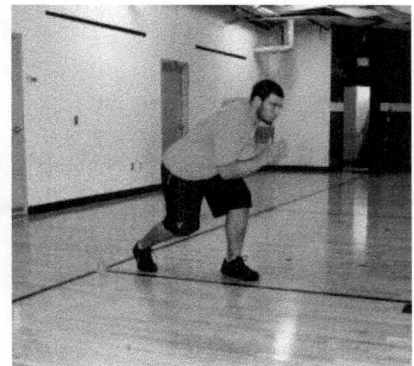

Stay low and drive off of cut leg

Speed & Power Cuts

Speed cuts develop the power, movement skills, and injury prevention of the body in the acceleration involving the inside cutting foot. In contrast, power cuts develop the power, movement skills, and injury prevention of the body in the acceleration involving the outside cutting foot. Coming out of each cut, the drive sprinting mechanics should be emphasized with the center of gravity out in front and good knee and hip angles to produce force into the ground for maximum acceleration.

Once through the agility progression, it is important to continue with at least one good transitional movement, a power cut, and a speed cut to provide repeated bouts of these for injury prevention and maximum performance when heading into the sports competition and practice season. Upon reaching this phase, you can incorporate any and all agility drills. The body should be prepared for all advanced movement as well as reaction agility drills. This is also the phase of the training program to take time to focus on position-specific drills.

Examples: Agility Progression and Quick Foot Drills

Agility Technique (2 or 3 cone) Drills

- *2 Cone Drill (Base Agility teaching drill):* Set up two cones no more than 5 meters apart. Athletes practice drop, stop, and drive techniques in forward, backward, and lateral movement patterns.
    - Narrow cones allow for increased number of direction changes (practice of key steps)
    - Drop body low and drive in new direction (drop and drive)
    - To stay low, you can have athletes reach down
    - Can do forward, lateral, and frontwards/backwards direction change

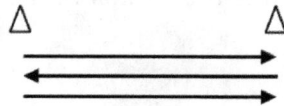

- *3 Cone Drill (5-10-5)*
    - Add a third cone 5m from the second cone.
    - Start from the middle cone and go either right or left to the outer cone.
    - Change direction and go to the farthest cone and then change direction and go back through the middle cone.
    - The longer 5-10-5 pattern allows for greater acceleration between cones which increases the challenge of changing directions.

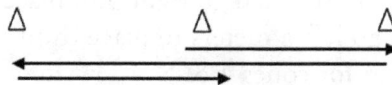

- *Forward/Backward 5-10-5 Drill*
    - Start straddling middle cone, then sprint 5 meters to the right
    - Decelerate, drop, and drive to change direction
    - Backpedal 10 meters to left side cone
    - Keep forward lean with chest over feet to keep balance
    - Decelerate, drop and drive to change direction
    - Sprint back through the middle cone

- *Forward/Backward Ladder*
    - Start at first cone, sprint 5 meters to the second cone
    - Decelerate, drop and drive to change direction
    - Backpedal 5 meters to back to first cone
    - Keep forward lean with chest over feet to keep balance
    - Decelerate, drop and drive to change direction
    - Sprint forward 10 meters to the last cone
    - Decelerate, drop and drive to change direction
    - Backpedal 10 meters through the first cone

Cutting Skills Drills

The speed cuts develop the inside acceleration foot and the power cuts develop the outside acceleration foot.

- *Speed Cut:* Sprint through the cones as fast as possible.
  - o Place five cones 5m a part in a straight line
  - o Perform the drill by just sprinting through the cones as fast as possible
  - o As you weave slightly through the cones, stay tight to the cones
  - o Stepping just to the side of the cone with the inside foot

- *Figure 8:* The Figure 8 is a more intense version of the speed cut that develops the inside acceleration foot.

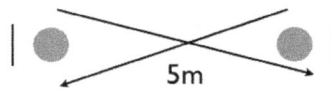

5m

- *Power Cut Phase I (3 cone drills):* Shuffle side to side, covering 5 meters and coming to a jump stop. Touch cones on each side with hand and keep hips low. The athlete should go back and forth four times to cover a total of 20 meters for the completion of one repetition of the drill.

- *Power Cut Phase II (5 cone drills):*
  - o Place five cones in a zig zag or W pattern
    - ▪ Set first cone at start, go 5m then go right 5m, place second cone
    - ▪ Go up 5 meters then go left 5 meters to place third cone
    - ▪ Continue same pattern for cones 4 & 5
  - o The zig-zag, five-cone pattern allows for practice of the inside and outside foot cutting skill.
  - o Sprint diagonally to the cone and then plant (using the drop, stop and drive technique), cut (inside or outside foot cut) and sprint to the next cone with the same acceleration technique as in sprinting.
  - o Repeat all the way through or line up one cone and work one cut at a time.
  - o This drill can be done utilizing sprinting, lateral, and forward/back movement patterns.
  - o Outside Foot Cut: Decelerate, drop, stop and drive off of the outside foot (the outside leg as you approach the cone) to change direction.
  - o Inside Foot Cut: Decelerate, drop and drive off of the inside foot (the inside leg as you approach the cone) to change direction (plant and drive), stepping over the top (cross over step).

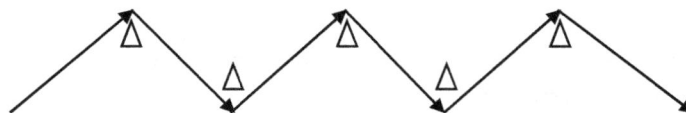

- *Power Cut Phase III:*
  - Perform at 50% or 75% to first develop the proper cutting technique.
  - These will be repeated cuts sprinting from one cone to the next.
  - Align five cones as described in "Power Cut Phase II."
  - Cuts should be made on the outside foot with an inside lean, plant and drive step with the outside toe pointed straight ahead.
  - Inside knee and toe should point in the direction of the cut
  - Hips and body lean should be so low that the athlete can touch their inside hand to the ground. The athlete re-accelerates (same acceleration technique as in sprinting) to the next cone and repeats the same cutting technique.

- *Power Cut Phase IV:*
  - Perform at 50% or 75% to first develop the proper cutting technique.
  - These will be repeated cuts sprinting from one cone to the next.
  - Align five cones as described in "Power Cut Phase II."
  - Cuts should be made on the inside foot, stepping up and over with an inside lean, plant and drive step with the outside toe pointed straight ahead.
  - Inside knee and toe should point in the direction of the cut
  - Hips and body lean should be so low that the athlete can touch their inside hand to the ground. The athlete re-accelerates (same acceleration technique as in sprinting) to the next cone and repeats the same cutting technique.

- *Lateral Shuffle*
  - Align five cones as described in "Power Cut Phase II."
  - Start at first cone and shuffle to second cone
  - Decelerate, drop and drive to change direction
  - Shuffle to third cone
  - Decelerate, drop and drive to change direction
  - Shuffle to fourth cone
  - Decelerate, drop and drive to change direction
  - Shuffle to fifth cone

- *Forward/Backward Drill*
  - Align five cones as described in "Power Cut Phase II."
  - Start at first cone sprint to second cone
  - Decelerate, drop and drive to change direction
  - Backpedal to third cone
  - Keep forward lean with chest over feet to keep balance
  - Decelerate, drop and drive to change direction
  - Sprint to fourth cone
  - Decelerate, drop and drive to change direction
  - Backpedal to fifth cone

Transitional Agilities

Transitional agilities start practicing and preparing the body to go from one movement into an entirely different movement. This is the phase where the coach can start using all their favorite agility drills after the speed and power cut base has been established.

- *Agility Square*

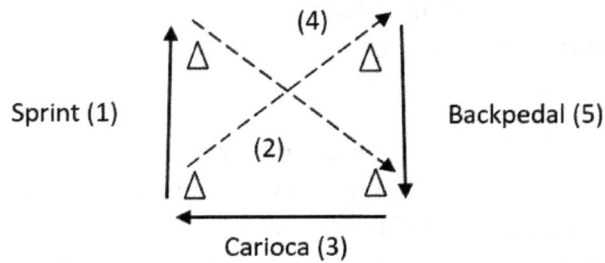

(Dashed lines – lateral shuffle 2 & 4)

- *U - Drill*

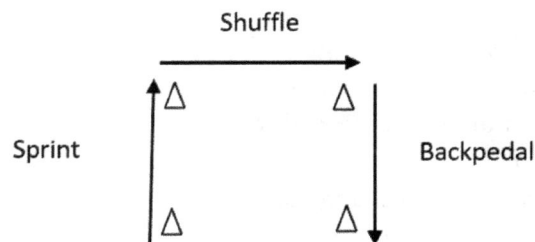

- *Sprint (Outside foot cuts)*
  - Place four cones in a square with 5 meters between cones
  - Sprint from cone 1 to cone 2 and drop, plant, and drive performing a 90-degree outside foot cut
  - Sprint from cone 2 to cone 3 and drop, plant, and drive performing a 90-degree outside foot cut
  - Sprint and stop at cone 4
  - Repeat drill starting with cone 4, going in opposite direction

- *Sprint (Inside foot cuts)*
  - Place four cones in a square with 5 meters between cones
  - Sprint from cone 1 to cone 2 and drop, plant, and drive performing a 90-degree inside foot cut
  - Sprint from cone 2 to cone 3 and drop, plant, and drive performing a 90-degree inside foot cut
  - Sprint and stop at cone 4
  - Repeat drill starting with cone 4, going in opposite direction

- *Sprint/Shuffle/Backpedal (Outside Foot Cut)*
  - Place four cones in a square with 5 meters between cones
  - Sprint from cone 1 to cone 2 and drop, plant, and drive performing a 90-degree outside foot cut
  - Sprint from cone 2 to cone 3 and drop, plant, and drive performing a 90-degree outside foot cut
  - Backpedal and stop at cone 4
  - Repeat drill starting with cone 4, going in the opposite direction

- *Sprint/Shuffle/Backpedal (Pivot)*
  - Place four cones in a square with 5 meters between cones
  - Pivot off inside foot, swinging outside foot in towards the cone (to change direction)
  - Sprint from cone 1 to cone 2 and drop, pivot, and drive, performing a 90-degree inside foot pivot
  - Shuffle from cone 2 to cone 3 and drop, pivot, and drive, performing a 90-degree inside foot pivot
  - Backpedal and stop at cone 4
  - Repeat drill starting with cone 4 going in opposite direction

- *Diagonal (Backpedal to Sprint)*
  - Place four cones in a square with 5 meters between cones
  - Backpedal diagonally from cone 1 to cone 3 and drop, plant and drive
  - Sprint from cone 3 to cone 2 and drop, plant and drive
  - Backpedal diagonally and stop at cone 4
  - Repeat drill starting with cone 4 going in opposite direction

- *Agility Square*
  - Place four cones in a square with 5 meters between cones
  - Sprint from cone 1 to cone 2 and drop, plant and drive
  - Shuffle diagonally from cone 2 to cone 4 and drop, plant and drive
  - Short Carioca from cone 4 to cone 1 and drop, plant and drive
  - Shuffle diagonally from cone 1 to cone 3 and drop, plant and drive
  - Backpedal from cone 3 to cone 4

Quick Feet Drills

Ladders and rope/line jumping are movement tools to get a lot of repetitions with the toes and heels up to work off the balls of the feet. As with the jump rope, just a handful of movements using the ladder should be picked out to maximize performance. Another technique to use is a slight forward lean when going through the ladder so your center of gravity is out in front. Remember the center of gravity creates movement, this will force your feet to be quicker off the ground.

- *Rope/Line Jump:* Emphasize toes up. Try jumping rope with the toes down and the toes up and compare. Notice how much quicker their feet are with the toes up.

    - Forward/Back Hops   - Crisscross Hops

    - Over and Back Runs   - Side to Side Hops

    - Heel Clicks   - and many more…

- *Quick Foot Ladder:* Use your imagination to add rotational movement as well. And emphasize toes up.

- *Forward Run*
    o Face the line or rope with toes positioned behind the line or rope
    o Using short quick steps run touching toes over and behind the line or rope without touching the line or rope
    o To improve foot speed, stay on toes and take short steps (stepping close to the line or rope)

    - One Foot Run   - One in, One Out

    - Two Feet Run   - Two in, Two Out

    - and many more

One Foot In

- Stand laterally to the left of the ladder, run laterally through the ladder placing one foot in each box (as diagram illustrates)
- Can be performed for speed using quick steps or can be done using high knee technique
- Run through leading with the right foot, then repeat standing on the opposite end of the ladder and leading with the left foot

One Foot In, One Foot Out Run

		R		R		R		R
		1		3		5		7
L	R	L		L		L		L
F	F	2		4		6		8

200

One Foot In Run

L	R	L	R	L	R
F	F	2	1	4	3

Two Feet In

- Stand laterally to the left of the ladder
- Run laterally through the ladder, placing both feet in each box
- Can be performed for speed using quick steps or can be done using high knee technique
- Run through leading with the right foot, then repeat standing on the opposite end of the ladder and leading with the left foot

Two Feet In Run

L	R	L	R	L	R	L	R	L	R
F	F	2	1	4	3	6	5	8	7

One Foot In, One Foot Out

- Facing the ladder, run through the ladder placing one foot in each box (as diagram illustrates)
- Can be performed for speed using quick steps or can be done using high knee technique
- Run through leading with the right foot, then repeat leading with the left foot

One Foot In, One Foot Out Run

LF				
RF	L2	L4	L6	L8
R1	R3	R5	R7	R9

One Foot In, One Foot Out Run

	R	R	R	R
	1	3	5	7
L R L	L	L	L	
F F 2	4	6	8	

Two In, One Out

- Face the direction of the ladder and stand to the left of the first ladder box
- Run through the ladder, placing both feet in each box and alternating the right and left feet outside the ladder (as diagram illustrates)
- Run through leading with the right foot, then repeat standing to the right of the ladder and leading with the left foot

LF

RF   L6   L12

L2	L4	L8	L10	L14
R1	R5	R7	R11	R13

       R3   R9

Two Feet In, Two Feet Out Run

		L	R	L	R	L	R	L	R
		2	1	6	5	10	9	14	13
L	R	L	R	L	R	L	R	L	R
F	F	4	3	8	7	12	11	16	15

Two In, Two Out

- Face the direction of the ladder and stand to the left of the first ladder box
- Run through the ladder placing both feet in each box and both feet outside the ladder, alternating to either side
- Run through leading with the right foot, then repeat standing to the right of the ladder and leading with the left foot

Two Feet In, Two Feet Out Run

LF   L8   L16

RF   R7   R15

L2	L6	L10	L14	L18
R1	R5	R9	R13	R17

      L4   L12   L20

      R3   R11   R19

- *Forward Hop*
  - Face the line or rope with toes positioned behind the line or rope
  - Using short, quick hops, touch toes over and behind the line or rope without touching the line or rope
  - To improve foot speed, stay on toes and take short hops (hopping close to the line or rope)

- *Lateral*

  - One in, One Out   - Two in, Two Out

  - One Foot In   - Two Feet In

  - Ali Shuffle   - and many more...

- *Lateral Hop*
  - Face forward with feet positioned to the side of the line or rope
  - Using short, quick, lateral hops, touch toes over and back without touching the line or rope
  - To improve foot speed, stay on toes and take short lateral hops (hopping close to the line or rope)

- *Cross Over*
  - Stand straddling the line or rope with your feet crisscrossed (right foot on left side in front and left foot on the right side back)
  - Hop and switch foot positions (right foot to the left back and the left foot to the right front)
  - To improve foot speed, stay on toes and stay close to line or rope
  - Keep doing the crisscross hops until the exercise time has been completed

- *Balance Training*
  These should be performed with an emphasis and concentration of the heels and toes up, balancing on the balls of the feet.

  - 1-Leg Balance
    - Balance on one leg for 30 seconds.
  - 1-Leg Bound and Balance
    - Jump laterally off one foot onto the opposite foot and hold balance for five seconds.
    - Repeat the other direction.

Reaction Agility Drills

- *5-10-5 Mirror*
  - Set up the drill in the 3 cone 5-10-5 format as described in Level 1
  - Two athletes face each other at the middle cone
  - One athlete is designated the leader and the other is the follower
  - The follower must mirror the leader's movements

5-10-5 Mirror Reaction

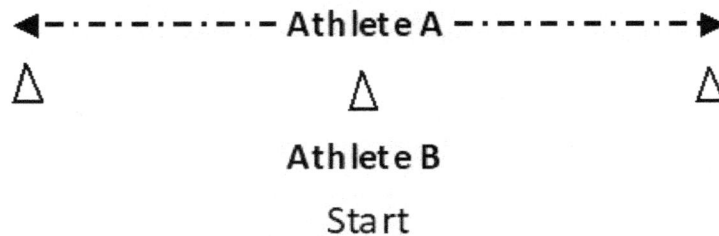

◄– · – · – · – · – Athlete A – · – · – · – · – ►

△   △   △

Athlete B

Start

- *Coach Reaction (5-10-5)*
  - ○ Set up the drill in the 3 cone 5-10-5 format as described in Level 1
  - ○ One athlete lines up across from the coach behind the middle cone
  - ○ The athlete reacts to the coach to determine which direction (R or L) to run the 5-10-5 drill

Coach 5-10-5 Reaction

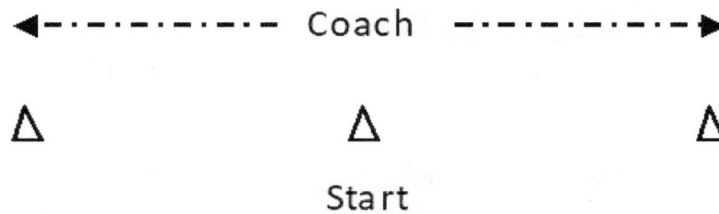

◄– · – · – · – Coach – · – · – · – ►

△   △   △

Start

- *Coach Reaction (T)*
  - ○ Using a "T" formation
    - ▪ The top of the "T" is spaced out like the 5-10-5
    - ▪ The tail if the "T" is placed 10 meters behind the center cone
  - ○ In the normal "T" drill, the athlete sprints from the starting cone to the middle cone
  - ○ Shuffle to the right cone
  - ○ Shuffle back across the top of the "T" to the far left cone
  - ○ Then shuffle back to the middle cone
  - ○ At the middle cone, backpedal past the starting cone
  - ○ In the Coach Reaction "T" drill, the athlete starts by sprinting to the middle cone and reacts to the coach's command to determine whether to shuffle to the right or to the left to execute the drill

Coach "T" Reaction

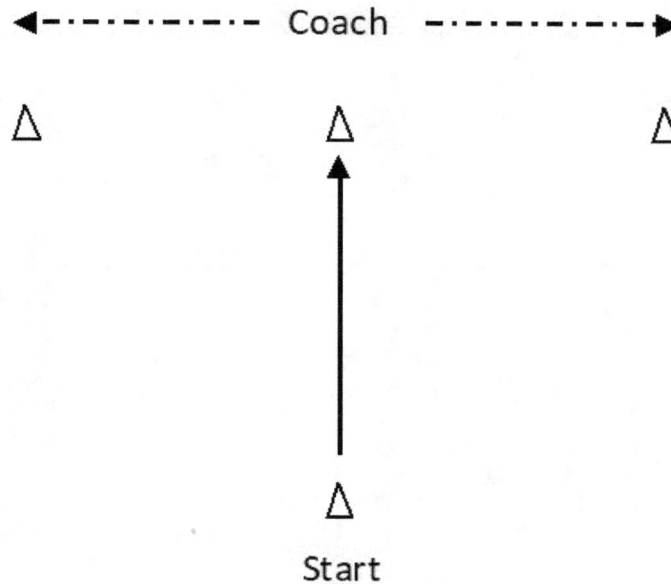

◄─·─·─·─·─ Coach ─·─·─·─·─►

△   △   △

△
Start

- *Multiple Direction Coach Reaction*
  - The athlete starts behind the first cone and sprints to the second cone 10 meters away
  - The coach will signal the athlete which direction to cut just before the athlete reaches the second cone
  - The coach can send the athlete:
    - To the right or left
    - Diagonally forward to the right or left
    - Diagonally backward to the right or left
  - The athlete has to react quickly and execute the correct one-step cut in the indicated direction
  - The coach can mix in different movements (shuffle, backpedal) as well

Coach Multiple Direction Reaction

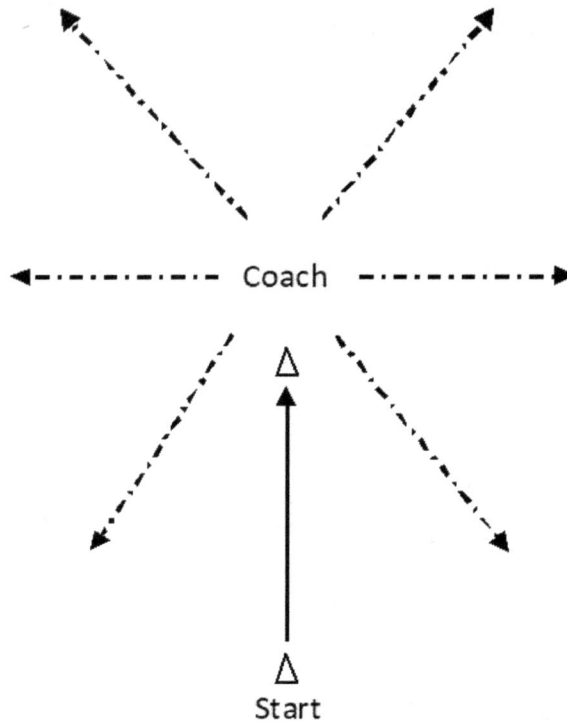

References: Chapter 8

1. Barnes, M., and J. Cissik. *Sports Speed and Agility*. Monterey, CA: Coaches Circle, 2004.

2. Brown, L., and V.A. Ferrigno. *Training for Speed, Agility, and Quickness*, 2nd ed. Champaign, IL: Human Kinetics, 2005.

3. Costello, F., and E.J. Kreis. *Sports Agility*. Nashville, TN: Taylor Sports,1993.

4. Foran, B. *High Performance Sports Conditioning*. Champaign, IL: Human Kinetics, 2001.

5. Halberg, G.V. *Relationships among power, acceleration, maximum speed, programmed agility, and reactive agility: The neural fundamentals of agility*. Masters thesis. Central Michigan University, Mount Pleasant, MI, 2001.

6. Radcliffe, J. C. *Functional Training for Athletes at All Levels*. Berkeley, CA: Ulysses Press, 2007.

Sections in this chapter are adapted from previously published books by Dornemann and O'Dell:

7. Dornemann, T. M. PowerRev *"Four Laws of Victory" Character Development Program: Build successful teams and athletes by teaching lessons that transcend sports*. Ronkonkoma, NY: Linus, 2015.

8. O'Dell, S. *The Power Revolution: A Sports Performance Guide to Achieving Maximum Power*. Monterey, CA: Coaches Choice, 2015.

9
SPEED TRAINING

By: Tim Dornemann, Ed. D., CES, PES, CSCS, OS Pro

Exercise Science Program & Kinesiology Director, Barton College
Associate Professor of Exercise Science, Barton College
&

Scott O'Dell

Director of Strength & Conditioning, East Central University

"SPEED KILLS." CHANCES are you have heard this more than one time in the sports world when referring to how one team can defeat their opponent. Next to head and heart, nothing is deadlier to the opponent than speed, regardless of the sport. When you beat your opponent from point A to point B, you are the one who gets the ball or keeps them from getting the ball or the one who steals a base or steals a double turning it into an out. The more speed you have behind you on the point of body-to-body impact with an opponent in a contact sport, then the more hurt and pain you inflict.

It does not take a lot to sell people on the importance of speed. Many believe that speed is strictly genetic, but as an effective sports performance coach you know this is false. With the appropriate integral approach that involves weight training, sprinting, plyometrics, dynamic flexibility and more, the physiological proponents of the body can be developed to make the body perform faster and more explosively.

Speed can also be taught in the form of technique. With no physiological change in the body whatsoever, the athlete can become faster by learning proper technique with the proper body angles and movement. Can you take the slowest person in town and have them competing in the next Olympic games in the 100-meter competition? Absolutely not, as this level of competition incorporates the proper physiological and biomechanical training of the body combined with genetics. But you can make anyone remarkably faster and take them to a whole new level of performance by appropriately training the physical makeup of the body and teaching the body correct biomechanics for maximum speed.

The bigger a muscle is, the more potential it has to generate force. Contrarily, some believe that the bigger the muscle, the slower the athlete, but that is false. The bigger the engine is in your car, then the faster the car is. The same applies here, it is just that this new bigger muscle must now be taught how to apply its new force potential. Training the muscles for increased force production, power, and speed will result in increases in muscle mass due to the fact that fast-twitch muscle fibers have much greater growth potential than slow twitch muscle fibers do.

The purpose of the speed program is to develop maximal speed in the forward direction. The speed training program consists of sprint technique, acceleration, resistance speed and maximum speed drills. As training progresses, the rest intervals are decreased from roughly a 5:1 to 3:1 rest-to-work ratio as conditioning improves. Since optimal performance is desired during maximum speed drills, time for full recovery between sprints is allowed. The number of repetitions performed for each drill is progressively increased as conditioning improves to maintain an adequate training stimulus. The sprint distance is also progressively increased in certain drills to increase the exercise demands.

There are two styles of sprinting: drive sprinting and reach and pull sprinting. Drive sprinting style uses the body's full potential for speed and acceleration. Drive sprinting uses triple extension (ankle, knee and hip) into the ground, therefore projecting the body across the ground to increase stride length. Drive sprinters also work for minimal "back-action" (this is where the heel goes through a butt-kicking motion and then the sprinter pulls their knee through, not wanting to waste valuable time in the hip cycle). Drive sprinters do their best to bring the knee straight up into position to drive off of the ground and avoid the wasted time of a butt-kicking motion and then pulling their knee through. Also, the toes and heels should be up, driving the balls of the feet into the ground.

An easy indication to tell if your athletes are drive sprinting is to look at their shin angles. When the knee is in front of the ankle, this is a positive shin angle. When the knee is behind the ankle joint this is referred to as a negative shin angle. When your athletes have positive shin angles they are drive sprinting, driving the force from the hip extension into the ground.

Reach and pull sprinting is still commonly used, but is an inferior style to drive-style sprinting. Reach and pull sprinters stand very upright and reach the foot out in front of the body to pull the body across the ground. There is a misconception that this is how to increase stride length; this is what we describe as over-striding. Over-striding is commonly associated with hamstring pulls. Reach and pull sprinters also have a tendency to run with very bad back action, hence wasting time in their hip cycle.

Many coaches also still like to teach a "velocity phase." This is a phase where the sprinter is trying to maintain their speed after reaching their full acceleration. Since sprinters sprint for distances long enough to require maintaining max speed, some feel this is necessary for actual sprinters in track and field, but as part of a sports performance program we must remember that our athletes are not just sprinters—we are developing the total athlete. Teaching only drive sprinting also minimizes the risk of hamstring injury due to over-striding. Most hamstring injuries occur when the hip is flexed and the knee is extended. Over-striding puts the hamstring in this position. Furthermore, good sprinters should be able to hold their acceleration mechanics for 40 meters or more (Seagrave, 2008); then why spend time on the complexity and injury risk of a velocity phase unless it is a 100 meter sprinter?

The only sport where the velocity phase is necessary is in track and field; since other sports require constant stop and go, acceleration and deceleration and change of direction, the majority of athletes never even have the chance to achieve a velocity phase. The only sprint components that are necessary to teach for effectiveness, time, efficiency and simplicity are acceleration, drive sprinting, and working to maintain drive sprinting through an entire sprint. Sprinting is one of many aspects of performance training needed by athletes and their chosen sport(s), therefore the velocity phase is not critical when training the total athlete in a sports performance program.

The most powerful body angle to accelerate from the ground is at 45 degrees. This was demonstrated in a very forceful way by the late Sean Taylor, of the Washington Redskins, in the 2007 National

Football League's (NFL) Pro Bowl when he hit the American Football Conference (AFC) punter Brian Moorman. It was an earth shattering hit in which Taylor had his body in a 45-degree angle from the ground upon the point of impact. This is the same thing with speed, the most powerful acceleration will take place when the body is at a 45-degree angle off of the ground. The 45-degrees from the ground for the take off point is the same angle airplanes and shot putters use, due to the power of the acceleration.

To see an example, view the NFL Films YouTube clip, "2006 PB - Sean Taylor hit on Brian Moorman HD." https://www.youtube.com/watch?v=SC7Wx3zCiQo

Also highly crucial—and far too often ignored—is the arm action. Usually, the faster the arms move, the faster the legs move (Bowerman & Freeman, 1991). Elbows should be locked at 90 degrees. Any longer of an arm extension than this and the arms will move slower. Any shorter than this diminishes any force production from the arms to transfer through the core to the legs. With a proper arm swing, driving the right elbow back will then transfer a force through the core to the left hip to make the left hip drive into the ground harder; the same takes place when you drive the left elbow back, transferring force into the right hip. Hands and shoulders need to be relaxed and moving straight forward and backward. This is another reason rotational strength is important: so the athlete has the strength to stop themselves from swaying with wasted lateral movement. The hands should travel from shoulder height to the glute.

Good posture is another point of emphasis as good posture produces 10-12% more force production (Farentinos & Radcliffe, 1999). Good posture will also help to ensure proper muscle firing sequence (Seagrave, 2008): (1) good posture activates the hip flexor, (2) the activated hip flexor activates the glute, (3) the glute must be activated before the hamstring. If any of these are thrown out of sequence, such as poor posture shutting down the hip flexor and therefore shutting down the glute, then the hamstrings become overloaded with work and pull during hip extension.

There should be no drills that focus or emphasize a butt-kicking motion. There are plenty of warm-up drills for the hip flexor and quads, so there is no need to practice a butt-kicking drill that provides repetition for poor sprinting mechanics.

Sprinter's Start (Seagrave, 2008): The sprinter's start can vary from coach to coach; the following coaching pointers are a starting point. Each individual athlete may have better acceleration with some minor changes, but this is a starting point to work from and will consistently be close, if not perfect, for most athletes' maximum acceleration.

- The front foot should be placed two feet from the starting line.
- The back toe is lined up with the front heel.
- The back knee is at about a 120-degree angle.
- Hips are higher than the shoulders.

- The front hand should be at the starting line.
- The front elbow should not be locked out but have a slight bend.
- Chin should be tucked down.
- Initial push should come from both feet. The back foot actually produces more force while the front foot takes longer to produce force. A good understanding is that the front foot is in the same position as the sticking point of a deep squat, producing slower movement, whereas the back foot is in a position similar to the higher point of a deep squat when speed through that range of motion is greater.
- The correct muscle firing sequence should be applied by focusing on the glutes first, then the hamstrings.
- Acceleration can take place for over 40 yards in good sprinters.

Two-point sprinter's start: Legs in the exact same positioning as the sprinter's start, only now lift the hand up and (as much as possible) attempt to keep the back parallel with the ground, both elbows locked at 90 degrees and the weight up on the balls of the feet leaning forward.

During training, things such as exactly how far the feet are from the starting line or the angle of the back knee can be experimented with for each individual athlete's best acceleration time. In discussing the sprinter's start, Seagrave went on to state that the smaller, quicker athletes may benefit more from being closer to the line for quicker more acute movements; versus the bigger, more powerful athlete's being a little further from the line for more sweeping power movements. Put a slight emphasis on the center of gravity being out in front of the body, while being careful not to be so far out in front that the athlete is out of control and fails to get hip and knee extension. Brandon Marcello and Mark Verstegan explain center of gravity in the book *High-Performance Sports Conditioning* (2001) with the following:

Center of mass is the hypothetical balance point of the body, which is located at 55 percent of height in women and 57 percent of height in men (Hay and Reid, 1988). The center of mass is a constant and will always lie within the body. Height, sex, and body type affect an athlete's center of mass.

In a static, erect position, the center of mass will be located at the same point as the center of gravity. The difference is that the location of the center of gravity shifts with movement; it will fluctuate within the body, and many sport actions will shift it outside the body. This shift of the center of gravity away from the center of mass creates movement.

This proper acceleration technique being practiced will translate through the field/court/track and all areas of movement. These are basic fundamentals of movement to get from point A to point B that should be taking place during all movement that involve an acceleration or re-acceleration such as: lateral cuts, diagonal cuts, rotation, linear sprints, and points of impact with another athlete during contact sports.

Speed training should also be progressed in the following order throughout the off-season plan: (1) resistance, (2) over speed, this phase will further be discussed, (3) maximum speed.

1. **Resistance** will overload the muscle and physiologically help the muscle develop more force production, along with teaching great technique with a forward body lean (lean should come from the ankles, not the waist) and positive shin angles. Using resistance training early in the off-season also "eases" the body into speed training by preparing the muscles in a slower movement and can also decrease the impact on the joints early in training, i.e. sprinting up an incline catches the foot at a higher point so it doesn't have the full force into the ground. Be careful not

to spend too much time in this phase, however, as it also teaches a slower movement with longer foot contact time with the ground, both of which are not what you want when heading into competition.

2. The **overspeed method** should be considered very thoroughly before performing in your program. This is a method where the athlete trains at speeds about 8-13% faster than their fastest speed. It is done to put the body in a position where it is moving faster than normal to help the body to adapt to the faster movement as a way to improve stride frequency while sprinting. Theoretically over speed makes great sense as it forces the hip cycle to go through faster than it can without any implementation. But the negative side to this is that it enforces terrible technique by causing braking (when the heel hits the ground first) and over-striding. Usually, the athlete ends up allowing themselves to be pulled, therefore losing their good technique and form. Seagrave (2008) warned highly against over-speed training, with the exception of elite athletes. If you must, then it would be most ideal to perform over-speed training down a hill with 1–2 degrees of downgrade (a very slight and gradual downgrade). Some coaches use bungees/resistance cords to provide resistance speed training; however, these should not be used if they negatively affect form. What all too often happens when using bungees is that athletes get pulled, their arm swing comes up too high and the braking and over-striding take place. No implement that can impair technique should ever be used. In speed training, technique should always be of first priority over all other training theories and implements.

3. In **max speed** sprints the athlete sprints for a given distance on flat ground with no implements on your playing surface with maximum traction, then allows for maximum recovery. The emphasis here is on speed, not conditioning. This is good to have last in the progression to head into competition since we are working on teaching our new potential for force production to now perform very acutely for maximum speed and power.

When training for speed, providing full recovery is essential. The goal of speed training is to increase how fast an athlete can go from point A to point B; the goal is not for energy system development. Not providing adequate recovery prevents the ability to optimally increase speed.

Speed Progression

Phase I: Resistance Speed

- Hills
  - Research shows that anything greater than an eight degree angle uphill sprinting has a negative effect on speed training due to too much resistance hindering technique, foot quickness and the speed of muscle contraction.
  - In resistance sprinting, you want to be able to maintain 90 percent or more of your maximum speed (Pearson, 2014).
- Partner Towing - 10 yards tow and then release for the second 10 yards
- Barefoot Striders
  - Good for learning technique, having shoes and socks off naturally causes the athlete to do a better job of keeping their heels and toes up giving them quicker feet off the ground. They also have a more natural tendency to bring their knees up higher.

Phase II: Over-Speed

- Downhill Running – On a 2-3% downgrade (any more slope will cause a loss of technique)
- Barefoot Striders

Note: bungee drills are often referenced with overspeed training; however, often athletes lose proper form due to being pulled, resulting in arms swinging too high, breaking and overstriding. All drills should emphasize and reinforce proper mechanics and drills that can result in promoting bad technique should be avoided.

Phase III: Max Speed Sprints

- No resistance or assistance
- Give full recovery time between sprints
- Goal is improving speed, <u>not</u> conditioning

Speed Drill Technique

Technique Drills

Arm Swing (seated or one knee)

1. Keep good posture
2. Elbows locked at 90 degrees
3. Relax hand, face and neck
4. Swing arms from facial check to back pocket
5. Body should start bouncing up and down (showing transfer of power from arms to legs)

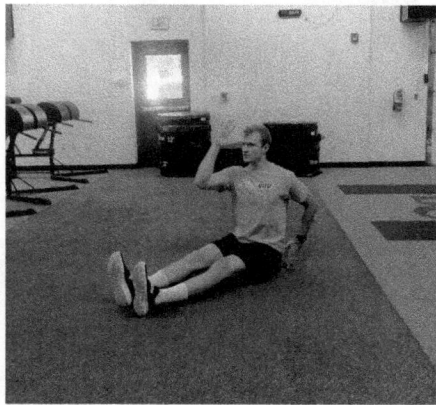

Arm Swings (Side View) – Elbow and hand position

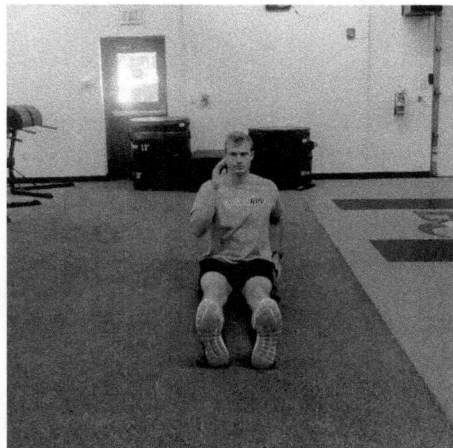

Arm Swings (Front View) – Arms tight to the body without rotating across body

Leaning Wall March

1. Keep body in a straight line at a 45 degree angle
2. Hands placed overhead, leaning on wall
3. Bring knee forward
4. Keep toe and heel up
5. Foot strike even with mid-foot of plant leg
6. Avoid any back action

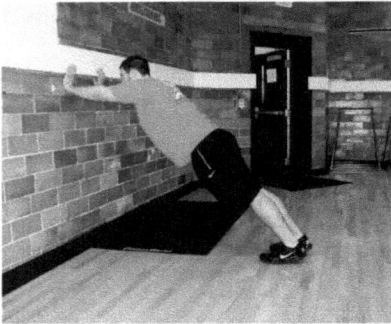

Wall March Starting Position   Wall March Knee Up Position   Wall March Foot Strike Position

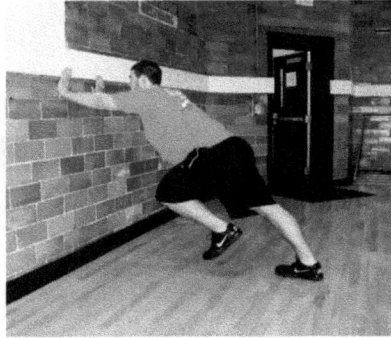

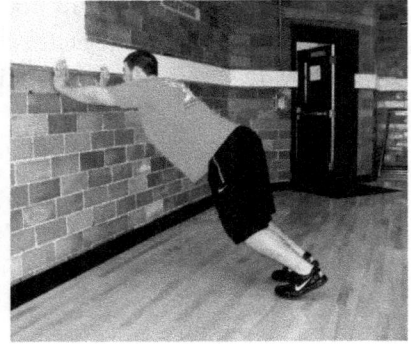

Acceleration Drills

Falling Start

1. Keep body in straight line
2. Lean forward as far as possible while keeping it in a straight line
3. At last moment, pull knee up to catch body
4. Accelerate for given distance
5. Emphasize high knee and toes
6. Avoid any back action

Kneeling Start

1. Start kneeling on one knee
2. As you start, forward, push off of kneeling leg, driving body forward
3. Push out, **not** up and push off both feet
4. Avoid back action, try to keep body in a straight line and at 45-degree angle

Push Up Start

1. Start laying stomach down
2. As you start forward, push upper body up like doing a push up
3. Pull one leg up under body

4. Push out, **not** up and pushing off both feet
5. Avoid back action, try to keep body in a straight line and at 45 degree angle

Sprinters Start/3 Point Start (right handed example)

1. Place both toes on a line
2. Step back to line up right toe with left heel
3. Turn on right heel 90 degrees, pointing toe to the side
4. Turn on right toes 90 degrees (feet should be about shoulder width apart)
5. Kneel down on right knee
6. Place right hand down to the side of right knee
7. Flatten back and raise hips (back leg at a 120-degree angle)
8. Lean body weight forward with pressure on the front hand and balls of feet
9. Push out, **not** up and pushing off both feet
10. Avoid back action, try to keep body in a straight line and at 45-degree angle

Two Point Starts

1. Same position as sprinter start, except slightly more upright
2. Hand is not on ground (only feet have ground contact)

Two Point Start Variations:

- Forward - Sprint forward, pushing off of both feet, coming out low and explosive with knees and toes up.
- Lateral - Push off of both feet, pick up and open the near knee and toe up and point to the direction you are sprinting, coming out low and explosive with knees and toes up.
- Reverse - Push off both feet towards the direction of sprinting while turning over the designated shoulder, opening up with the same leg as the shoulder, turning and pivoting off of the opposite leg. With the leg opening up as the body is turning, the knee and toe should point in the direction being sprinted towards as you are coming out low and explosive with knees and toes up.

Build Up Sprints

- Building up speed gradually, emphasizing arm-swing build up as speed builds up
- Cones can be used to indicate speed changes
  - Example: Cones at 10, 20, 30 and 40 yards
    - 0 to 10 yards – Walking pace
    - 10 to 20 yards – 25% run or jogging pace
    - 20 to 30 yards – 50% run
    - 30 to 40 yards – 75% run
    - 40 yards – 100% sprint for a couple strides
- Emphasize breakdown technique to slow down and stop
  - Drop hips and widen feet
  - Use short, choppy steps to stop under control

Resistance Drills

Sled Walk

- This is more of a leg strength exercise than a running form exercise (therefore greater loads can be used)
- Using resistance from a sled or other apparatus (e.g., tire), have a hip or upper body harness linking athlete to the sled
- Have athlete start far enough in front of the sled so that there is no slack in the rope from the sled to the harness
- Start in a three point start
- Walk forward using good form (arm swing, body angle), pulling the sled 20-40 yards
- Emphasize staying on toes to accentuate working the calf muscles

Sled Pull

- Using resistance from a sled or other apparatus (like a tire), have a hip or upper body harness linking athlete to the sled
- Have athlete start far enough in front of the sled so that there is no slack in the rope from the sled to the harness
- Start the athlete in a three point start
- Sprint forward using good form (arm swing, body angle) pulling the sled 20-40 yards
- Generally, it is best to use up to 10% of the athlete's body weight for resistance
- If resistance causes the athlete to use bad form, stop and lower resistance

Parachute

- Start with the parachute chord extended behind the athlete
- Have a partner hold the parachute up so that it can catch air once the athlete starts moving
- Start in a 3 point stance
- Partner releases the parachute when the runner starts moving
- Sprint forward against the resistance of the parachute using good form (arm swing, body angle) for 20-40 yards or longer (parachute works well for longer distances)

Partner Tow

- Using partners, have one athlete stand behind the runner and have a towel placed around the runner's waist with the ends held by the athlete in back
- The runner starts in a staggered stance and leans forward against the resistance from behind
- The runner drives knees up, going forward against the resistance using proper arm swing
- Don't let the front runner lean too far forward (if they are leaning too far, have partner lessen resistance)
- Partner allows runner to move forward against resistance for 5-10 yards, then lets go of one end of the towel to release the runner
- The runner continues to sprint, using good form, for a total of 20-40 yards

Uphill Running

- Use a hill with up to a 2-3% upgrade (any more slope will cause a loss of technique)
- Run uphill using good form (if form is broken, then hill is too steep and bad habits are introduced or reinforced)
- The slight uphill slope provides resistance, which increases strength as a means to help increase stride length

Over Speed Drills

Release Harness

- Using equipment like a bullet belt, have a partner provide resistance for the sprinter
- The sprinter cycles their legs as fast as they can while using good form
- The partner provides resistance from behind over the first 5-10 meters and then releases the partner by pulling back the handle, causing the Velcro to detach to let the sprinter go

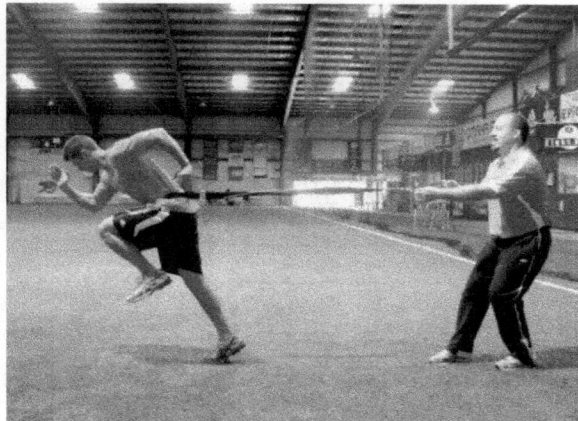

Downhill Running

- Use a hill with up to a 2-3% downgrade (any more slope will cause a loss of technique)
- Run downhill using good form (if form is broken, then hill is too steep and bad habits are introduced or reinforced)
- The slight downhill slope quickens the stride turnover rate as a means to help increase stride frequency

References: Chapter 9

1. Bowerman, W.J. Freeman, W.H. (1991). High Performance Training for Track and Field. Champaign, IL: Human Kinetics.

2. Farentinos, R. Radcliffe, J. (1999). High Powered Plyometrics. Champaign, IL: Human Kinetics.

3. Foran, B. (2001). High Performance Sports Conditioning. Champaign, IL: Human Kinetics.

4. Hay, J.G. Reid, J.G. (1988). Anatomy, Mechanics, and Human Motion, 2nd ed. Englewood Cliffs, NJ: Prentice Hall.

5. Pearson, C. (2014). National Strength and Conditioning Association Minnesota Sports Performance Clinic. University of Minnesota.

6. Seagrave, L. (2008). United States of America Track and Field Level I Certification Workshop. The University of North Carolina-Chapel Hill.

Sections in this chapter are adapted from previously published books by Dornemann and O'Dell:

7. Dornemann, T. M. *POWERREV Youth Athletic Development Program: Building Champions in Sports and in Life*. Ronkonkoma, NY: Linus, 2016.

8. O'Dell, S. *The Power Revolution: A Sports Performance Guide to Achieving Maximum Power*. Monterey, CA: Coaches Choice, 2015.

10
PLYOMETRIC TRAINING

By: Tim Dornemann, Ed. D., CES, PES, CSCS, OS Pro
Exercise Science Program & Kinesiology Director, Barton College
Associate Professor of Exercise Science, Barton College
&
Scott O'Dell
Director of Strength & Conditioning, East Central University

THE TERM PLYOMETRICS first came about in the 1970s after the success of Russian high jumpers using this training philosophy in competition. Previously, some say it was called "shock training" and some say it was called "jump training." The actual starting point of plyometrics, no matter what the name was, is not completely known. What is known is that it has worked well for athletes that need to develop power, speed, and explosion.

Remember the stretch reflex in the body discussed earlier? When hip and knee flexion take place, the quadriceps, hamstrings and glutes are all being stretched and the muscles want to reflex back powerfully. Remember how your muscles are like a rubber band? When they are stretched they want to pop back with power and speed. Training the stretch reflex will aid in the development of your muscles doing this more efficiently, which means more powerful and with more speed. When a joint is being flexed, a muscle is being stretched and training the stretch reflex will make the extension of the joint more powerful.

The *Essentials of Strength Training and Conditioning* (1994) defines the three main components of a plyometric drill with the following:

The three main components of a plyometric drill are the eccentric phase, the amortization phase, and the concentric contraction. The amortization phase is the period of time from the initiation of the eccentric phase (touching the surface) to the initiation of the concentric phase contraction (start of the upward motion of the jump). As a result, the muscles in the leg become like a rapidly stretched rubber band. The "stretched rubber band" will result in a greater ability to develop power. In other words, the muscles are being trained to become more explosive. To take advantage of the stretch reflex, keep the amortization phase as brief as possible. Remember, the rate of stretch is more important than the magnitude. Greater power is produced when the depth of the countermovement is short and rapid rather than large and slow.

Plyometrics are not just for increasing power, jumping ability, and speed. This training is also highly effective for teaching deceleration (Bompa & Carrera, 2005). Therefore, it can also play an important role in injury prevention: teaching the body how to stay under control during deceleration. As mentioned by Ditiman and Ward (2003) "explosive stopping is the key to quickness."

Pre-training Evaluation

There is a belief that you have to squat 1.5 to 2.5 times your body weight in pounds before performing plyometric movement. However, at a 2009 Bar-B-Que, I observed a 5-year-old boy performing single leg speed hops (a very high intensity plyometric movement), and I am convinced he could not squat 1.5 times his body weight. Yet he performed this exercise repeatedly over and over while playing around without getting injured. And how many 5-year-olds that cannot squat 1.5 times their body weight do you see bounding up the stairs, or bounding across a creek or puddle? It happens all the time without an over-training effect or injury. Add to that, everyone has a different definition of squats with various depths. Everyone also has a different method for a 1-rep max using single repetition testing maxes or multiple rep maxes. So I am not sure how this could be the rule of thumb to follow before allowing an athlete to perform plyometric training, as everyone's definition of a squat max is different.

A proper pre-training evaluation to enter plyometric training would be the following:

1. The athlete is able to exercise with their own bodyweight over the course of the time spent on the training.
2. Appropriate flexibility in the ankle joints (this can be developed during the first phase discussed later in the chapter).
3. Appropriate flexibility in the shoulders, hips and spine for proper hip set and absorption of impact (this can also be developed during the first phase of plyometric training and will be discussed later in the chapter).
4. Proper balance (this can also be developed in the first phase and is discussed in the agility chapter).

The plyometric training program is designed to teach proper jump technique and to improve power production through use of the stretch-shortening cycle. Plyometrics are a quality over quantity workout. The volume of foot contacts is controlled and longer rest periods are used to promote maximal effort training and prevent fatigue, which can lead to injury. The PowerRev plyometric program uses specific program progressions to produce safe and effective training.

The basic level concentrates on teaching proper jump landing and jump technique. Single response jump drills incorporating different types of jumps (squat, tuck, split, scissor, etc.) are used to teach basic jump technique and body control. Then, multiple response jumps are added in using the jumps learned previously. In the next exercise progression, horizontal jumping drills and single-leg drills are incorporated. Next, jumping over objects, transitional power drills, and rotational hops are added to the program. These more advanced drills provide a way to mimic sport movements. The 180-degree-hurdle-hop drill might be similar to a baseball movement a second baseman uses to avoid a runner while turning a double play. A squat jump to sprint drill is similar to a basketball player jumping for a rebound and then immediately sprinting to the other end of the court on a fast break.

Total Torso Movements (Single Response) involve the entire body and an increased amount of flexibility, balance and basic overall body strength. Single Response refers to performing one repetition at a time, reloading and resetting the body and then performing the next repetition. Technique, flexibility, balance and overall body strength should be emphasized and developed in this process. Once the athlete has these qualities developed to be able to perform these repetitions with good technique at pace with single response, then they may advance to multiple response. Multiple Response consists of the same exercises but now performing the repetitions continuously.

Plyometric Basics

Plyometric Progressions

- In-Place Jumps
  - Single Response (single jumps - teaching technique and safety)
  - Multiple Response (continuous jumps – true plyometrics)
- Horizontal Jumps
- Jumping over objects
- Transitional Plyometrics
- Rotational Movements
- Box Jumps
  As athletes advance, movements can progress from double to single leg activities

Plyometric Forms

- Upper Body
- Lower Body
- Core/Torso

Safety

- Proper Progression
- Proper Warm-up
- Proper Equipment (footwear)
- Proper Volume
- Proper Surface
- Grass, track, wood court

Basic Jumps

- Landing drill (safety check)
- Rocket Jump
- Tuck Jump
- Squat Jump

Horizontal Jumps

- Broad Jump
- Zig/Zag, Ice Skaters

Jumping over Objects

- Forward/Back Hops
- Lateral Hops

Landing Drill Technique

- Step off of a box or elevated surface
- Land softly on balls of feet, then lower heels to ground
- Land feet shoulder width apart into a squat position with feet pointed straight forward
- Knees should track over toes
    - Knees should not angle in (knee valgus)

Lateral View

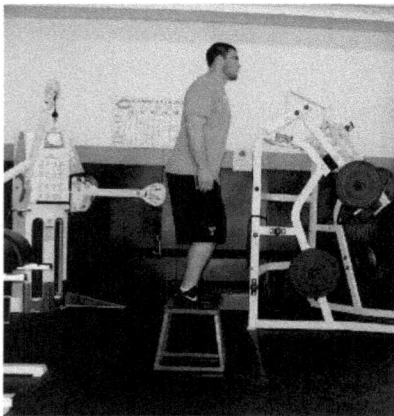 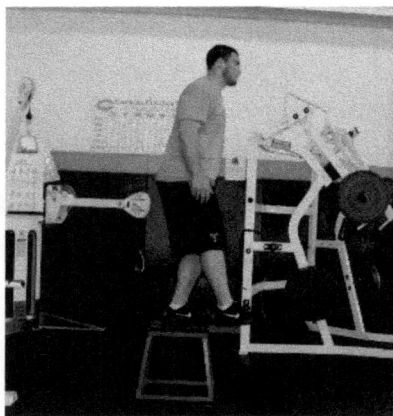 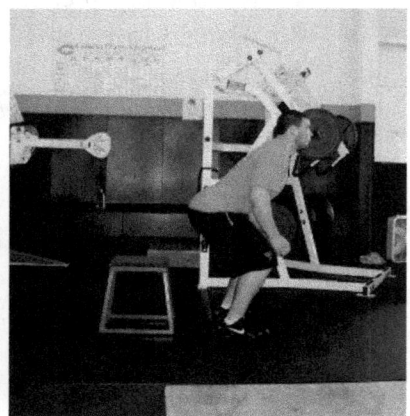

Front View

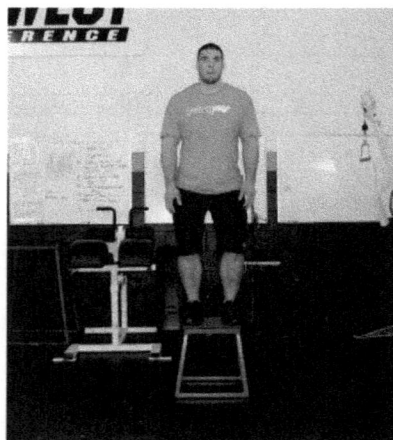 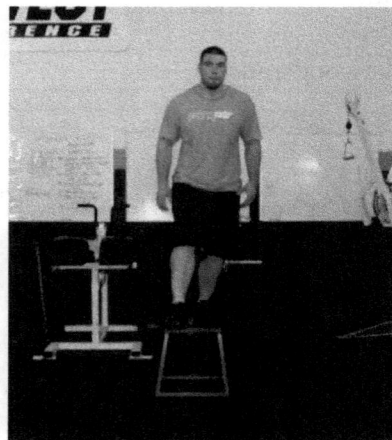

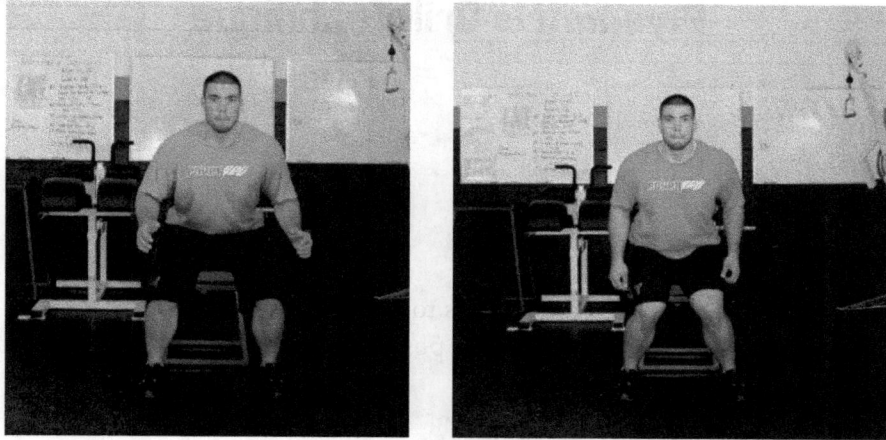

Guidelines for Plyometric Training

1. Use a progression, such as progressing from single response to multiple response.
2. The athlete needs to be able to exercise continuously for several minutes and have the strength to handle their own body weight.
3. Flexibility in the ankle joints and calf muscles for proper foot mechanics is a must. Teach exercises first that are centered around the ankle joint (can also be utilized in warm-ups).
   - Ankle Hops
   - Ankle Flips
4. Flexibility in the shoulders, hips and spine for proper hip set and segmental cushioning should also be assessed.
5. Proper balance for proper torso tilt and joint alignment.
6. Athlete must be able to maintain proper stability of the foot as it is in contact with the ground along with firmness of stance, joint tension, and coordinated control.
7. Maximum of 8-10 repetitions/set or 20 yards.

Plyometric Technique

- Toe Up Rule - Emphasize toes up. Try jumping rope with toes down and then toes up and compare. Notice how much quicker their feet are with their toes up.
- Heel Up Rule - Emphasize heels up. Try jumping rope with heels down and then heels up and compare. Notice how much quicker their feet are with their heels up.
- Knee Up Rule - Bring the knee up with no back action (as discussed in the speed and acceleration section).
- Hip Up Rule - Exaggerating the hip extension
- Thumbs Up Rule (Blocking) - Forcefully using the arms ahead of the body will increase posture and therefore increase force production of all the body's limbs.
- Joint Tension Upon Landing - Land with ankles, knees and hips flexed. Land quietly, "like a ninja."

Plyometric Drill Technique

Single Response Drills

Squat Jump

- Start in squat position
- Jump up, blocking up with arms
- Land softly on balls of feet, then lower heels to ground
- Land feet shoulder width apart into a squat position, feet pointed straight forward
- Knees should track over toes

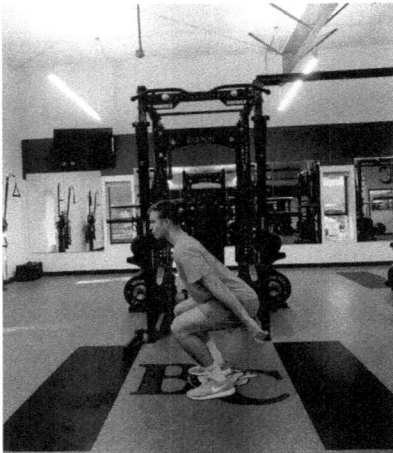

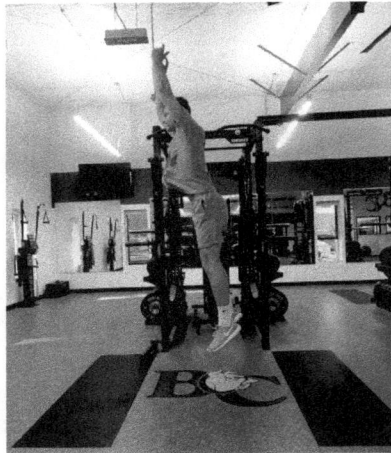

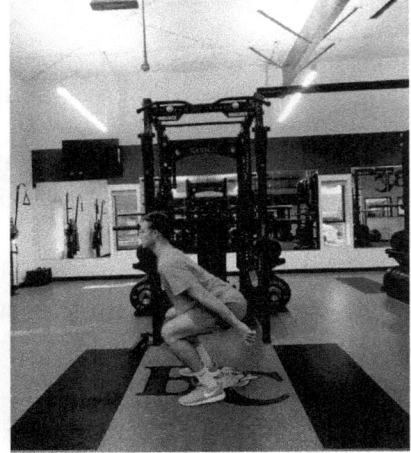

Tuck Jump

- Start in 1/4 squat position
- Jump up, blocking up with arms
- Drive knees up to hip or even chest height during jump
- Land softly on balls of feet, then lower heels to ground
- Land feet shoulder width apart into starting position

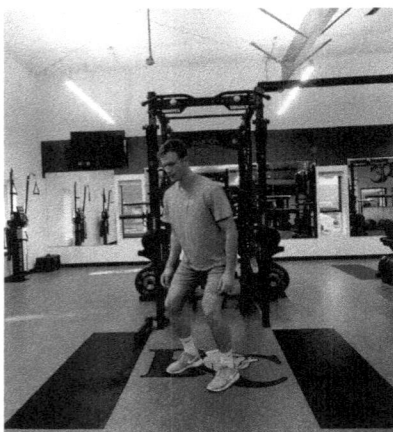

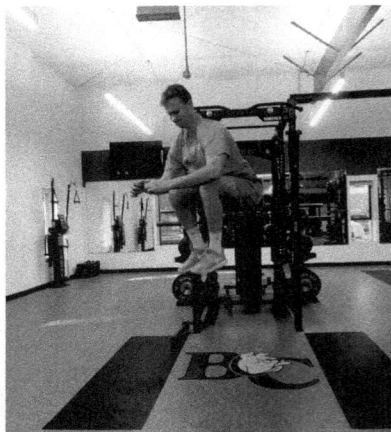

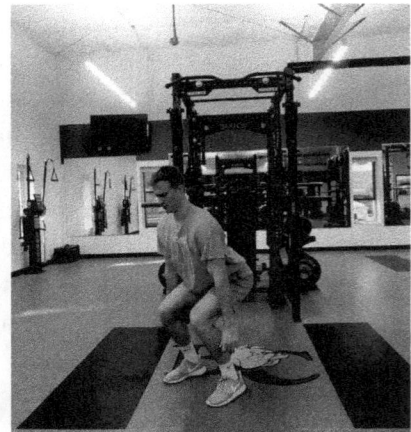

Rocket Jump

- Start in 1/4 squat position
- Jump up, blocking up with arms
- Extend arms reaching as high upwards as possible during jump
- Land softly on balls of feet, then lower heels to ground
- Land feet shoulder width apart into starting position

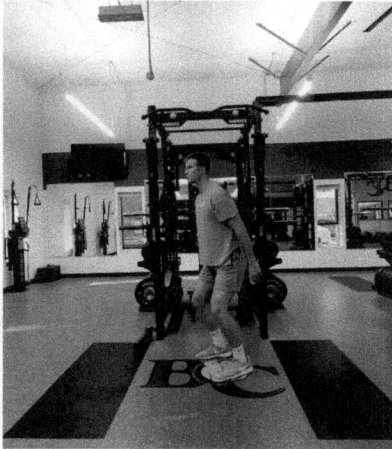

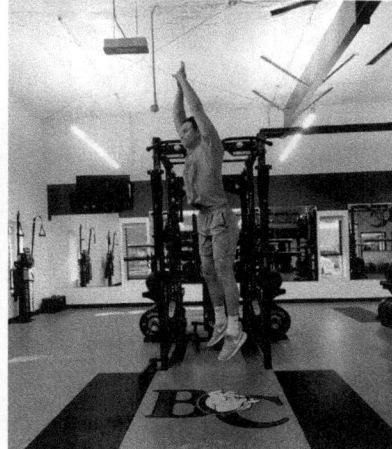

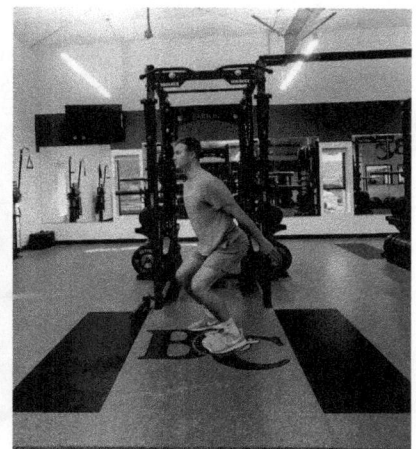

Split Squat Jump

- Start in bottom lunge position
- Jump up, blocking up with arms
- Landing in lunge position with same legs in front and back
- Land softly on balls of feet, then lower heels to ground

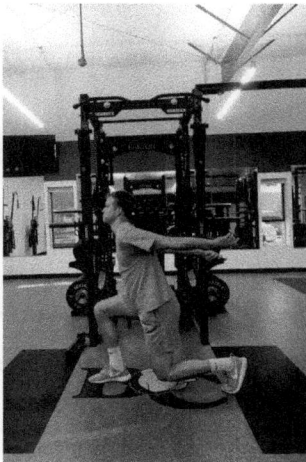

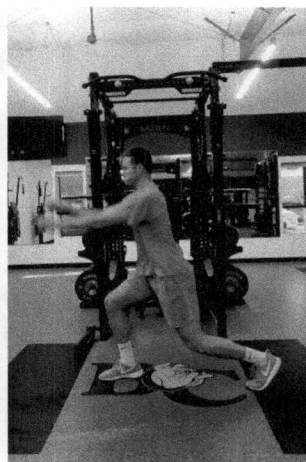

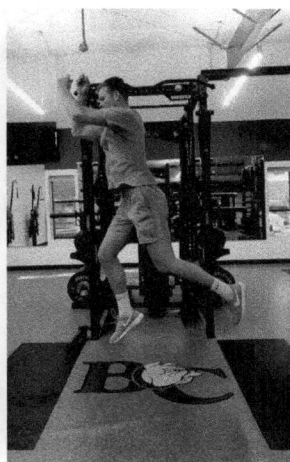

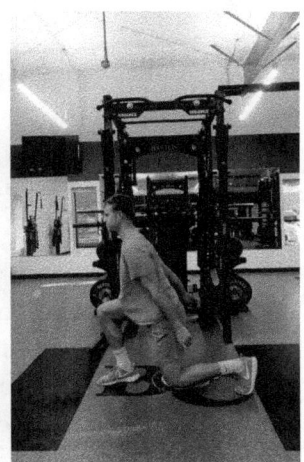

Scissor Jump

- Start in bottom lunge position
- Jump up, blocking up with arms
- Switch leg position during jump, landing in lunge position with opposite legs in front and back
- Land softly on balls of feet, then lower heels to ground

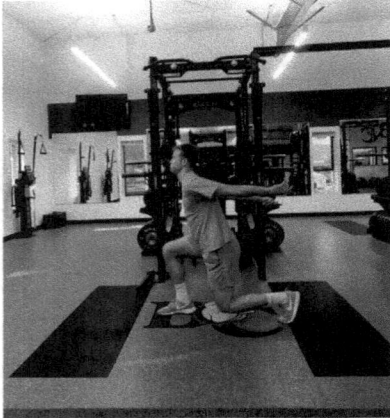

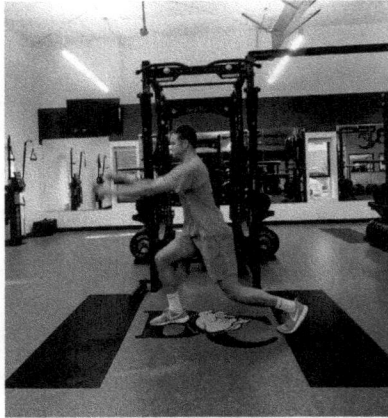

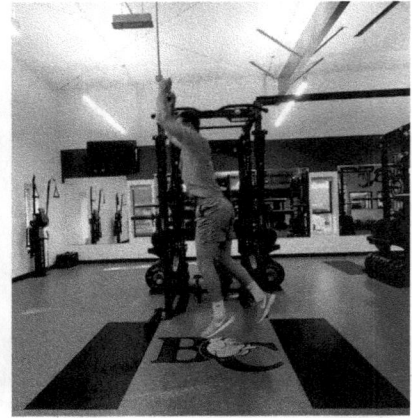

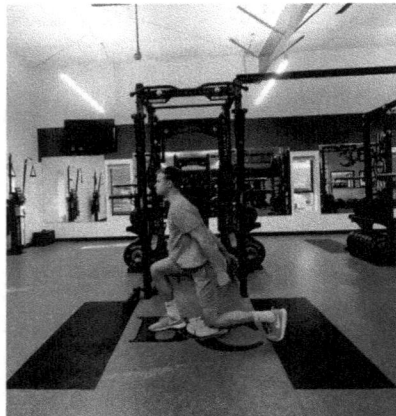

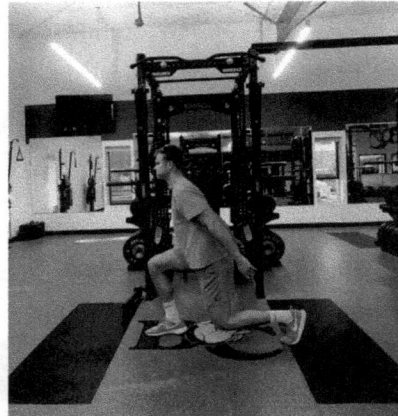

Multiple Response Drills

Squat Jump

- Start in squat position
- Jump up, blocking up with arms
- Land softly on balls of feet
- Land feet shoulder width apart into a squat position, feet pointed straight forward
- Knees should track over toes
- Perform multiple jumps consecutively as fast as possible (minimizing landing/ground contact time)

Tuck Jump

- Start in 1/4 squat position
- Jump up, blocking up with arms
- Drive knees up to hip or even chest height during jump
- Land softly on balls of feet
- Land feet shoulder width apart into starting position
- Perform multiple jumps consecutively as fast as possible (minimizing landing/ground contact time)

Rocket Jump

- Start in 1/4 squat position
- Jump up, blocking up with arms
- Extend arms reaching as high upwards during jump
- Land softly on balls of feet
- Land feet shoulder width apart into starting position
- Perform multiple jumps consecutively as fast as possible (minimizing landing/ground contact time)

Scissor Jump

- Start in bottom lunge position
- Jump up, blocking up with arms
- Switch leg position during jump, landing in lunge position with opposite legs in front and back
- Land softly on balls of feet
- Perform multiple jumps consecutively as fast as possible (minimizing landing/ground contact time)

Horizontal Drills

Broad Jump/Double Leg Bound

- Start in ¼ squat position, feet shoulder width apart
- Jump outwards, using arms to throw body forward
- Land softly on balls of feet
- Land feet shoulder width apart into a ¼ squat position, feet pointed straight forward
- Knees should track over toes
- Perform first as a series of single response jumps
- Then progress to doing multiple jumps consecutively as fast as possible (minimizing landing/ground contact time)

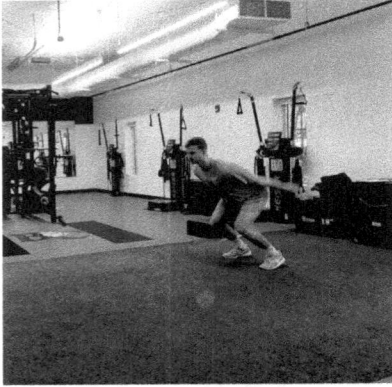

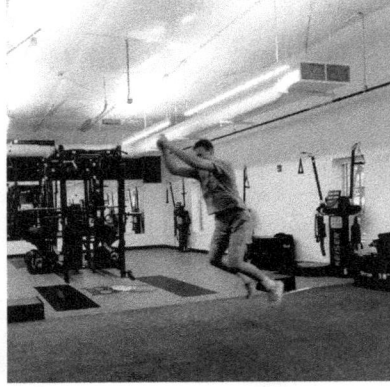

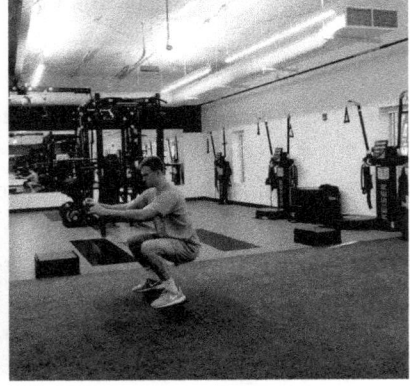

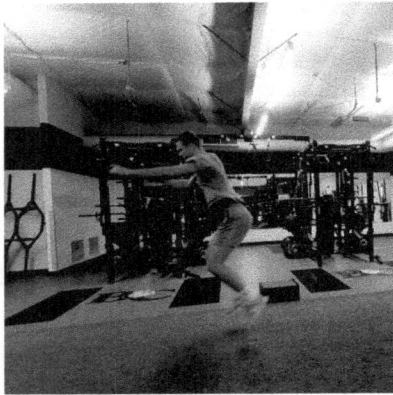

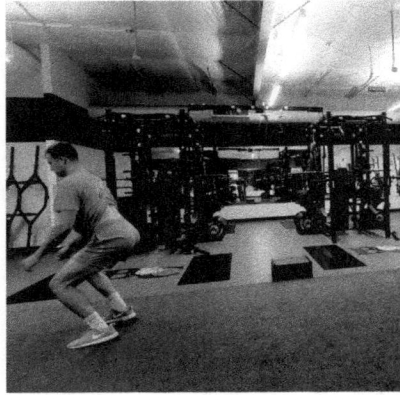

Single Leg Bound/Skip (Alternate leg Bound)

- Start in 1/4 squat position, feet shoulder width apart
- Jump/skip forwards for distance off of one leg, driving the opposite arm forward to throw the body forward
- Drive knee up, keeping front toe up (dorsi flex)
- Land softly on ball of foot and alternate legs
- Perform first as a series of single response jumps (slow but continuously)
- Then perform multiple jumps consecutively as fast as possible (minimizing landing/ground contact time)

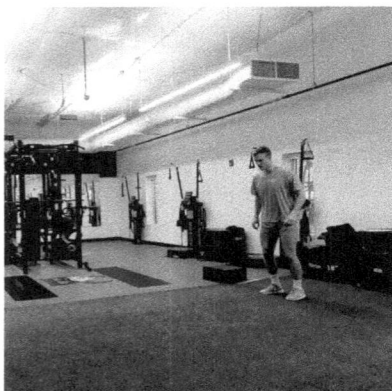

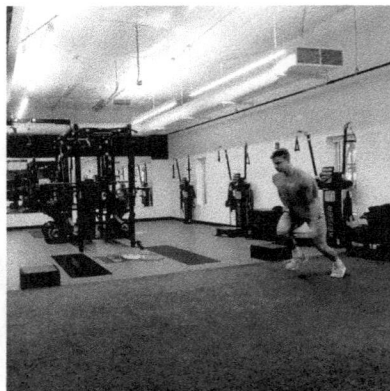

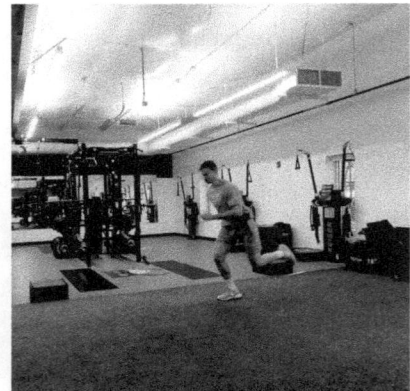

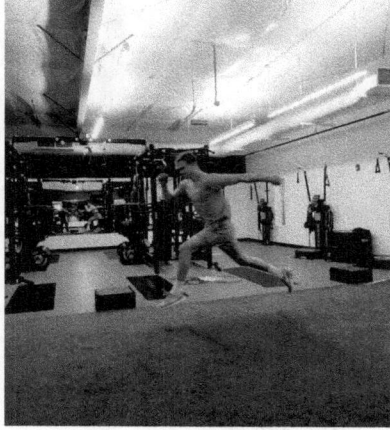

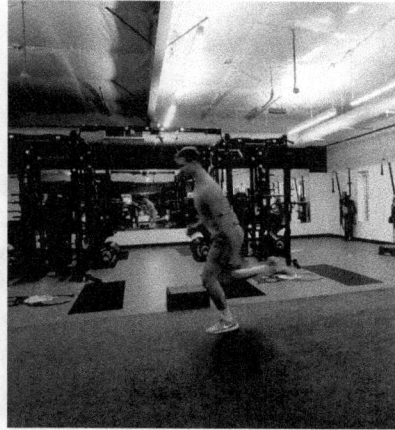

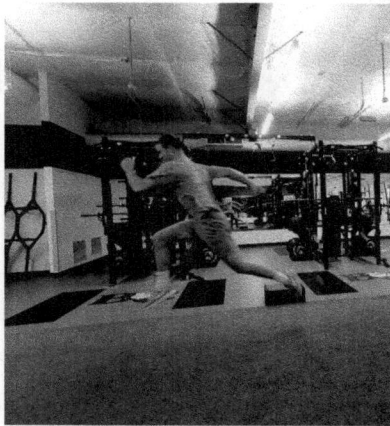

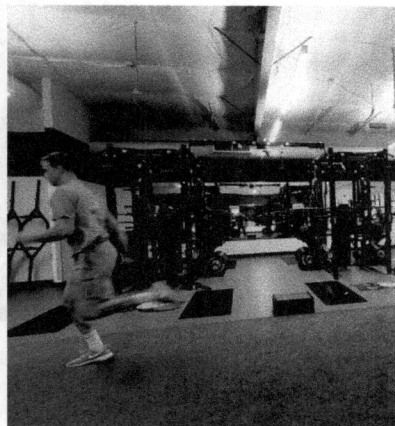

Ice Skater Skip

- Start in 1/4 squat position, feet shoulder width apart
- Jump / skip forward and laterally, at a 45-degree angle off of one leg, driving the opposite arm to throw the body in the direction of the skip
- Drive knee up, keeping front toe up (dorsi flex)
- Land softly on ball of foot and alternate legs
- Perform first as a series of single response jumps (sticking landing to build stability and to strengthen ankle and knee joints)
- Then perform multiple jumps consecutively as fast as possible (minimizing landing/ground contact time)

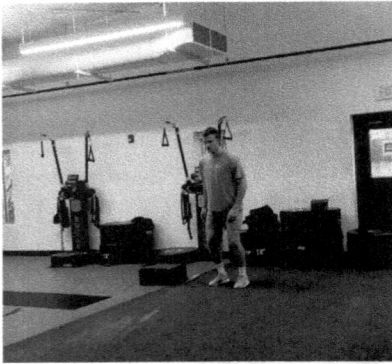

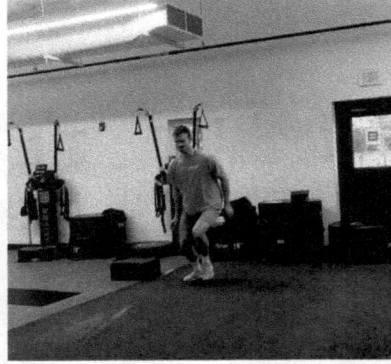

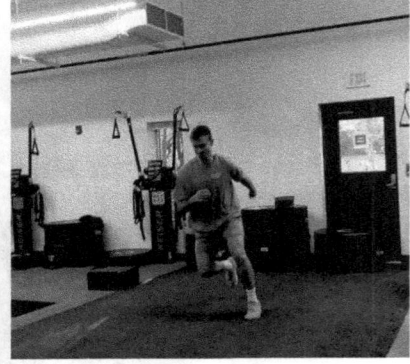

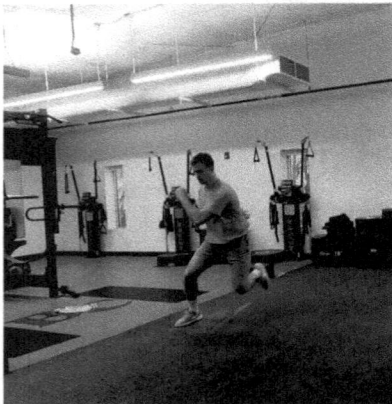

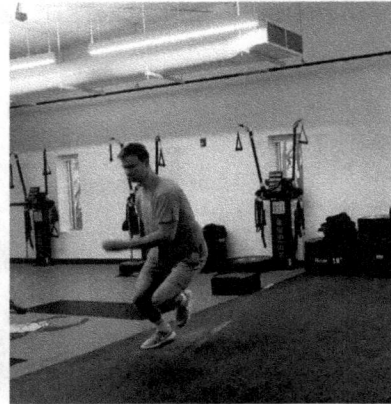

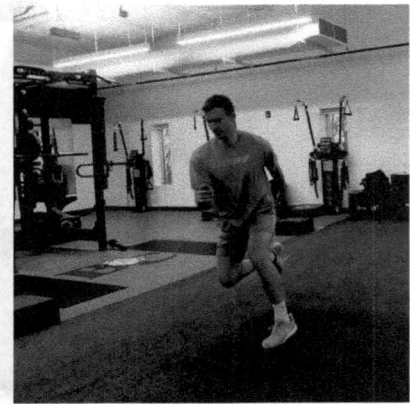

Lateral Hop (Right)

- Start with feet close together
- Going Right
  - o Drop right leg behind left leg, perform single leg squat with left leg
  - o Then drive, jumping off left foot and land softly on right foot
  - o Touch right foot down and repeat moving right
- Perform first as a series of single response jumps (sticking landing to build stability and to strengthen ankle and knee joints)
- Perform multiple jumps consecutively faster (minimizing landing/ground contact time)

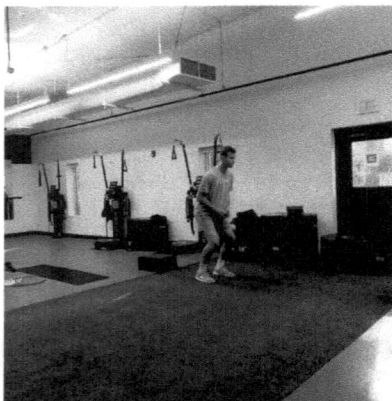

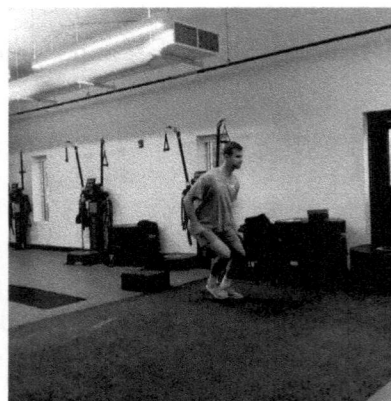

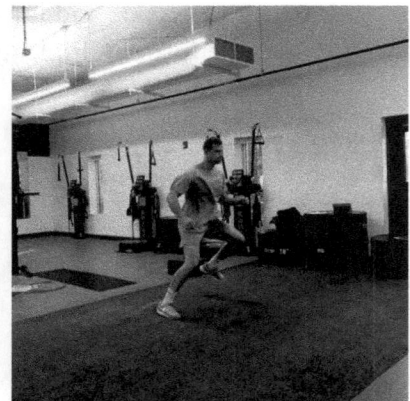

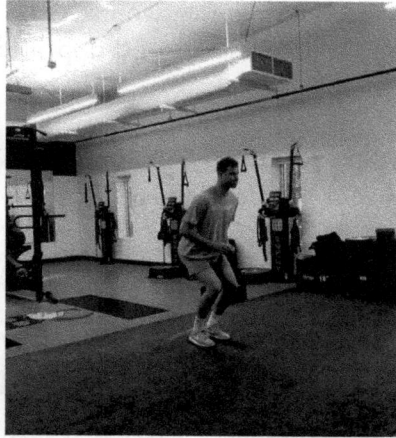

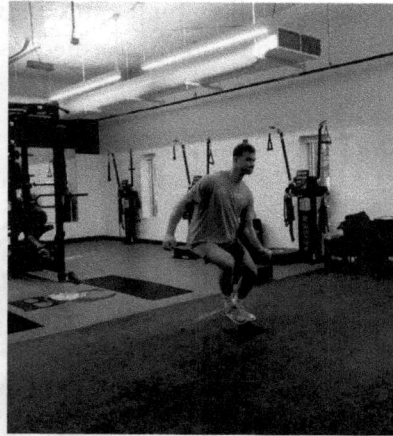

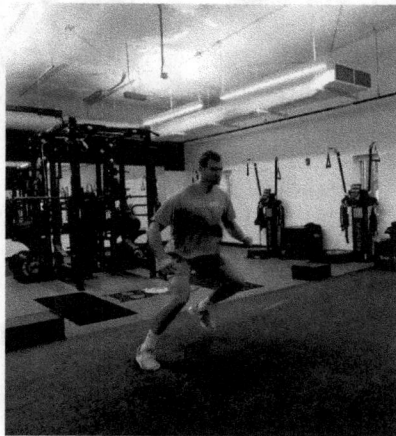

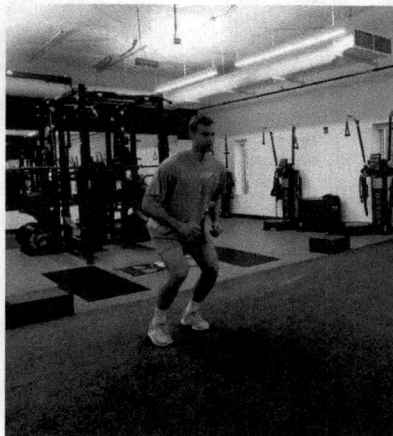

Lateral Hop (Left)

- Start with feet close together
- Going left
  - Drop left leg behind right leg, perform single leg squat with right leg
  - Then drive, jumping off right foot and land softly on left foot
  - Touch left foot down and repeat moving left
- Perform first as a series of single response jumps (sticking landing to build stability and to strengthen ankle and knee joints)
- Perform multiple jumps consecutively faster (minimizing landing/ground contact time)

Jumping Over Objects

Forward Hurdle Hops

- Start in ¼ squat position, feet shoulder width apart with barrier or hurdle placed in front of both feet
- Hop forward and back with both feet all the way over the barrier and back for the assigned repetitions

- Single-response hops allow for a pause between each hop to reset yourself
- Multiple-response hops are performed as quickly as possible, one hop after another (touch and go)

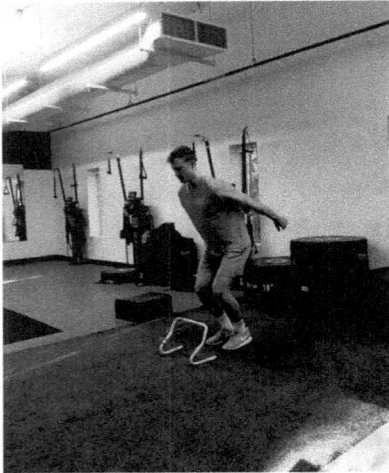

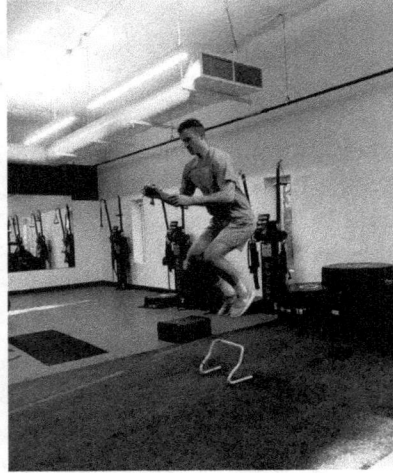

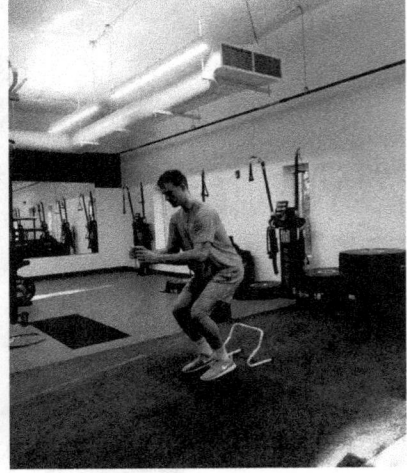

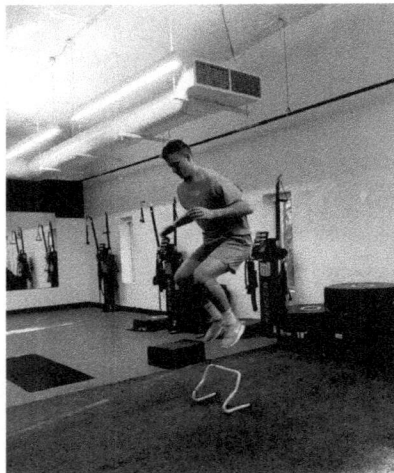

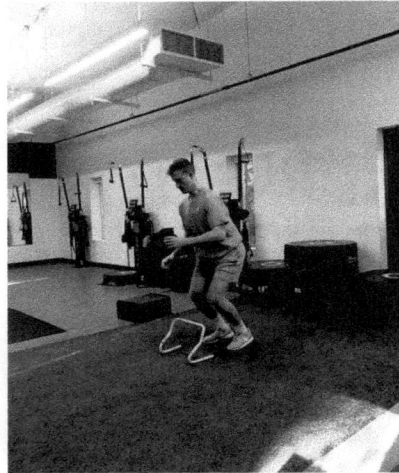

Side / Lateral Hurdle Hops

- Start in ¼ squat position, feet shoulder width apart with barrier or hurdle placed to the right or left side
- Hop laterally with both feet all the way over the barrier and back for the assigned repetitions
- Single-response hops allow for a pause between each hop to reset yourself
- Multiple-response hops are performed as quickly as possible, one hop after another (touch and go)

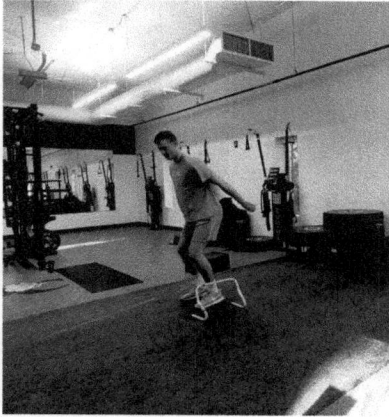

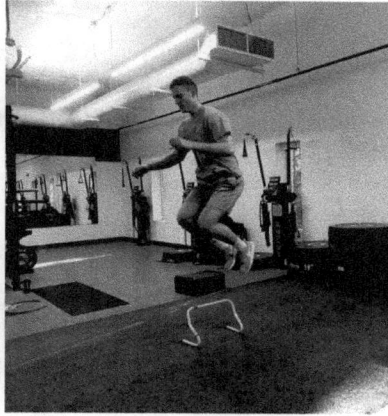

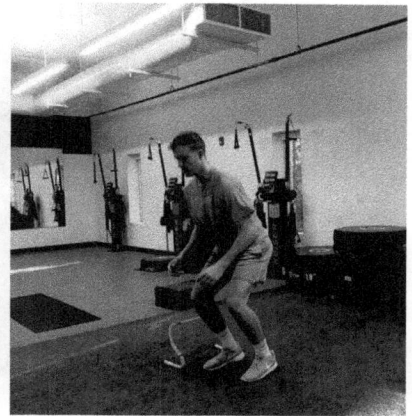

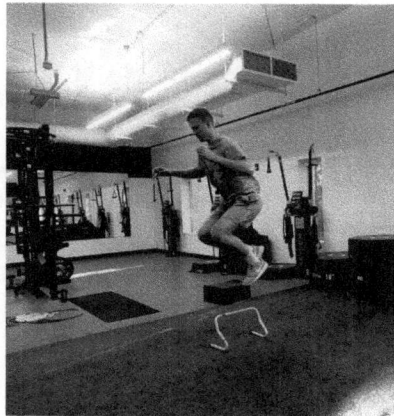

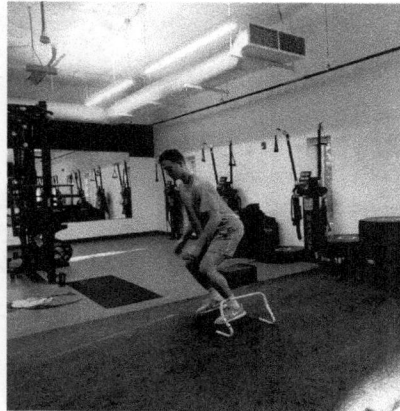

Multiple Hurdle Hops

- Start in ¼ squat position, feet shoulder width apart with a series of two or more barriers or hurdles lined up in front or laterally to the side
- Hop forward or laterally with both feet all the way over the series of barriers for the assigned repetitions
- Single-response hops allow for a pause between each hop to reset yourself
- Multiple-response hops are performed as quickly as possible one hop after another (touch and go)

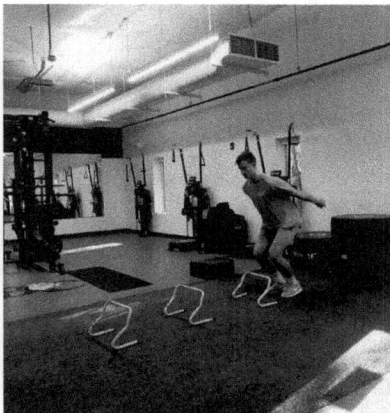

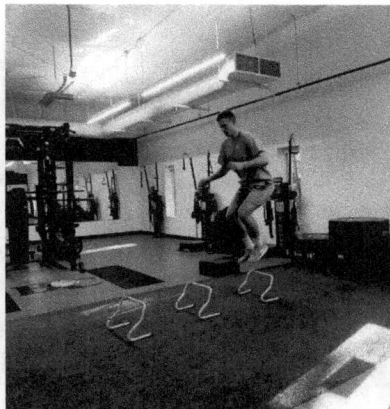

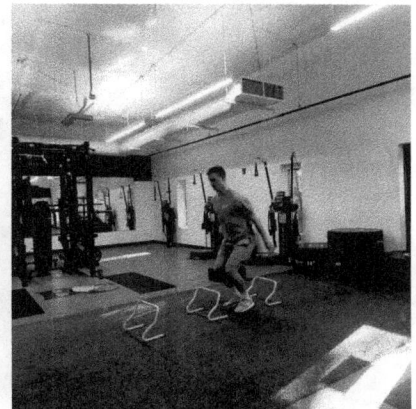

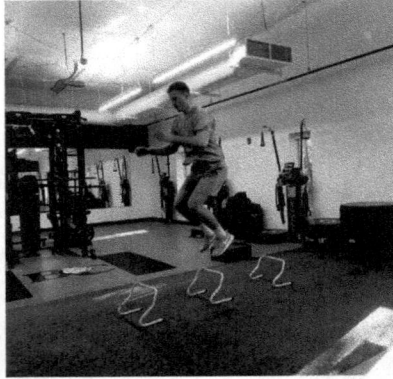
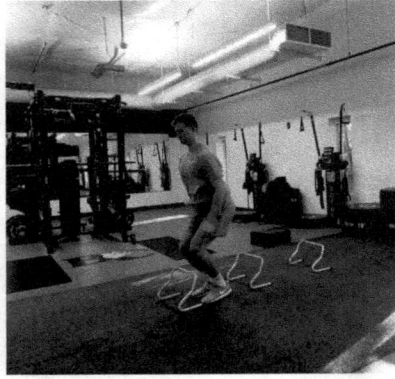

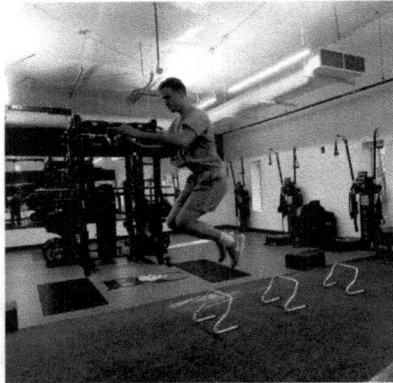
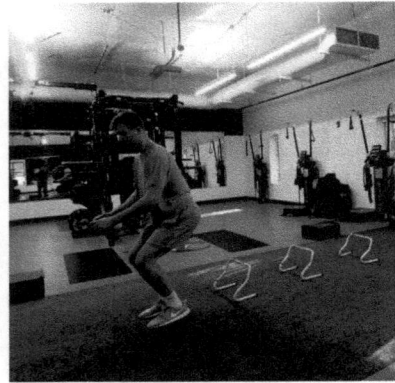

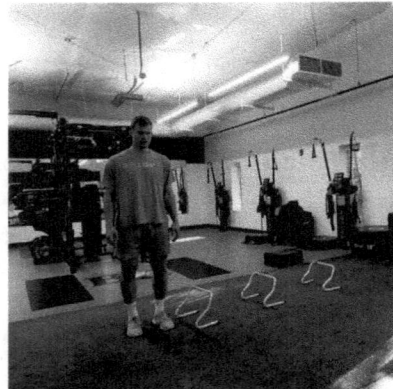
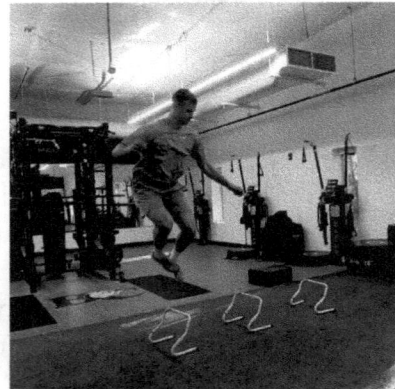

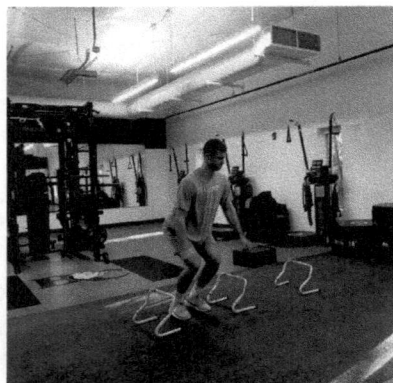
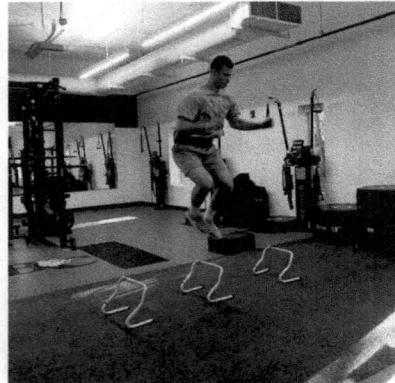

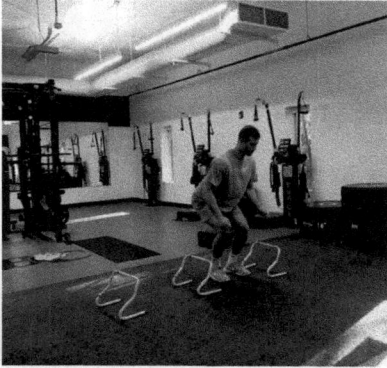

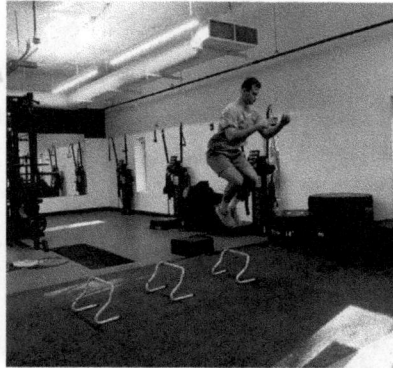

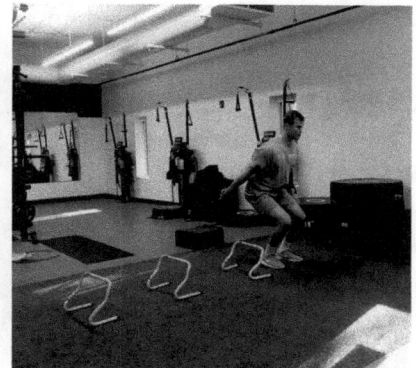

Single Leg Hurdle Hops

- Single leg hurdle hops can be performed using single or multiple hurdles placed to the front or to the side.
- Single leg hurdle hops are a higher intensity exercise with the athlete hopping and landing on the same foot.
- Single-response hops allow for a pause between each hop to reset yourself
- Multiple-response hops are performed as quickly as possible one hop after another (touch and go)
- Hurdle height can be altered to match an athlete's ability. Height can be increased appropriately as athletes improve.
- As with other plyometric drills, once double-leg options have been mastered, progression can be made to single leg drills.

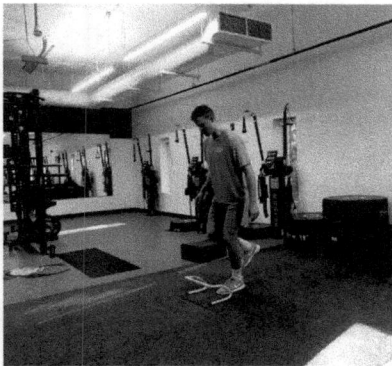

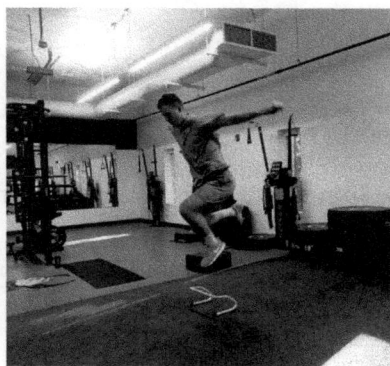

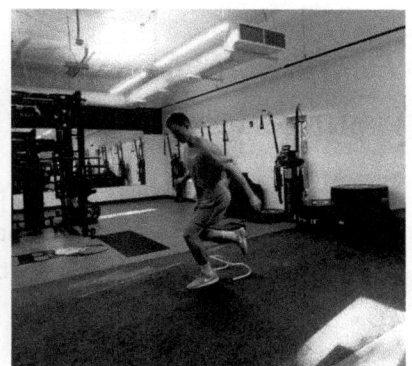

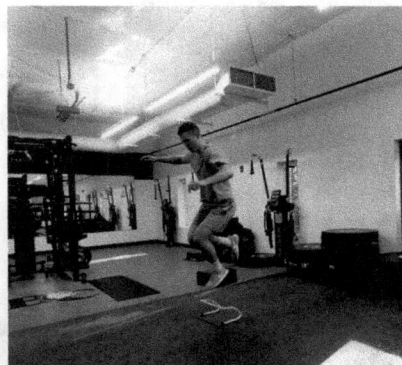

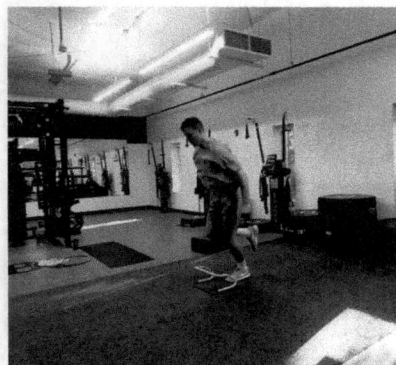

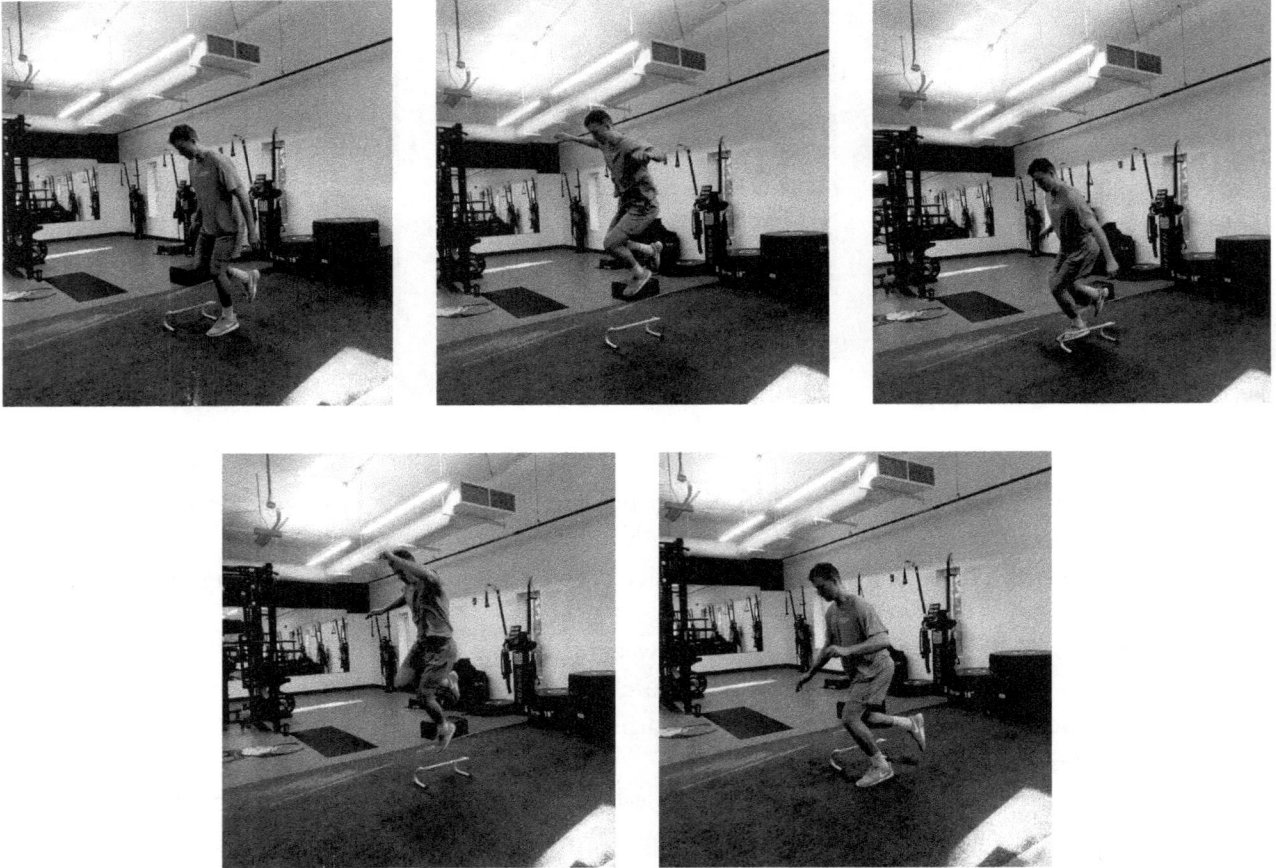

Transitional Plyometrics

In-place Jumps to Transition

- Perform one or more in-place jumps (squat jump, rocket jump, scissor jump or tuck jump) in a single- or multiple-response format
- Immediately after performing the last jump transition to another movement (like sprint, shuffle, backward or diagonal run)

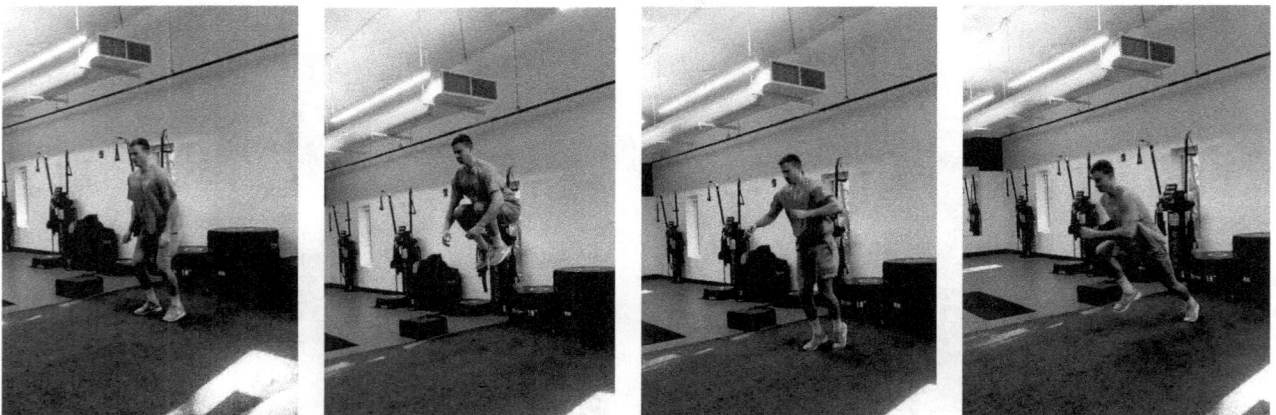

Horizontal Jumps to Transition

- Perform one or more horizontal jumps (broad jump, bound/skip, ice skater or lateral hop) in a single- or multiple-response format
- Immediately after performing the last jump transition to another movement (like sprint, shuffle, backward or diagonal run)

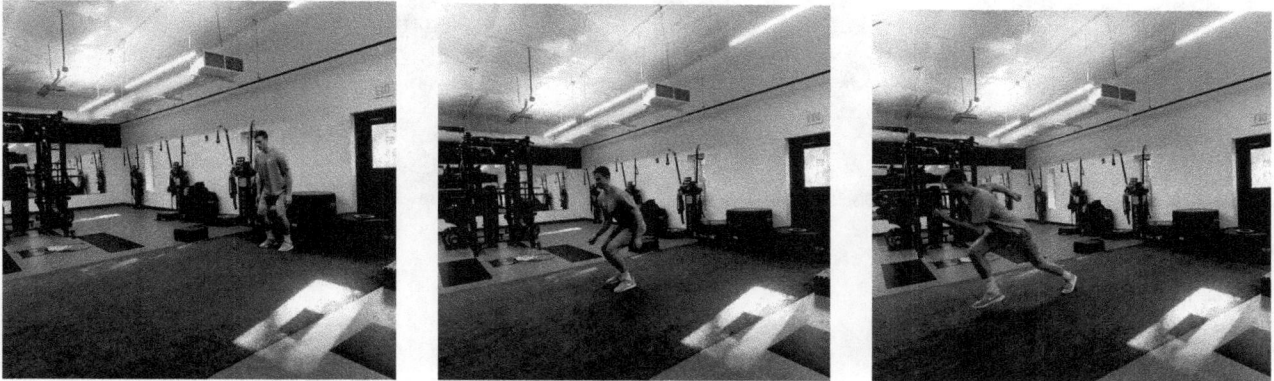

Barrier Jumps to Transition

- Perform one or more Level 4 barrier jumps (forward hurdle hops, side hurdle hops, multiple hurdle hops or single leg hurdle hops) in a single- or multiple-response format
- Immediately after performing the last jump transition to another movement (like sprint, shuffle, backward or diagonal run)

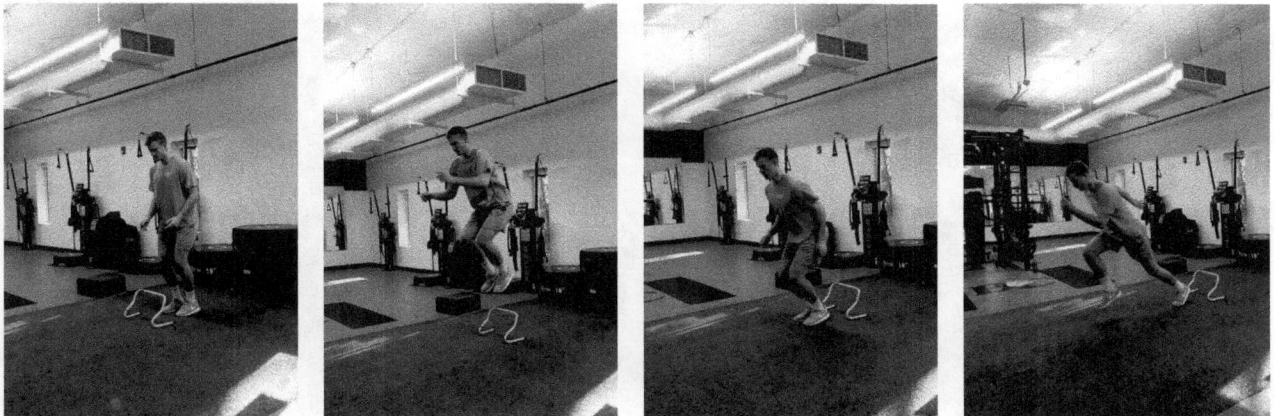

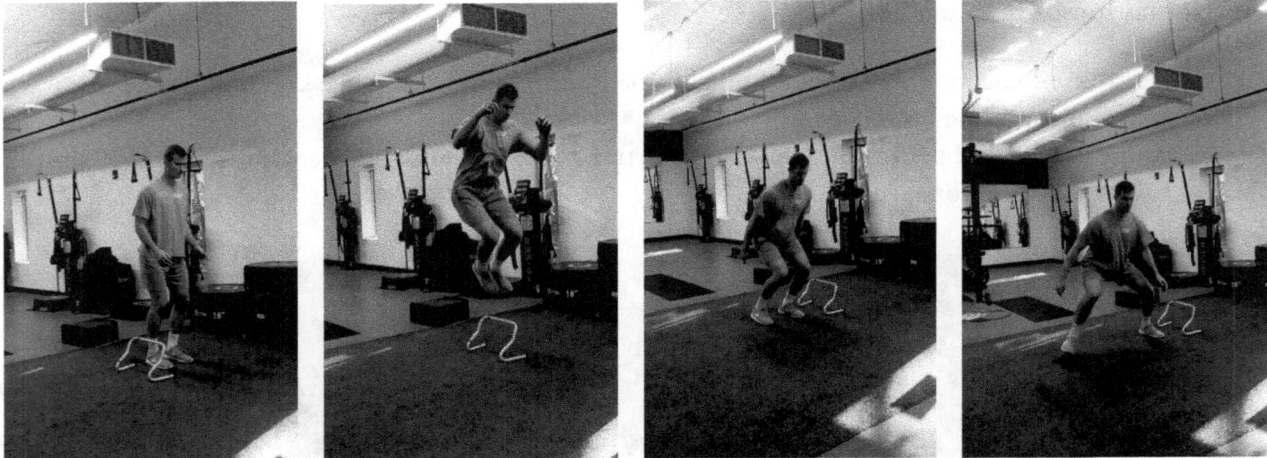

Box Jumps

Jump to Box

- Start on the ground, behind the box, in good athletic position
- Drive up with your arms to assist your lower body as you jump to the top of the box
- Land with both feet firmly on the box using good landing technique
- Knees in line with feet and not extending out over the toes (as taught in the landing drill)
- Jumping onto a box lowers the intensity of the landing since the athlete does not descend as far under the force of gravity (can be progressed to single leg jump)

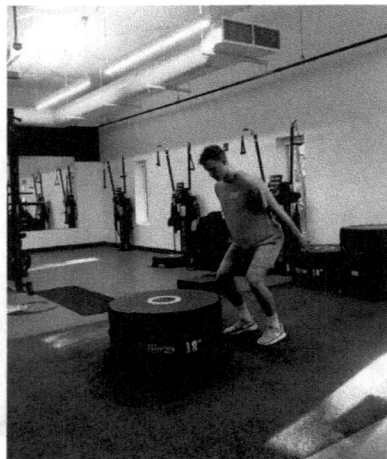

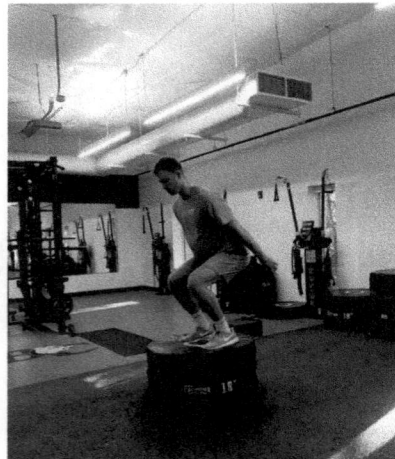

Depth Jump

- Stand on top of the box with feet shoulder width apart in good athletic position
- Step off the box and use good landing technique when feet hit the ground
- Then drive the arms upwards as you jump upwards
- This can be done initially using a slight pause at the bottom as athletes learn the technique

- Ideally, a true depth jump is performed as a "touch and go" movement where the athlete tries to jump upwards as quickly as they can after touching the ground

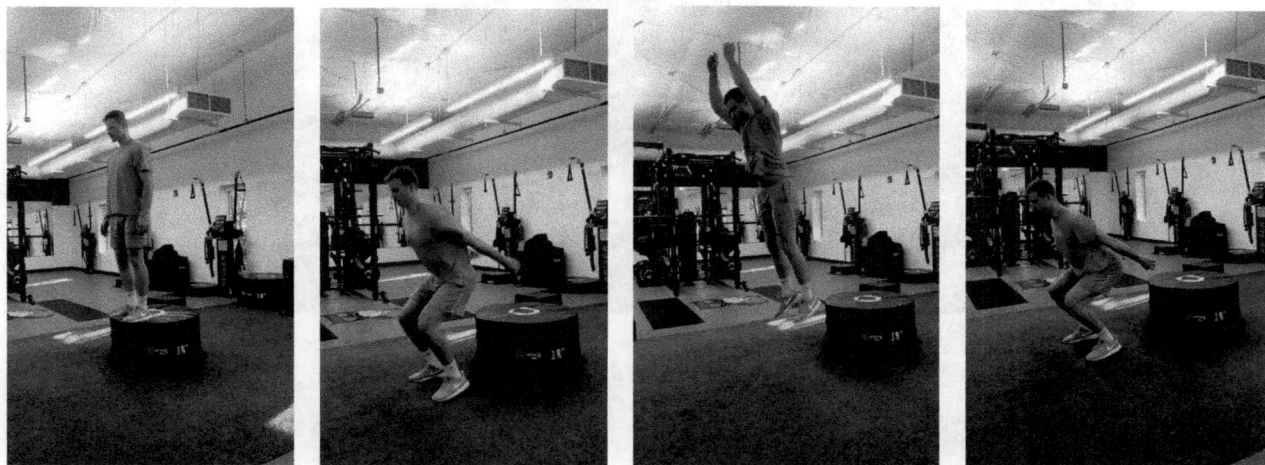

Multiple Box Jumps

- Using multiple boxes, the athletes combine the jump to a box and depth jump movements
- A two box series example would be starting on top of the box then stepping off the box into a depth jump onto a second box
- Numerous combinations of jump to boxes and depth jumps can be performed with multiple boxes
- For safety, when jumping onto a box, land firmly and pause before next movement
- With depth jumps, try to transition as fast as possible from the landing into the next jump

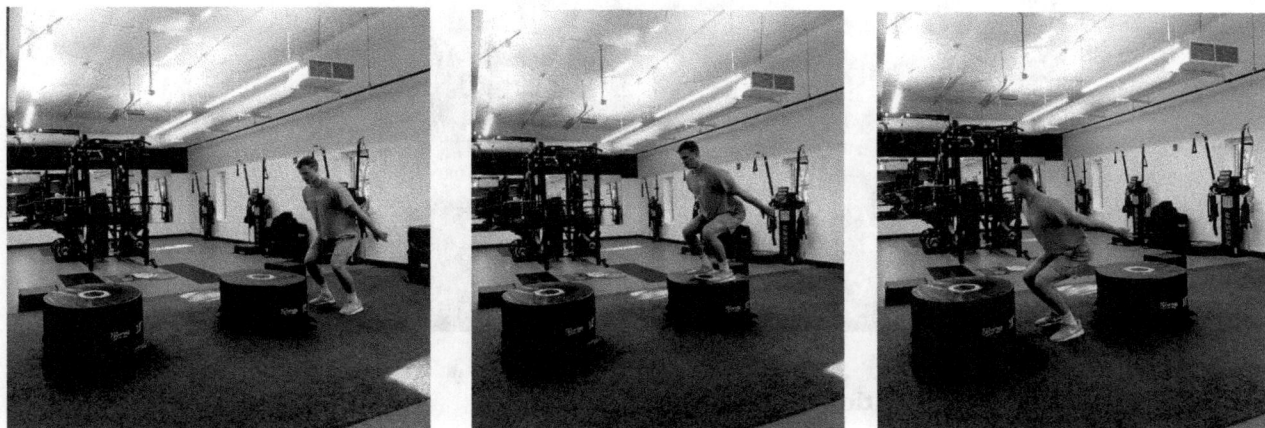

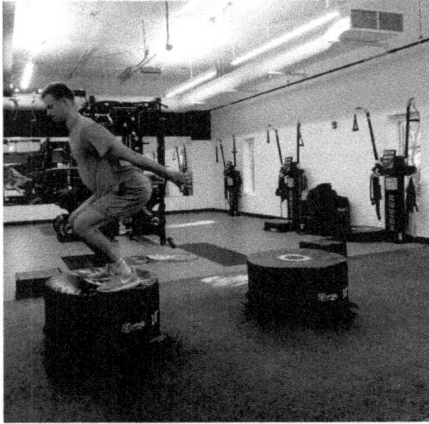

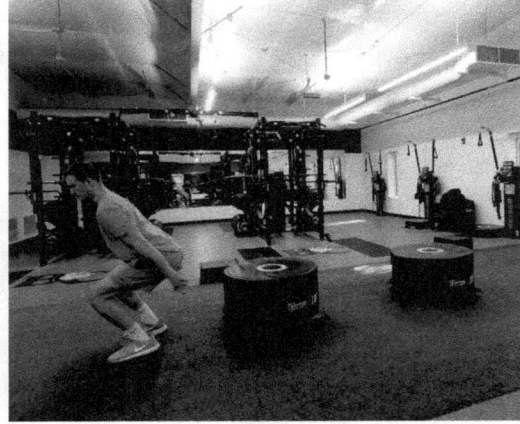

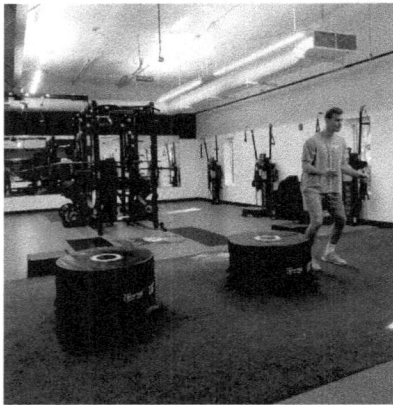

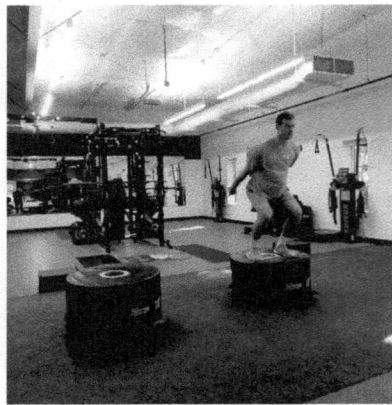

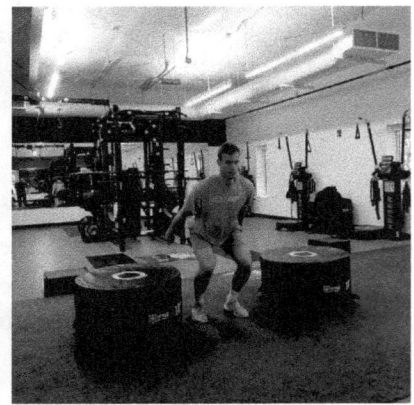

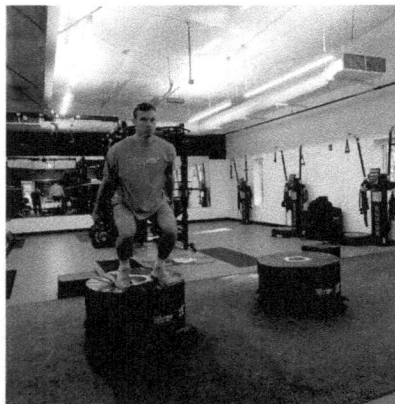

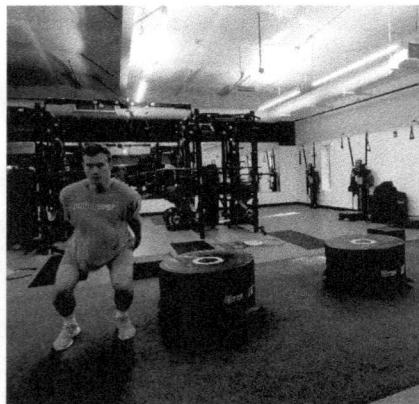

Multiple Box Jumps with Rotation

- A rotational element can be added to the multiple box jump format by executing 90-degree turns as the athlete steps off or jumps up to a box
- This added challenge helps develop body awareness and control
- A two box series example would be:
- Starting on top of the box then stepping off the box and turning their body 90 degrees before they touch the ground

- Then the athlete makes another 90-degree turn with their body as they jump up to the next box
- Be sure correct landing technique is used and ground transitions are made as quickly as possible

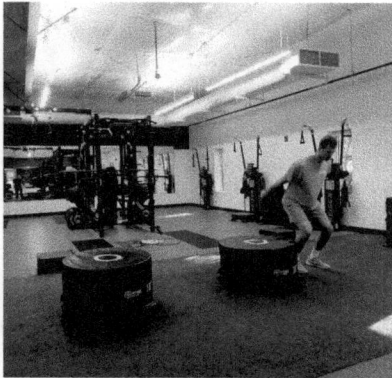

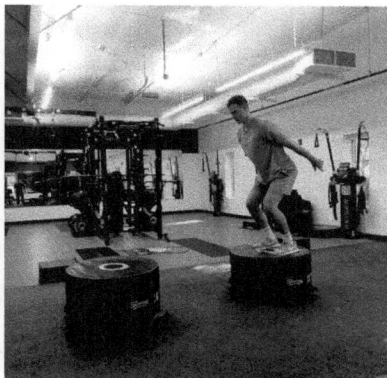

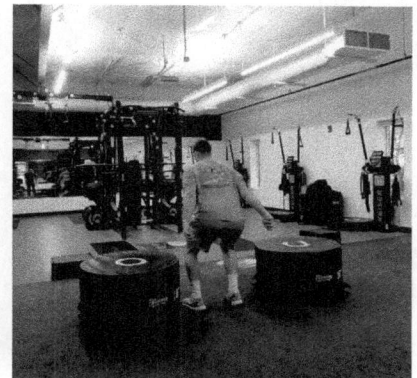

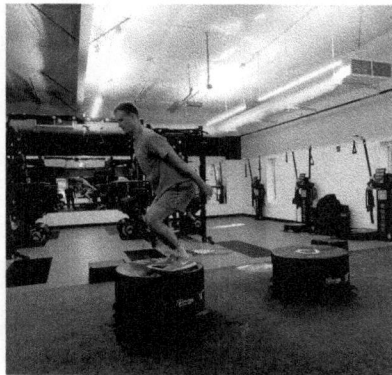

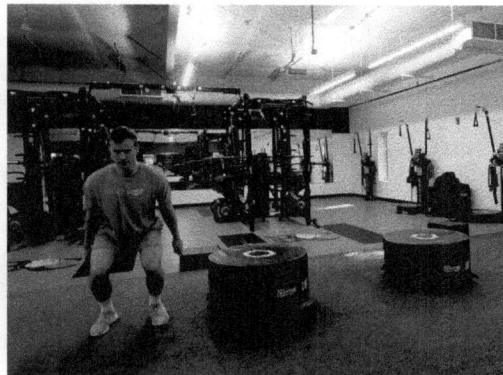

References and Suggested Reading: Chapter 10

1. Baechle, T.R., and R.W. Earle. *Essentials of Strength Training and Conditioning (3rd ed.).* Champaign, IL: Human Kinetics, 1994.

2. Bompa, T.O., and M. Carrera. *Periodization Training for Sports.* Champaign, IL: Human Kinetics, 2005.

3. Dintiman, G., and B. Ward. *Sport Speed.* Champaign, IL: Human Kinetics, 2003.

4. Farentinos, R. and J. Radcliffe. *High Powered Plyometrics.* Champaign, IL: Human Kinetics, 1999.

5. Radcliffe, J. *A Power Perspective. Strength and Conditioning Journal.* 46-47. October, 1994.

Sections in this chapter are adapted from previously published books by Dornemann and O'Dell:

6. Dornemann, T. M. *POWERREV Youth Athletic Development Program: Building Champions in Sports and in Life.* Ronkonkoma, NY: Linus, 2016.

7. O'Dell, S. *The Power Revolution: A Sports Performance Guide to Achieving Maximum Power.* Monterey, CA: Coaches Choice, 2015.

SECTION 3

CREATE YOUR PROGRAM

11
ENERGY SYSTEM DEVELOPMENT

By: Phillip Bishop, Ed. D.
Professor Emeritus of Exercise Science, University of Alabama

FUNDAMENTAL TO ALL sport movement is muscle contractions, and fundamental to muscle contractions is energy production. For anyone to move at all, they must have the ability to generate energy and that energy must ultimately be in the form of adenosine triphosphate (ATP). Because athletes often need to generate a LOT of energy either all at once or spread out over an entire match or game, developing a lot of energy is essential to good performance.

Energy Comes from Food

There are two major sources of energy in the body: carbohydrates and fats. For sports purposes, it is useful to think of carbohydrates as "fast performance fuel" and fats as "slow and steady fuel." Our ability to produce energy very rapidly is limited by the amount of oxygen we can mix with the fuel to produce energy. Carbohydrates are high performance because our bodies break them down partially without oxygen. A sprinter running very fast for 50 or 100 meters can do it without stopping. This is because the energy to run very fast (but not very far) can come from breaking down carbohydrates and utilizing the small amount of energy stored. We typically have about 10 seconds worth of all-out energy stored in our bodies.

To sprint 200 meters, our stored energy will get us about halfway, and then our bodies will break down stored carbohydrates for the rest. If we sprint 400 meters, then we can use all of our stored energy, plus our energy from breaking down carbohydrates, but we can get even more energy by breaking down carbs and recycling that process. This produces the chemical lactic acid. Lactic acid, sometimes called lactate, is good in this scenario. By producing lactic acid our body makes more energy for our legs to carry us to the 400-meter finish line.

To run (not sprint) 800 meters or further, our body first uses our stored energy and the energy our body makes from the non-oxygen breakdown. When we need to go this far we need even more energy, so our body will begin to combine oxygen with our carbohydrate fragments to produce a LOT of energy.

In fact, as long as our need for energy per minute stays low enough, our bodies can combine oxygen with both carbohydrates and fats to give us the energy to run 160 kilometers. We run more slowly per meter at 160 kilometers partly because the process of transporting oxygen from the air around us all the way down to our leg muscles takes longer than producing energy in the muscles.

Stored Energy

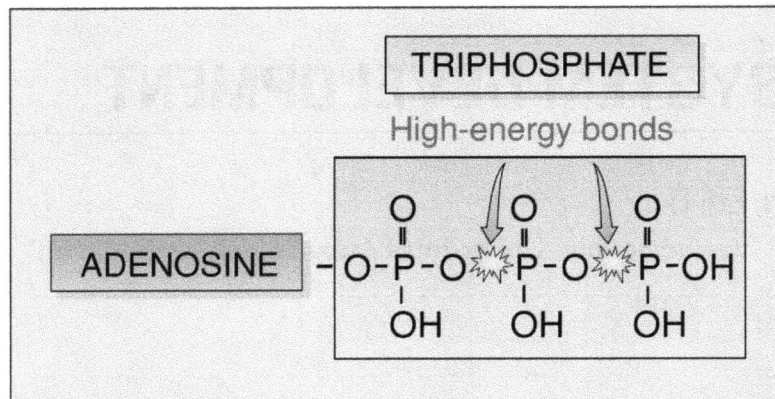

Copyright © 2011 Wolters Kluwer Health | Lippincott Williams & Wilkins

Because ATP is essential for so many vital functions, God gave our bodies the ability to store up ATP. We have ATP ready for use already in our cells, particularly muscle cells. ATP is used by stripping off a phosphate - adenosine triphosphate becomes adenosine diphosphate (ADP) and, when necessary, can release even MORE energy by releasing another phosphate to produce adenosine monophosphate (AMP). Energy is required to attach these phosphates to adenosine and that energy is released when it is broken down. This energy is used in contracting muscles and operating the body.

Our bodies also have a chemical called creatine phosphate (CP), which can help regenerate ATP without oxygen. CP is another form of stored energy and when the phosphate is stripped off, energy is released, which causes AMP to gain an energy-rich phosphate to become ADP and then causes ADP to gain an energy-rich phosphate to become ATP. These reactions can move in either direction and the same ATP/ADP/AMP/CP is recycled over and over again, in God's very conservative recycling program within our bodies.

There is one catch here. Although we have energy available for emergency and short-term use, there is not a lot of energy stored up and quickly available. We have roughly enough stored energy for about 10 seconds of all-out effort by a muscle. This amount of energy is enough to keep us operating routinely at a low-energy-demand state, and can get us out of an emergency, but when we have to run 200 meters, we will need more energy, as we will for 1600 meters or 160 kilometers. And this is where oxygen comes in.

Why We Need Oxygen

For the moment, let's only consider how we turn carbohydrates into energy to power leg muscles, or any other muscles, plus power our heart, lungs, brains, nerves, kidneys, liver, stomach and most everything else. The most basic carbohydrate in our body is glucose, which has the formula: 6 Carbons, 12 Hydrogens, and 6 Oxygens ($C_6H_{12}O_6$).

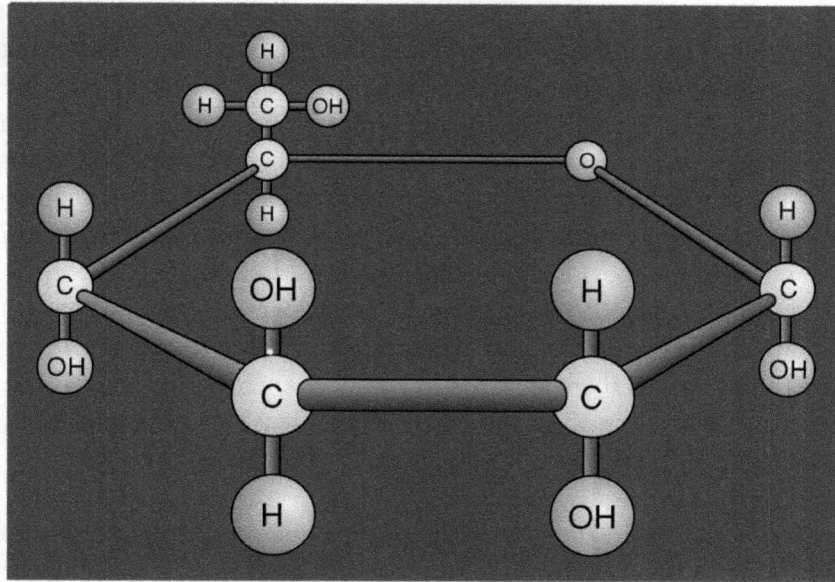

Copyright © 2011 Wolters Kluwer Health | Lippincott Williams & Wilkins

Before we go any further, take a look at those oxygen atoms in glucose. There are the same number of oxygens as there are carbons. This means that these carbons bring some of their own oxygen with them. But more oxygen is needed. Transporting extra oxygen from the local air to our calf muscles is a long, and fairly slow, trip simply because of the many steps involved in this journey.

Producing Energy in the Human Body

Energy (E) is stored in food and our bodies are good at extracting that energy. In the reverse of a manufacturing assembly line, our body has three connected disassembly lines; our bodies break down the food to make energy. Our body uses three main steps in supplying the internal energy needed to recombine our ADP and ATP over and over again.

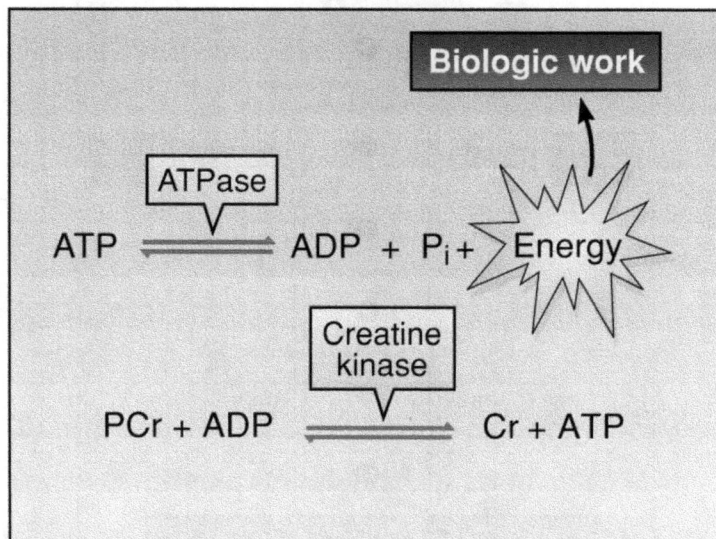

Copyright © 2011 Wolters Kluwer Health | Lippincott Williams & Wilkins

1. **Glycolysis**

   Glyco refers to "glucose," and lysis means "splitting." Our cells, especially our muscle cells, can do a lot of glucose disassembly, or splitting, in the interior of the cell. The first step in disassembly of glucose to retrieve the stored energy requires that we supply a little energy. Yes, we have to spend a little energy up front to extract the rest of the energy stored in glucose. During glycolysis, $C_6H_{12}O_6$ is split in half to make two molecules of $C_3H_6O_3$. This requires us to invest two ATP. Ultimately, the energy from food will come from combining the hydrogen atoms with oxygen atoms to release a lot of ATP energy and produce H_2O (water). The carbons will ultimately be expelled as carbon combined with oxygen, in the form of carbon-dioxide (CO_2). Oxygen is needed for both producing energy and expelling the carbon, so this is an oxygen-intensive process. But, for a short sprint, there are ways to get some energy with no oxygen required. So if our bodies operate glycolysis very rapidly, then considerable ATP can be produced without oxygen.

   A Little More Energy without Oxygen!

   In the first part of glycolysis, the glucose is split into two matching parts which requires using, rather than producing, energy. In extracting the energy from the half-glucose, we can get ATP by removing a H- and storing the hydrogens in a storage molecule called nicotinamide adenine dinucleotide (NAD+). The NAD+ can pick up and release hydrogens (H-) readily, however the NAD+ is in limited supply. Because NAD+ is in limited supply, our ability to disassemble glucose molecules is limited by how much NAD+ is available.

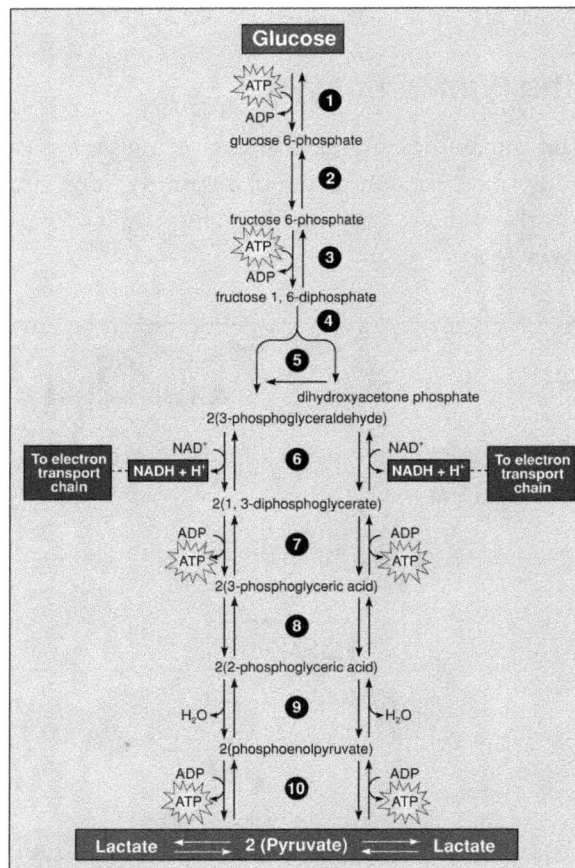

248

2. **Lactic Acid System**

Lactic acid may be the most misunderstood chemical compound in the body. The final product of glycogen splitting is pyruvate, a 3-carbon molecule. If we take a H- off of NADH, we get NAD+ and a free H-, which allows us to regenerate NAD+ for continuing glycolysis to produce ATP. Those free H- cause the pH level to drop, meaning the tissues and blood become more acidic. Our body chemistry, including energy production, operates best in a neutral (non-acidic, non-basic) environment. We need a place to store these extra H- while our bodies are continuing the process of glycolysis. We need oxygen to produce a lot of ATP, but it takes time to get additional oxygen into our cells. Therefore, we need to run glycolysis very rapidly, which exhausts our supply of NAD+, and we need a place to store H- so we can get more NAD+, which is in limited supply. The end product of glycolysis is pyruvate, $C_3H_4O_3$. The two H- were collected by NAD+ to form NADH.

Our excess H- can combine with our excess pyruvate to temporarily produce the substance lactic acid. Lactic acid is sometimes misunderstood as a problem or waste, but it is a clever means to temporarily store troublesome H- so we can produce more ATP and NAD+ without needing oxygen. Lactic acid is temporary.

Each of these processes is reversible. The lactic acid we produce is eventually reconverted during times of lower exercise intensity, back into pyruvate and the H- are eventually combined with O_2 once there is ample O_2 available. But pyruvate still contains a lot of energy in those 4 hydrogens it contains, so we need to get those out. And that brings us to the Citric Acid Cycle, also called the Krebs Cycle, or the 3-Carbon Acid Cycle.

3. **Citric Acid Cycle (aka Krebs Cycle or 3-Carbon Acid Cycle)**

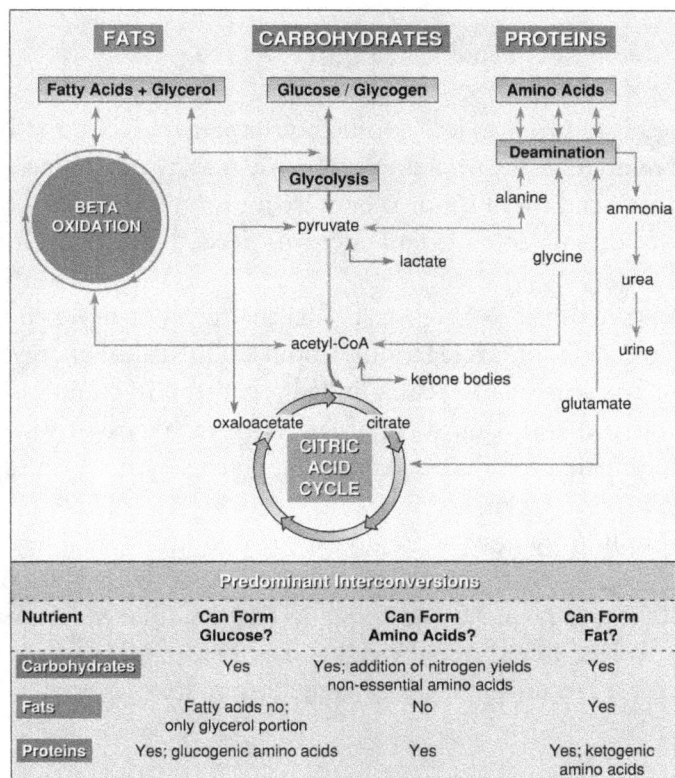

Predominant Interconversions			
Nutrient	Can Form Glucose?	Can Form Amino Acids?	Can Form Fat?
Carbohydrates	Yes	Yes; addition of nitrogen yields non-essential amino acids	Yes
Fats	Fatty acids no; only glycerol portion	No	Yes
Proteins	Yes; glucogenic amino acids	Yes	Yes; ketogenic amino acids

A Little more ATP without Oxygen

Since pyruvate still contains a lot of energy in the 4 hydrogens that are part of it, our body wants to get those out. This brings us to the third disassembly cycle, the citric acid cycle. This is also referred to as the Krebs Cycle or the 3-Carbon Acid Cycle. The Citric Acid Cycle is the last step in getting some ATP out of our old glucose molecule, which you will recall was cut in half in the early stage of glycolysis. The Citric Acid Cycle (CAC), takes place inside the mitochondria, a special compartment inside the muscle cell. In the CAC, the pyruvate first loses a H- to NAD+, then combines with a substance in the cell's fluids, acetyl. The acetyl combines with the pyruvate to form acetyl Coenzyme-A. This acetyl-CoA combines with another chemical that naturally occurs in cells, oxaloacetate, to form citric acid, which is where the CAC name originated. The CAC is a disassembly line. The acetyl-CoA simply serves as a delivery vehicle for the pyruvate to be totally disassembled so that the 3 remaining H- can be eventually combined with O_2 to make water and reform ATP from ADP and AMP.

The good news about the CAC is that it is also the key means by which we can break down fats and, in emergency, proteins to provide ATP.

Fat Metabolism

Fat is a great way to store lots of energy in a light-weight, small container. Carbohydrates are always stored with water, but fat is stored dry, which makes it lighter. This is important when we need to store a lot of energy. Fats are typically triglycerides which is a glycerol (similar to glucose) with three (i.e., tri) free fatty acids attached. There are many different types of fatty acids, but for illustration purposes consider my favorite one, palmitic acid, which is:

C_{16}, H_{32}, O_{11}.
Now compare palmitic acid to Glucose at $C_6H_{12}O_6$.

Clearly in Glucose the H- to O_2 ratio is 2 to one, but in palmitic acid it is almost 3 to one. The palmitic acid contains 1.5 as many C as O, whereas the glucose is a 1:1 ratio. These O_2 molecules are useful regardless of whether we breathed them in, or they were already in the cell. Looking at the (relatively) O_2-rich glucose, you can see that when a LOT of energy is needed quickly, glucose will contribute more O_2 than fats do.

So, we can think of carbohydrates as "high-test" fuel that gives us more energy per unit of breathed O_2. The one hitch is that we store, on average, only about 2000Kcal of energy in the form of glycogen (glycogen is just long chains of glucose molecules linked together). In comparison, the fat stores of even a very lean person at 4% fat and 100 Kg is 4 Kg of fat. With each g of fat worth about 9 Kcal we have 36,000 Kcal in stored fat compared to 2000Kcal of stored glycogen, or 18 times as much even for a very lean person.

Then why don't we simply store a lot more glycogen? Because it is so heavy. We only get about 4 Kcal per gram of stored glycogen. Each gram of glycogen is stored with 3-4 g of water, so our 500 g of glycogen requires 1500-2000 g of water! If we stored 36,000 KG like we estimated for a very lean athlete, that would be about 36 KG of additional weight to carry around. Keep in mind too that only our leanest male athletes are at 4% fat, most of us carry much more fat than that!

Getting ATP out of fat

Those fatty acids can be broken into pieces, pieces that are identical to, in fact are, acetyl-CoA. Our mitochondria will treat these acetyl-CoAs the same regardless of whether they come from a pyruvate or free fatty acids, so the CAC runs as well on one as the other. There is only one small caveat: if we are metabolizing a LOT of fat, and little glucose, our body will need to make a bit more oxaloacetate to accept the acetyl-CoAs. That's no problem for a body as well-designed as ours!

Recall that triglycerides also have a glycerol, and this glycerol is handled as if it were glucose, so that gives us a bit more ATP.

Getting ATP out of Protein

Protein's job is to build muscle and other tissue, but in emergencies it can be used as fuel. Protein is composed of long chains of amino acids. Each amino acid has different compositions and some amino acids can enter the metabolic pathways as glucose, and some as various parts of the Citric Acid Cycle, including as acetyl-CoA.

When you see pictures of starving people and notice the loss of muscle mass, it's often because the body is using protein for fuel and the muscles are being metabolized.

The FINAL step

So far we have NOT required any O_2, since all of our reactions thus far have been anaerobic (without oxygen). So why did I make the BIG deal about O_2? Because we also haven't gotten very much ATP generated yet, despite breaking glucose (and acetyl CoA from fats) down totally to C+, H-, and O_2.

So our last step in the process is to take all those H- ions, that were stripped off in Glycolysis and CAC, and combine those with O_2. If you are old enough to have seen a NASA space shuttle launch, you might remember the huge cloud of white that accompanied the acceleration of the shuttle from 0 mph to 180,000 mph. This cloud was water vapor produced when that HUGE brown silo attached to the bottom of the shuttle combined the Hydrogen in the top with the Oxygen in the back to produce a LOT of energy and a lot of water vapor. Inside our body this is called oxidative phosphorylation, and occurs in the Electron Transport Chain.

This last step of energy production produces a LOT of energy in combining those H- with O_2 to give us LOTS of ATP plus H_2O!

If we do a little accounting, we find that:

1. Glycolysis gave us 2 ATP * 2 (and two 3-C chains), minus 2 ATP to get started = net of 2 ATP total. But also gave us 2 H- which we will use in step 3 below.
2. Two puruvates going through 2 CAC gave us 2 GTP (similar to ATP) plus 10 H-.
3. The Electron Transport Chain took all the 12 H- generated in the previous steps and combined these with O_2 to give us 28 ATP!

So, when time is available to transport all the H- to the Electron Transport Chain, and to transport the O_2 to the mitochondria to combine with the H-, we can get a LOT of energy out of a single glucose molecule! So when we can generate ATP with oxygen, we can get a LOT of ATP, but it does take time.

For example, in a 100-meter sprint the race is over before we can get all this going, so we must rely on the energy we have quickly at hand.

But why does it take so long to get O_2 to the mitochondria? Because it takes a lot of steps. Here are the steps:

1. We expand our chest to create a lower pressure in our lungs to draw in air. The oxygen in the air must cross from the lung tissue (alveoli) which has a little film of fluid on it.
2. The O_2 then encounters a little more fluid before it then has to cross the capillary wall outside the alveoli.
3. Once inside the capillary, the oxygen must cross the blood plasma.
4. It next encounters the red blood cell wall, which it must cross to attach to hemoglobin.
5. The blood from the lungs is then carried to the left atrium, from here to the left ventricle.
6. The blood then must flow all the way down to our leg muscles.
7. Once in the legs, the oxygen must leave the hemoglobin, and cross the red cell wall into the blood plasma.
8. It must then cross the capillary wall through a bit of fluid into the muscle cell.
9. Inside the muscle cell, glycolysis takes place, but the O_2 is not involved and must cross the muscle fluid and enter the mitochondrial wall.

Whew! It is a long trip and a LOT of things can go wrong along the way. Yet, this system works remarkably well. But, you can see why production of LOTS of ATP by oxidation takes longer than simply running glycolysis and producing a little ATP very rapidly.

So, the Glycolysis system and the Citric Acid Cycle can run fast and produce enough ATP to get us ahead of that saber-toothed tiger, but we will have slow our pace to continue to generate enough ATP to run down that jack rabbit, like I once did in Corpus Christi, TX.

Energy System Integration

It is easy to be misled by our way of discussing these energy production systems. We sometimes falsely think that ATP and CP produce some energy, then glycolysis, then the Critic-Acid cycle, then Oxidative Phosphorylation produce the rest. NOT so! All of these are running ALL of the time!

Whereas we could hold our breath whilst sprinting 100 meters, we already have a small quantity of oxygen stored in our muscles and our blood has oxygen in it when we begin the sprint. So, oxygen is utilized even in a sprint, but it combines with the stored ATP and CP, which make up the bulk of the ATP utilized to complete the run. As you go up in run distance, the amount of ATP generated by using oxygen increases in proportion to the distance.

We started at 100 meters, let's go to the other extreme, a 42-kilometer marathon. To run this distance takes a tremendous amount of energy expended over the run duration. The amount of energy is fairly constant regardless of the speed of running, with running faster only taking a little more energy per kilometer (but it has to be produced faster). But to complete this run, a LOT of ATP must be generated, so a lot of oxygen is consumed. But regardless of how much ATP is needed and how much oxygen is used, our muscles still run on ATP, and glycolysis and all the other energy systems contribute to producing ATP.

Keep in mind too, that glycolysis is not just running one time in one muscle cell. Glycolysis is going on in many reactions in all working muscles. Similarly, the Citric Acid Cycle does not exist in little circles like you have seen it drawn (because it IS a cycle). The CAC is running multiple times in multiple mitochondria, simultaneously. One adaptation we see in sportsmen who need to expend a LOT of ATP (distance events) is that their muscles will produce MORE mitochondria to produce more ATP than those who don't need as much total energy (e.g. pole vaulters, sprinters, throwers, weight lifters).

Coaching Applications

So what? I'm just trying to produce elite athletes. Who cares about all of this? Well, to be a top athlete requires genetics and effective training in addition to desire and hard work. Genetics are crucial because some athletes were gifted by God with muscles designed to contract fast and produce energy very rapidly, but not very long. Recognizing that you cannot make a gifted distance-runner into a sprinter because the muscle fibers and needed energy system capacities aren't suited is obvious. And neither can we convert an explosive-gifted sportsman into a long-distance runner. God gives different gifts to the body of Believers as outlined in Romans 12 and I Corinthians 12.

The next issue is the fuel in what we feed our athletes. Recall that our glycogen stores are limited, whereas our fat stores, for practical purposes, are practically unlimited. So, if our athletes are using a LOT of glycogen in repeated sprinting, over the course of 4 or 5 or 6 consecutive days of hard training, they may use up almost ALL their stored glycogen. Our nervous system prefers to use glucose to generate ATP to keep firing, so when glucose is in short supply our sportsmen may suffer mentally as well as having slower performance due to the lack of "high-test" fuel.

So, in these cases we need to make sure our athletes are resting and consuming high carbohydrate diets. We also would want to try to give our sportsmen some recovery days where technique was emphasized instead of using so much fuel.

The most important application for coaching would be in energy specificity. Our body adapts to the stressors placed on it, and our metabolic systems adapt to the demands placed on them. Sportsmen like American football linemen expend a lot of ATP very rapidly, but only for about 5-6 seconds, then they get almost a minute, or sometimes MORE to recover. Plus, after a few plays, they usually are replaced by another part of the team or there is a time-out or other interruption. In this sport, the old practice of requiring these players to run a mile or more to train their aerobic system makes little sense. Even with our so-called "hurry-up" offense, there is still considerable time between plays.

On the other hand, the average world football (soccer) player covers about 10,000 meters in the course of a game. Fortunately, this is spread over 90 minutes, unlike in a 10-kilometer race, but the need for oxygen to generate ATP is obvious in both situations.

An athlete running all-out for about a minute or less needs to train their glycolytic and CAC systems by stressing THOSE systems primarily. Recall that the generation of lactic acid is a means for making MORE ATP available, so these sportsmen need to generate as much lactic acid as they can in training and in competition! It's good to generate lactic acid, so let's train our athletes to generate even more!

So, what does this look like in training applications? Those needing lots of ATP generation will need to maximize their ability to capture oxygen. This means they will do training that taxes their hearts to maximize their heart's ability to pump blood. Doing intermittent high intensity interval training (HIIT) will truly tax their heart and result in training adaptations. Likewise, if they keep running, or swimming, or rowing, or cycling between HIIT cycles, they will train their muscles to adapt to this situation, which is remarkably similar to how many soccer players have to move in a game.

Fat Control Applications

In some sports, such as wrestling, boxing, gymnastics and others, keeping body fatness low provides some advantages. It is extremely rare for anyone to want to lose muscle, but most everyone, at some point, would be happy to lose some fat.

Fat loss is accomplished when the energy expended in 24 hours is greater than the energy absorbed from the food and beverage consumed. Some folks suggest that "fat-burning" exercise is the way to lose fat; but now that you know the basics, you realize that low-intensity exercise (more time between repetitions) uses fat, whereas high-intensity, fast energy expenditure uses more carbohydrates.

Our body keeps up with energy accounting very well. If we are eating a mixed-diet of carbohydrates and fats, then it does NOT matter what we burn during an exercise bout, because we will burn fat most of the day, and in the end what matters is the difference between calories expenditure and absorption.

Some well-meaning folks have suggested that if we want our athletes to lose fat, we need to help them put on a LOT of muscle, because during any 24-hour period, all other things being equal, muscle will burn a lot more energy than fat. What these folks forget is genetics. Whereas some athletes can put on muscle mass, others are extremely limited in their ability to add substantial muscle. Plus, the total energy expenditure from ONLY weight training, except in extreme situations, is much lower per unit time than continuous exercise such as running, cycling and swimming, primarily because of the short duration of a set and the time between sets.

After doing research in exercise physiology for many years it has become apparent the enormous variability that God has instilled in creating each person in the image of God. This becomes apparent in fat control and in training. What produces good results in one person may be totally worthless in other people. As a coach, or trainer, it is your duty and opportunity to observe each sportsman or woman individually, what works for one will not be optimal for all, and what fails for one, may succeed for another.

There are sometimes reasons for treating a team as one unit, but it will be rare when any one person benefits maximally from any one diet, training regimen, or treatment. Be an "investigator" and an "experimenter" as you work with people and do NOT be afraid to try different things with different athletes. Be aware in reading research reports and research interpretations, because MOST research will ONLY report group average values, which fails to consider individuality. Because of this, many years back I created a statistical approach for identifying individual sportsmen's responses to experimental treatments.

For an example, take a look at our paper, *Bosak AM, Bishop Green JM. Active vs. passive recovery in the 72 hours after a 5km race. *The Sport Journal* 11 (3), 2008.availabe at: http://thesportjournal.org/article/active-versus-passive-recovery-in-the-72-hours-after-a-5-km-race/).

Reference: Chapter 11

1. Katch, McArdle, & Katch. *Essentials of Exercise Physiology* (4th ed.). Baltimore, Maryland: Lippincott, Williams, & Wilkins, 2011.

12
RESISTANCE TRAINING PROGRAM DESIGN

By: Tim Dornemann, Ed. D., CES, PES, CSCS, OS Pro

Exercise Science Program & Kinesiology Director, Barton College
Associate Professor of Exercise Science, Barton College

Program Design: Art or Science?

IS DESIGNING RESISTANCE programs an art or a science? This has been a long-time question. True program design has elements of both art and science. There are many tactics and approaches to designing great programs. Numerous combinations of sets, repetitions and loading can lead to similar outcomes– which is where the creativity or art of programming happens. Science provides a framework in which to be creative in developing training programs.

Observation that has led to research has helped establish a series of best practices in the designing of resistance training programs. These best practices shape programs so that the desired outcome of the program can be achieved. Using both a needs analysis and established programming guidelines helps strength coaches develop sports-specific programs to enhance the physical abilities of their athletes. A good program targets the specific needs of a sport. Using a target as an example, the goal is to hit the bullseye (specific characteristic of the sport) and not just hit the target.

The needs analysis is what provides direction to a good training program. Manipulation of the acute program variables (exercise selection, exercise order, number of repetitions, number of sets, training frequency, intensity/loading and length of rest periods) is what determines how effectively a program achieves its desired outcomes.

Needs Analysis

The needs analysis is the first and most important step in the process of designing a resistance training program. It is the foundation on which you build the specifics (acute program variable manipulation) of your program. The stronger the foundation, the stronger the program will be. To conduct a needs analysis, in the words of Stephen Covey, you need to "begin with the end in mind." To begin with the end in mind you must have a clear picture of what you want your program to accomplish and, more specifically, what attributes you want to physically develop in your athletes. Note that in this book, athlete refers to participants of any sport. Sometimes programs will refer to athletes as track and field participants and then use the term sportsmen for participants across sports.

To know what you want to accomplish in your program and to successfully accomplish the desired outcomes, you need two things: the sport you are programming for and the athletes that you will be training. A good needs analysis provides a systematic approach to knowing your sport and knowing your athletes at the level needed to develop a successful training program.

Sport Evaluation

A complete sport evaluation includes a sport movement analysis, physiological analysis and an injury analysis. More specialized strength coaches or sport coaches that are also responsible for strength and conditioning may already have an in-depth knowledge of the sport they are programming for. Strength and conditioning coaches that are responsible for training multiple sports cannot be experts in every sport they work with. Coaches that are less familiar with the sports they are programming need to study up on the sport they are programming for and use the resources that they have available. Sport coaches and athletic trainers/sports medicine professionals can be valuable sources of the information needed to conduct a thorough evaluation of a sport.

The sport movement analysis of a sport can start with general analysis of movement used in a sport and can be as specific as examining the joint movement used in a sport. One aspect of the principle of specificity, mentioned in chapter one, is the inclusion of movements that are similar or specific to movements used in a sport. General movements can include the directional movements involved in a sport. For example, basketball utilizes multi-directional movement with players being required to move forwards, backwards and laterally. Jumping and change of direction are also physical characteristics that are important to the game of basketball. Sprinting and jumping are powerful movements that involve triple extension, which refers to the extension of the ankles, knees and hips. Sports that utilize throwing, kicking or striking often incorporate rotation. The sport movement analysis provides information that guides the choices of exercises used in a program. The more complete the movement analysis is, the more sport specific the program can be.

When conducting a physiological analysis, think about the physical characteristics that you want to develop in your athlete and what physical abilities are needed to thrive in this specific sport. Does your sport need attributes like speed, power, strength (force production), agility, stamina or quickness? Basketball players need to be agile, powerful and have stamina. Power is how quickly one can produce force. As a result, strength or the ability to produce force is the foundation of power. Developing power is actually developing coordination of the neuromuscular system. The muscular system is primarily responsible for force production, but the nervous system plays a key role in determining how fast that force can be produced. Two common forms of power training that are discussed in detail in other areas of this book are plyometric and explosive lifting.

In addition to the physical attributes of a sport, there is a second element to the physiological analysis of a sport: the conditioning needs of the sport. In simple terms, what sort of stamina is required to succeed in a certain sport? Specifically, what are the primary energy systems used in the sport? There are three systems that provide energy to the body:

1. Aerobic system - uses oxidation to produce energy

2. Phosphagen system - one of the two anaerobic energy pathways, sometimes referred to the ATP-CP system
3. Glycolytic system - the second anaerobic energy pathway

While all three systems work together and are utilized to some extent, sports tend to heavily focus on utilizing one or two of the systems. To best train athletes, identify the common energy systems used and coordinate training to develop those systems. For example, baseball and softball often incorporate short bursts of energy that would utilize the phosphagen system. In contrast, soccer (or football outside the U.S.A.) requires a great deal of endurance. While the aerobic oxidative system provides a foundation for the endurance required to play soccer, when analyzed closely, one sees that sport is played in spurts (intervals of slower and faster paced movement). With the game being played in intervals and not continuously maintaining an elevated heart rate, the primary energy system in soccer would be the anaerobic glycolytic system and not the aerobic oxidative system. As a result, training utilizing repetitive sprint intervals should be the conditioning focus and traditional aerobic conditioning.

The last aspect of the sport evaluation is the injury analysis. A good resistance training program should not only focus on the physical development needed to excel while playing a sport but should also include injury prevention. Injury prevention helps athletes stay healthy and in the game, allowing the improvements made in other areas of the program to be utilized in competition. If you do not have a deep understanding of the sport that you are programming for, athletic trainers and sports medicine professionals are valuable resources for conducting an injury analysis. For example, throwing sports often have higher incidences of rotator cuff injuries. Rotator cuff strengthening exercises–like internal and external shoulder rotation exercises–can be incorporated into programs to prevent rotator cuff injuries. Programs for sports where anterior cruciate ligament (ACL) injuries are common should feature ACL prevention techniques. This could include teaching proper jump landing techniques and change of direction or cutting techniques.

Athlete Assessment

The athlete assessment is an evaluation of the realities of your training situations. The facilities available and the experience of your athletes are parameters that influence the design of your program. The equipment you have available to you for training, such as the number of rack spaces, types of weights available and number of bars dictate the types of exercises that can be performed and how a program is executed. For example, to perform explosive lifts correctly, proper equipment like bumper plates and platforms or specialized flooring is needed. However, basic weighted triple extension movements can be performed with kettlebells or dumbbells if that is what is available. Facilities, space and time to train are all administrative variables that shape how programs are designed.

A true athlete assessment also examines the athletes you will be training. You need to know the training experience or "training age" of the athletes you are training. To a strength and conditioning coach, the experience an individual has playing their sport is not as important as what their physical training experience is. The physical training experience refers to how long the athletes that you are working with have been resistance training or in a strength and conditioning program. You also want to know what training activities and exercises the athletes are familiar with. The time your athletes have played a sport is not important in your planning, because your sport evaluation has provided you with the physical direction of your program (what the physical attributes are that are important to your target sport that you want to develop). While the sport evaluation shapes what goals you are training to achieve, the athlete assessment shapes how you are going to achieve those goals.

The National Strength and Conditioning Association (NSCA) defines three levels of training experience: beginner, intermediate and advanced. In general, these levels will influence the frequency and complexity of the training program. Beginners are not as physically prepared to train as frequently as advanced athletes and will require more recovery time to benefit from the training. More advanced athletes have been exposed to a wider variety of exercises and are capable of performing the more complex exercises that they have already learned. This provides a coach with more freedom in selecting exercises when working with more experienced athletes.

With the end in mind, a coach may want to design training to increase power. How the coach accomplishes that can be very different based on the experience of the athletes. Progression is a key to training; however, an athlete's experience level will dictate the proper progression that is needed. A coach may want to use explosive lifting with beginners, but due to the complexity of explosive lifting it can take a long time to learn, which means explosive lifts might not be the best place to start developing power. Use of body weight plyometric exercises or less complex dumbbell or kettlebell exercises, like swings and snatches, might be a better way to introduce triple extension movements and power development with beginners. In contrast, when a coach is working with experienced athletes that have experience with complex movements, explosive lifts might be an appropriate starting point.

Physical Testing and Evaluation

Physical testing and evaluation is the final element of the athlete assessment. Testing provides the last piece of the puzzle needed to develop a safe and effective training program. You need to know where you are starting from and what your athlete's capabilities are when you start your program. Good programs are never static; they constantly evolve based on the feedback provided by physical testing. Initial testing provides a baseline or a starting point for your training program. Testing conducted during or after a training program indicates how well the program worked. Regular testing tells a strength coach what worked and what did not work, allowing for you to keep what worked and change what did not work so that the next training cycle can be more effective.

How and what you test should mirror your sport evaluation. If your goal is to produce power, then you can use a vertical jump test to assess vertical power or a standing long jump test to assess horizontal power. If agility is a key element of your program, you can use a pro-agility (5-10-5) test to measure change of direction, but if your sport involves multiple direction agility, then a test like the T-Test that features use of multiple directional movement might be better. Sprint tests of varying distances can be used to assess speed, but you need to look at the realities of your court or field space to pick the appropriate sprint distance for your sport. When assessing stamina or conditioning, you want to match the tests with the primary energy systems used in the target sport. For sports that utilize the aerobic pathway, an aerobic capacity test like the beep test would be appropriate. Sports that utilize anaerobic glycolysis heavily would want to utilize an anaerobic capacity test like the 300-yard shuttle test. The key point is that you want to match up the tests performed with the physical attributes that you are trying to develop in your program. Specific information on physical testing and evaluation is covered in more detail later in this book.

Acute Programming Variables

While the needs analysis provides the foundation and direction that the resistance training program is built upon, the acute program variables are the specific decisions made that will shape the program so it accomplishes the training goals. Manipulation of the six acute programming variables—exercise selection, training frequency, exercise order, training load/repetitions, volume and rest periods—determine which of the training goals of developing muscular strength, power, hypertrophy or muscular endurance occur. All the program variables must be coordinated toward the training goal for training to be optimized. The NSCA provides program variable guidelines to give a framework for the development of a successful program.

Know the Training Goals

Before reviewing the program variables and the guidelines, one needs to have a clear understanding of the four training goals.

- **Muscular strength** targets the development of maximal or absolute strength. The goal of muscular strength training is maximal force production.
- **Power development** seeks to produce force as quickly as possible. The equation for power is force or work divided by elapsed time ($P = W/\Delta t$). Whereas force production relies primarily on the muscular system, power results from the coordination of the muscular and nervous systems to produce force as quickly as possible.
- **Hypertrophy** refers to the growth of the muscle fibers. Hypertrophy training increases muscle size, which in turn increases the capacity of the muscle to produce strength.
- **Muscle endurance** focuses on the ability of a muscle to sustain a submaximal effort.

The NSCA guidelines provide recommendations for how to manipulate each of the six-training variables to produce four different training goals.

Exercise Selection

Selecting exercises used in a program should be done strategically based on common sports movements, training experience of the athletes, equipment availability and common injury sites. Linking the sport movement analysis to exercise selection makes programs more sport specific. Exercises can be chosen based on movement patterns, muscles used and joint actions utilized in a sport. Choosing the exercises to be used in a resistance training program is an excellent example of how a good news analysis shapes decisions made in designing a program. For example, tennis players need to be able to move well laterally. To help enhance lateral movement, frontal plane exercises like a side lunge or lateral step up can be incorporated in a program. Tennis strokes use upper body musculature including the shoulders, chest and back. A chest fly trains the chest muscles while horizontally adducting the arms similar to a forehand stroke. Rotation is heavily utilized in tennis and can be included in abdominal training to target the oblique muscles through twisting exercises like the Russian twist or cable chop.

Training experience and equipment availability can also dictate exercise choices. In basketball, increasing power plays an important role in increasing jump height and speed. Not every facility is equipped with bumper plates and platforms or specialized flooring to do explosive lifting like power cleans. Similarly, athletes with little training experience would not be prepared to attempt complex lifts safely, like the power clean. If proper equipment is not available, then coaches need to select exercises that produce similar adaptations using equipment that is available. In the case of training for power using triple extension movements, plyometric exercises or kettlebell/dumbbell swings could be used. If proper equipment is available, but experience is lacking, then coaches need to take time to progress their athletes properly before using complex exercises. With power cleans, it could take months to progress athletes through clean variations from basic movements like a power shrug or a high pull at different heights or from a rack before ever attempting a full power clean from the floor.

Another factor that needs to be considered when selecting exercises is common injuries. Using tennis as a continued example, rotator cuff injuries are common in sports that feature overhead movements. Band internal and external rotation exercises can be incorporated to help prevent shoulder injuries. Promoting muscle balance is an important factor in injury prevention. Muscles work together in pairs. Too much emphasis on one side creates an imbalance on the opposite side, which can easily lead to an injury. Performing too many quadriceps dominant exercises can create a situation where the hamstrings muscles can be overpowered and injured. That is why posterior chain exercises like Romanian deadlifts need to be included to strengthen the hamstrings and promote muscle balance.

Training Frequency

Frequency of resistance training is a key to effectively achieving the desired training outcome. When training the muscular system, pushing the muscle past its normal limits (the overload principle) signals the body that it needs to get stronger to be able to handle similar taxing demands in the future. To do this, the muscle is broken down and built back stronger. Training too frequently places the muscle in a situation where it is constantly broken down and never has a chance to rebuild or recover. That is why it is generally recommended to allow 24–48 hours of recovery between training sessions for the same muscle group. Adequate recovery time needs to be taken to allow the muscle to build back stronger. This is the key to the principle of use and disuse, if the muscle is overloaded appropriately and given enough rest to rebuild, an athlete will continue to get stronger. However, if too long is taken in between training sessions then the body begins to lose the gains that had been made.

How long it takes the body to adapt to training is directly related to the amount of physical training experience an athlete has. Athletes that have been training longer have prepared their bodies to be able to adapt to a training stimulus quicker. As a result, they can train more frequently. Inexperienced athletes have not developed the ability to recover as quickly and need more time between sessions to improve optimally. The NSCA defines beginning or untrained athletes as having a physical training age of two months or less, intermediate athletes have two to six months of training experience and advanced athletes have training for a year or more (Haff & Triplett, 2016). The training frequency recommendations by the NSCA are two to three sessions a week for beginners, three to four times a week for intermediate and four to seven times a week for advanced.

It is important to note that with higher frequencies of training the body still needs time to adapt and the same muscle group should not be trained two days in a row. Full-body training programs that include all major muscle groups should not be performed more than three days a week. One day of rest is needed in between each training session. More frequent training utilizes what is referred to as a split routine where muscle groups are strategically rotated so that the same muscles are not training on consecutive days. A common split routine is a four-day upper/lower body split. In a four-day routine the upper body would be training twice a week, such as Mondays and Thursdays, then the lower body would be training two days a week on Tuesdays and Fridays. The more frequent the training, the more complex the split routines become so that muscle groups have adequate rest before they are trained again.

Sport season is another factor that influences training frequency. The pre-season or first transition phase is a period when sport training demands an increase in preparation for competition and physical training is peaked. During the in-season of competitive training phase, sport practice and competition are the priority and physical training is continued in a decreased capacity to maintain training gains throughout the competitive season. The postseason or second transition phase (often referred to as an active rest period) is a time of recovery that provides time for rest and recuperation after the heavy demands of competition. Off-season or the preparation phase of training is the period of time between the postseason (about four weeks after competition ends) to the preseason (about six weeks prior to the first competition) when physical development is the primary goal. The NSCA recommends resistance training frequencies of four to six sessions per week during the off-season, three to four sessions per week during the preseason, one to three sessions per week during the in-season and zero to three sessions (informally) during the postseason.

Exercise Order

Exercise order can be a key factor in optimizing training to produce desired results. In general, exercises should be ordered from large to small because smaller muscles work together with larger muscles in exercises involving the large muscle groups. Small muscle group exercises can often be trained using isolation exercises like biceps curls for the biceps or triceps extensions for the triceps. However, training small muscles first can have a negative effect on the performance of large muscle group exercises. For example, the triceps are incorporated in the bench press. If the triceps are trained before the bench press, then the triceps can become fatigued which limits the effectiveness of the bench press to train the chest. Fatiguing the triceps creates a weak link in the chain of muscles used in the bench press. This can result in preventing the right amount of overload in the chest to produce improvement. When training athletes, training small before large muscles (pre-fatiguing) is not recommended.

Being able to categorize exercises helps coaches order exercise properly. Primary exercises are exercises that generally involve multiple muscles and multiple joints like squats, deadlifts, lunges and leg presses for the lower body and bench/chest press, shoulder press, pull ups and lat pulldowns for the upper body. Secondary exercises use one joint and focus on one muscle group to isolate specific muscles. Power exercises that utilize triple extension are a special type of primary exercise and should always go at the beginning of a workout. Since these exercises are complex and involve maximal effort, power exercises need to be performed when the body is fresh at the beginning of a workout. This will promote optimal technical performance and reduce injury risk. As a general rule, power exercises should be performed first, followed by primary exercises and then secondary exercises.

Within the strategy of progressing from power, to primary, to secondary exercises, exercise order can strategically be arranged to increase or decrease the demands of the workout. Alternating upper and lower body exercises can be less taxing due to the extra recovery time provided by alternating. Pushing and pulling movements use similar muscles, like upper body pushing muscles use the chest, shoulders and triceps while upper body pulling movements use the back and biceps.

Examples of Upper/Lower Body Exercise Order while Progressing from Primary to Secondary Exercises

Alternate upper and lower body:	Alternate pushing and pulling within the upper or lower body:
• Bench press • Back squat • Bent over row • Alternating lunge • Shoulder press • Leg curl • Biceps curl • Leg extension • Triceps extension	• Bench press • Bent over row • Shoulder press • Biceps curl • Triceps Extensions

Loading and Repetitions

The intensity of a set of repetitions is based on the loading or number of repetitions used. Lighter, sub-maximal weights can be used for a higher number of repetitions. As the weight increases and gets closer to a maximum amount that can be lifted, the repetitions decrease. Loading intensity is often related to the percentage of a one-repetition maximum (1RM) lift. Procedures for determining the 1RM load are explained in the testing section of this book (on page 369-370). In general, heavy loads are used to overload the muscle to stimulate maximal or absolute strength gains, and more repetitions with lighter loads are used to produce gains in muscular endurance and hypertrophy.

The NSCA provides recommendations for the 1RM loading percentages and goal repetitions for strength, single-effort power, multiple-effort power, hypertrophy and muscular endurance (see table below). The NSCA recommendation for maximal or absolute strength gains is six or less repetitions at a load of 85% or more of 1RM (Haff & Triplett, 2016). Single-effort power loading should be between 80-90% of 1RM for one to two repetitions and multiple effort-power should utilize 75-85% of 1RM for three to five repetitions (Haff & Triplett, 2016). Between six and 12 repetitions at between 67-85% of 1RM is recommended for hypertrophy training (Haff & Triplett, 2016). 67% or less of 1RM with 12 or more repetitions should be used to promote muscular endurance (Haff & Triplett, 2016).

Load and Repetition Assignments Based on the Training Goal

Training Goal	Load (%1RM)	Goal Repetitions
Strength	≥ 85	≤ 6

Power:
   Single-effort event
   Multiple-effort event
	
	80 - 90
	75 - 85
		
		1 – 2
		3 - 5

Hypertrophy	67 - 85	6 - 12
Muscle endurance	≤ 67	≥ 12

Essentials of Strength Training and Conditioning – NSCA (4th ed.)
Table 17.9 (Haff & Triplett, 2016)

Based on the SAID principle (detailed in the first chapter of this book), after overloading the body utilizing the NSCA guidelines for strength, power, hypertrophy and muscle endurance will provide the body with stimulus needed to produce the targeted training adaptation. However, once the body adapts to a stimulus, the stimulus must be changed or increased for improvement to continue, as is explained in the principle of progressive resistance in the first chapter. The NSCA provides guidelines for increasing weight based on the strength, size and training level of the athlete and the area of the body being trained. Larger, stronger, more experienced athletes can handle larger increases in weight than smaller, weaker, less experienced athletes. Since lower body muscles are generally larger than upper body muscles, the lower body can handle larger increases in weight (see table below). For smaller, weaker, or less experienced athletes the NSCA recommends increasing by 2.5–5 pounds (1-2 kg) for upper body exercises and 5-10 pounds (2-4 kg) for lower body exercises (Haff & Triplett, 2016). Upper body exercise increases of 5-10+ pounds (2-4+ kg) and lower body increases of 10-15+ pounds (4-7+ kg) are recommended for larger, stronger, or more experienced athletes (Haff & Triplett, 2016).

Examples of Load Increases

Description of Athlete	Body Area Exercise	Estimated Load Increase
Smaller, weaker, less trained	Upper body Lower body	2.5 – 5 lb. (1 – 2 kg) 5 – 10 lb. (2 – 4 kg)
Larger, stronger, more trained	Upper body Lower body	5 – 10+ lb. (2 – 4+ kg) 10 - 15+ lb. (4 – 7+ kg)

Essentials of Strength Training and Conditioning – NSCA (4th ed.)
Table 17.10 (Haff & Triplett, 2016)

Rest Periods

The time taken to recover between sets or exercise is an important factor that is often overlooked. When training for maximal strength and power, athletes have a tendency to rest to little, which will reduce the effectiveness of the training. Both maximal strength and power training require full recovery; put the body in a position where energy stores have been fully recycled to optimize each training set. The longer the rest periods are, the more energy or ATP that the body is able to recycle. This allows the body to use maximal effort to lift heavier, high-intensity loads for the targeted number of repetitions. The NSCA recommends two to five minutes of rest between sets when training for maximal strength, single-effort power and maximal-effort power (Haff & Triplett, 2016).

When training for hypertrophy and muscular endurance, rest periods are shortened to intentionally challenge the body by creating a situation where the body is working from behind in its energy production. Shorter rest periods do not allow all the energy to be recycled. For example, an athlete may start out at 100% energy capacity during the first set, but the shortened recovery only allows 75% of the energy to be recycled for the second set. Then, when the shorter rest is repeated, the lifter could be at 50% for the third set. This energy deficit stimulates the body to increase muscle endurance and size and challenge the anaerobic glycolytic system to generate energy to make up the deficit. The NSCA recommends using rest periods between 30 to 90 seconds when targeting hypertrophy and 30 seconds or less when training for muscular endurance (Haff & Triplett, 2016).

Volume

Volume refers to the total amount of work performed in a workout. Volume can be indexed using the total amount lifted in the workout, which is a product of the combination of the sets, repetitions and weights used in a workout; or by the total sets and repetitions used in a workout. Training status can influence the volume needed to produce improvements. Beginners will show gains using lower volumes of one to two sets. Research has shown that beginners can get a majority of gains produced with three sets of training when using just one set of an exercise. Beginners have not built up as much tolerance to training as experienced lifters and, as a result, beginners can overload muscles with lower volumes of training. Knowing this can help a coach ease new athletes into a training program safely.

Experienced lifters have built up a tolerance to training that requires a higher volume of training to produce results. The NSCA recommends use of two to six sets when training for maximal strength and three to five sets for either single-effort or multiple-effort power training (Haff & Triplett, 2016). Three to six sets are recommended when targeting hypertrophy and two to three sets are recommended for muscular endurance training (Haff & Triplett, 2016).

Summary

The development of resistance training programs starts with a sports needs analysis consisting of a sport evaluation and an athlete assessment. The sport evaluation explores what you want to accomplish through your program by examining the movements, physiology (including energy systems utilized) and common injuries related to the sport targeted. The athlete analysis provides the realities of the athletes you are training by examining the training level (physical training experience and experience with exercises) and the current capabilities (determined from baseline testing) of your athletes. The needs analysis, along with the administrative variables of time and equipment available for training, provides a foundation and direction for designing sport-specific resistance training programs.

The plan for achieving the goals outlined through the needs analysis is developed by properly manipulating the acute training variables. Choices made in exercise selection, training frequency, exercise order, loading/repetitions, duration of rest periods and training volume all need to be coordinated towards the common goal of increasing muscular strength, power, hypertrophy or endurance. The NSCA provides training guidelines for coaches to coordinate these program variables towards the desired training outcome.

In general, training for maximal strength requires heavy loads with a lower number of repetitions and full recovery. Muscular endurance improvements can be produced using lighter loads, more repetitions and shorter rest periods. The combination of light to moderate loading, a moderate number of repetitions and shorter rest periods stimulates production of growth hormone and testosterone, which stimulates muscle growth.

To maximize power production, power exercises should always be placed at the beginning of the workout (following a proper warm-up) when the body is fresh and technique and effort can be maximized. Full recovery needs to be allowed whenever training for power to reduce chance of injury and maximize levels of performance. This means that two to five minutes of rest should be used with power exercises even when training for muscular hypertrophy and endurance that normally require shorter rest periods. The number of repetitions and training volume should also be reduced following NSCA power guidelines, even if the rest of the workout targets muscle endurance or hypertrophy. The key to power production is moving the weight as fast as possible; following these special power recommendations will help optimize power training while reducing injury risk.

The table below provides a summary of the NSCA recommendations for repetitions, loading, number of sets and rest intervals for developing maximal strength, hypertrophy, muscle endurance and single-effort and multiple-effort power.

NSCA Recommendation Summary

Training Goal	Load (%1RM)	Goal Repetitions	Sets	Rest Interval
Strength	≥ 85	≤ 6	2 – 6	2 – 5 min.
Power: Single-effort event	80 - 90	1 - 2	3 - 5	2 – 5 min.
Power: Multiple-effort event	75 - 85	3 - 5	3 - 5	2 – 5 min.
Hypertrophy	67 - 85	6 - 12	3 - 6	30 sec. – 90 sec. (1.5 min.)
Muscle endurance	≤ 67	≥ 12	2 - 3	≤ 30 sec.

Essentials of Strength Training and Conditioning – NSCA (4th ed.) (Haff & Triplett, 2016)

Reference: Chapter 12

1. Haff, G. G., and Triplett, N. T. *Essentials of Strength Training and Conditioning-NSCA* (4th ed). Champaign, IL: Human Kinetics, 2016.

13
ATHLETIC DEVELOPMENT & SPORT-SPECIFIC DESIGN

By: Scott O'Dell

Director of Strength & Conditioning, East Central University

Energy Systems

There are three energy systems the body uses (Wilkins):

1. The Adenosine Triphosphate (ATP) energy system, which provides instant energy for intense exercise such as that used by a powerlifter performing a 1-repetition maximum.
2. The Non-Oxidative/Glycolytic energy system, which starts to be used after the first 2-3 seconds of exercise such as that used by a 100 meter sprinter.
3. The Oxidative energy system, which is used for events lasting longer than 2 minutes.

Weight training is beneficial in any type of training program for any type of sport. However, it is still common to see people running long distances with the belief it will make them faster or more in shape. The following factors take place when using long distance running as the only training technique: the muscle learns to be slow, the foot learns to maintain a longer contact time with the ground, it does nothing to teach sprinting mechanics, it can lead to overtraining symptoms such as shin splints and joint tendinitis, and it diminishes any power and speed development gained from other areas of training. Abernathy, et al (1999) studied this directly and found that "concurrent strength and endurance training appears to inhibit strength development when compared with strength training alone." There are major benefits to building a training program that includes weight training for strength and power with your endurance training.

Kraemer and Fleck (2004) have found the following when strength and endurance training are used concurrently:

1. High-intensity endurance training may compromise strength, especially at high velocities of muscle actions.
2. Power capabilities may be most affected by the performance of both strength and endurance training.
3. High-intensity endurance training may negatively affect short-term anaerobic performance.
4. The development of peak oxygen consumption is not compromised by a heavy resistance training program.
5. Strength training does not negatively affect endurance capabilities.
6. Strength and power training programs may benefit endurance performances by preventing injuries, increasing lactic acid threshold and reducing the ground contact time during running. Strength training can positively affect endurance training but endurance training negatively affects strength training.

If you have any questions about this as a coach, try filming one player for an entire game or practice. When watching the film, hold a stopwatch in your hand. Write down the length of time for every period of seconds your athlete is standing or out of the game in black ink. Then also write down the length of time for every period of seconds your athlete is in movement in red ink. And keep in mind that, for most sports, when movement is taking place, your athlete is moving in a powerful, high-speed fashion to make a play. Now, at the completion of the game or practice, take a look at your sheet and you should have numbers recorded alternating back and forth between black and red ink. The results are typically surprising for many coaches as to how much time the body is not in movement compared to how much time the body is involved in a powerful, fast movement. For many coaches who played their sport this is shocking because as players your mind is constantly working, so it feels as though you are moving non-stop. Even though your mind may be working, your body is not always working. If you condition your athletes using the appropriate energy systems for their sport, then not only will their body perform better, but their mind will perform better as well.

Here is an example of results you would likely see. The following chart showing the percentages of energy systems are used for each sport is taken from *Essentials of Strength Training and Conditioning* (1994):

Sport:	(ATP) (Anaerobic)	Non-Oxidative/Glycolytic (Anaerobic & Aerobic)	Oxidative (Aerobic)
Baseball	80	20	-
Basketball	85	15	-
Fencing	90	10	-
Field Hockey	60	20	20
Football	90	10	-
Golf	95	5	-
Gymnastics	90	10	-
Ice Hockey			
Forward, defense	80	20	-
Goalie	95	5	-

Sport:	(ATP) (Anaerobic)	Non-Oxidative/Glycolytic (Anaerobic & Aerobic)	Oxidative (Aerobic)
Lacrosse			
Goalie, def, att	80	20	-
Midfielders	60	20	20
Rowing	20	30	50
Skiing			
Slalom, jump, down	80	20	-
Cross-country	-	5	95
Pleasure skiing	34	33	33
Soccer			
Goalie, wings, strik	80	20	-
Halfbacks or link men	60	20	20
Swimming and diving			
50 yd, diving	98	2	0
100 yd	80	15	5
200 yd	30	65	5
400 yd, 500 yd	20	40	40
1500 yd, 1650 yd	10	20	70
Tennis	70	20	10
Track and Field			
100 yd, 220 yd	98	2	-
Field Events	90	10	-
440 yd	80	15	5
880 yd	30	65	5
1 mile	20	55	25
2 miles	20	40	40
3 miles	10	20	70
6 miles (cross country)	5	15	80
Marathon	-	5	95
Volleyball	90	10	-
Wrestling	90	10	-

Taking a look at the energy systems definitions in the first paragraph and looking at the percentage of energy systems used in the chart should give you an idea of your ideal work-to-rest ratio to be working towards as you get to a pre-competition phase. You should also look at the amount of change of direction and the most common sprinting distances covered in your sport. This also shows that if you play a sport such as softball where athletes are in an anaerobic state for over 75% of the time, then testing the mile is more detrimental than positive.

If you are in softball your athlete's sit in the dugout, then they get up and hopefully make contact and sprint to first base. If they are a great hitter then 3 out of 10 times they will stay at first base for a period of minutes before sprinting for maximum speed again. A pitcher might throw 100 pitches a game; this is 100 repetitions of maximum power (e.g., a plyometrics workout). Therefore teaching the body to perform slower by running a mile is not beneficial to the sport performance. If you want to increase your chances of winning, concentrate more on speed and agility training to create more infield hits, turn singles into doubles and field more balls, therefore decreasing the chances your opponents have to get on base.

Conditioning Drills

Conditioning drills are important to condition the athlete for optimal performance during the competition. When designing your program, consider how long the drill takes your team or athlete to perform and then decide the rest intervals, with the goal to make them as sport specific as possible. For example, if you are spending 10 minutes on the conditioning drills for softball or baseball players, replicate the percentages of time they spend in an anaerobic state—eight minutes total of slower conditioning to keep them in anaerobic state and two minutes total of aerobic state. Do condition at the end of your field/court work. If you are conditioning at the end of a speed/agility/plyometric session, keep in mind that your athletes have already been through a workout by the time you get to this point. It is easy to do too much; be aware of overtraining and be patient knowing you have an entire off-season to get to where you want to be. For most sports, a dose of repeated bouts of speed and explosion without full recovery are going to define sport-specific conditioning. And remember that 60 seconds, or 400 meters of a linear sprint is the standard breaking point when sprint mechanics turn into distance mechanics. It should be a goal of the conditioning to not drive the athlete to losing sprint mechanics.

Fast Pace 20s   • Repeated twenty-yard sprints with minimal recovery time.
Forward and Backs (5 yards)   • Sprint forward 5 yards and backpedal five for a total of twenty-five yards of work.

Forward and Backs (20 yards)
   • Sprint forward 5 yards
   • Backpedal 5
   • Sprint forward 10 yards
   • Backpedal 10
   • Sprint forward 15 yards
   • Backpedal 15
   • Sprint forward 20 yards

150-yard shuttles
- Sprint 5
- Cut and sprint back to the starting point
- Sprint 10
- Cut and sprint back to the starting point
- Sprint 15
- Cut and sprint back to the starting point
- Sprint 20
- Cut and sprint back to the starting point
- Sprint 25
- Cut and sprint back to the starting point

300-yard shuttles (25-yard distance)
- Sprint 25 yards
- Cut and sprint back 25 yards to the starting point
- Repeat 5 more times for a total of 12 25-yard sprints

300-yard shuttle (50-yard distance)
- Sprint 50 yards
- Cut and sprint back 50 yards to the starting point
- Repeat 2 more times for a total of 6 50-yard sprints

Extra Cardio

If your athletes are doing extra cardio workouts to lose some fat, help them understand that is not the most efficient way to burn fat. Compare the body of a world class distance runner with a world class sprinter and just with the naked eye one can see the sprinter has a much leaner build with lower body fat. The long-distance runner trains with a very long, steady state of running. The sprinter trains with bouts of speed, explosion and power, thus creating more of an increase in testosterone levels (Copeland, et al, 2004). Hackney, et al (1995) found the same results stating, "the present findings suggest the relationship between testosterone is affected by anaerobic exercise but not aerobic exercise." Gray, et al (1993) took eight trained male athletes through an intense interval exercise protocol to exhaustion and immediate post-tests showed a 38% increase in testosterone and a 2000% increase in growth hormone. Testosterone promotes fat loss (Bonifacio et al, 2005), muscle strengthening (Fleck and Kraemer, 2004), and bone mineral density (Bonifacio et al, 2005). If athletes want to have extra workouts to burn fat, they should continue in the same style of conditioning training for more testosterone stimulation and maximum effectiveness for their time, while also not compromising any increases in power and speed.

References: Chapter 13

1. Abernathy, P.J., Barry, B. K., Leveritt, M., Logan, P.A. "Concurrent Strength and Endurance Training: A Review." *Sports Medicine* 28, no. 6 (December, 1999): 413-427.

2. Baechle, T.R. *Essentials of Strength Training and Conditioning.* Champaign, IL: Human Kinetics, 1994.

3. Barnes, M., Cissik, J. *Sports Speed and Agility.* Monterey, CA: Coaches Circle, 2004.

4. Bompa, T.O., Carrera, M. *Periodization Training for Sports.* Champaign, IL: Human Kinetics, 2005.

5. Bonifacio, V., Fabbri, A., Gianfrill, D., Gianetta, E., Greco, E., Isidori, A., Isidori, A. M., Lenzi, A. "Effects of Testosterone on Body Composition, Bone Metabolism, and Serum Lipid Profile in Middle-Aged Men: A Meta-Analyses." *Clinical Endocrinology* 63, no. 3 (September, 2005): 280-293.

6. Bowerman, W.J., Freeman, W.H. *High Performance Training for Track and Field.* Champaign, IL: Human Kinetics, 1991.

7. Brown, L., Ferrigno, V.A. *Training for Speed, Agility, and Quickness, 2nd ed.* Champaign, IL: Human Kinetics, 2005.

8. Brughelli, M., Cronin, J. Preventing Hamstring Injuries in Sport. *Strength and Conditioning Journal* 30, no. 1 (February, 2008): 55-64.

9. Costello, F., Kreis, E.J. *Sports Agility.* Nashville, TN: Taylor Sports, 1993.

10. Dintiman, G., Ward, B. *Sport Speed.* Champaign, IL: Human Kinetics, 2003.

11. Farentinos, R., Radcliffe, J. *High Powered Plyometrics.* Champaign, IL: Human Kinetics, 1999.

12. Fleck, S. J., Kraemer, W. J. *Designing Resistance Training Programs Third Edition.* Champaign, IL: Human Kinetics, 2004.

13. Foran, B. *High Performance Sports Conditioning.* Champaign, IL: Human Kinetics, 2001.

14. Gray, A. B., Telford, R. D., Weidemann, M. J. "Endocrine Response to Intense Interval Exercise." *European Journal of Applied Physiology* 66, no. 4 (April, 1993): 366-371.

15. Hackney, A. C., Premo, M. C., McMurray, R. G. "Influence of Aerobic Versus Anaerobic Exercise on the Relationship Between reproductive Hormones in Men." *Journal of Sports Sciences* 13, no. 4 (August, 1995): 305-311.

16. Halberg, G.V. "Relationships among power, acceleration, maximum speed, programmed agility, and reactive agility: The neural fundamentals of agility." Master's thesis, Central Michigan University, Mount Pleasant, MI, 2001.

17. Hay, J.G., Reid, J.G. *Anatomy, Mechanics, and Human Motion, 2nd ed.* Englewood Cliffs, NJ: Prentice Hall, 1988.

18. Helgurud, J., Hetland, E., Hoff, J., Rognmo, O., Slordahl, S. "High Intensity Aerobic Exercise in Superior to Moderate Intensity Exercise for Increasing Aerobic Capacity in Patients with Coronary Artery Disease." *European Journal of Cardiovascular Prevention and Rehabilitation* 11, no. 3 (June, 2004): 216-222.

19. Landin, D., Nelson, A. G., Schexnayder, I. C., Winchester, J. B., Young, M. A. "Static Stretching Impairs Sprint Performance in Collegiate Track and Field Athletes." *Journal of Strength and Conditioning Research* 22, no. 1 (January, 2008): 13-18.

20. Pearson, C. *National Strength and Conditioning Association Minnesota Sports Performance Clinic.* University of Minnesota, 2014.

21. Radcliffe, J. C. *Functional Training for Athletes at All Levels.* Berkeley, CA: Ulysses Press, 2007.

22. Radcliffe, J. "Getting into Position." *Training and Conditioning* 9, no. 3 (April, 1999): 38-47.

23. Seagrave, L. *United States of America Track and Field Level I Certification Workshop.* The University of North Carolina-Chapel Hill, 2008.

24. Wilkens, K. J. "Endurance Training: Intervals Versus Long-Slow/Steady Distance." DragonDoor.com. https://www.dragondoor.com/articles/endurance-training-intervals-vs-long-slow/steady-distance/.

14
PERIODIZATION OF EXERCISE

By: Ben Cook

Author & Director of Programming and Pit Crew Recruiting, PIT Instruction & Training

PERIODIZATION HAS BECOME the principal method of organizing sports training plans. Periodization is a model of training that has shifted from an emphasis on work, to work recovery. This subtle shift in thinking is now so ingrained in athletic training plans that coaches and trainers sometimes confuse what portion of training is periodization and what is programming choice. To understand periodization, it helps to think about simple physical adaptations to stress. The formation of a callus on the hand is one simple example. The body is introduced to an abrasion caused by friction. The irritating abrasion forms a blister. Allowed to heal, the blister hardens into a callus. The hand is now stronger and better prepared for future, heavier work. The work in this example is not defined. The

- Programming applies changes/manipulation to various training variables at a particular time in the training.
- Periodization establishes the total arch of time for training and the divisions of that arch to best optimize recovery.
- Before you can periodize any program of training you need to understand the training variables.

work is the programming establishing the stress of callus formation, and even though programming is significant, the time allowed for recovery is when the callus actualizes. Work in the bench press exercise may be used by a powerlifter, a bodybuilder and a volleyball player, but how each athlete's recovery may be structured is vastly different.

The History of Periodization

When the body is confronted with any type of physical stress, it responds by either getting better at managing the stress or becoming worse at managing the stress. Periodization is simply a plan of recovery implemented over time that manages physical stress for improved performance outcomes. The benefits of a proper recovery plan can reduce fatigue and injury while enhancing peak power, strength, and athletic performance.

Periodization principals are not exclusively a modern idea. A myriad of thought dating nearly 4,000 years has formed the foundations of our modern training concepts. Li Ji, Confucius, Plato, Galen and even Leonardo Da Vinci considered the human body's adaptable qualities and the need for rest after work. [8] Massachusetts physician Henry Gassett Davis saw the human body's protective remodeling abilities against physical forces. In the late 1800s, while using traction to lengthen shortened tendons in clubfoot patients, Davis formulated ideas about imposed demands and tissue adaptations. Davis' work would give rise to a cornerstone of exercise science known as Specific Adaptations to Imposed Demands or the SAID principle, which supports the use of controlled forces to coax the body into making favorable adaptations.

In 1936 McGill University's Hans Selye proposed the General Adaptation Syndrome (GAS), a three-stage theory for how the body responds to stress. [2] Although Selye's research was focused primarily on the endocrine system's response to extreme deprivation and environmental conditions, it had many similarities to the SAID principle. Soon other scientists around the world began formulating the GAS model's theories, applying it to other stressful events like sports training. Exercise physiologists would eventually adapt Selye's three stages theory to sports training plans to incrementally introduce work intensity while controlling for fatigue.

In the United States during the 1970s, UCLA's John Garhammer began his initial investigations of traditional periodization, introducing it to American athletes. [19] During the 1980s, Mike Stone and Harold O'Bryant teamed to examine periodization principles. Their various research articles and an eventual book "The Scientific Approach to Strength Training" [18] finally gave tactical ways to adopt periodization into athletic training programs.

Stone and O'Bryant's Periodization Stages

- Stage 1 Hypertrophy Stage – Fatigue to muscle exhaustion induced by high repetitions and shorter rest intervals between sets of exercise. Intended for increasing muscle endurance, size and creating a well-conditioned muscular foundation for the strength and power work that would follow.

- Stage 2 Basic Strength Stage – Six to eight weeks of heavier work. Repetitions are incrementally reduced while using greater resistance. Intended to increase both the muscles' leverage potential and neural drive.

- Stage 3 Strength and Power Stage – The load continues to increase as the repetitions drop in number down to 2 or 3 repetitions. Here, the movement speeds are increased to positively affect the reflex components of the nervous system.

- Stage 4 Peaking or Maintenance Stage – The repetitions in the core lifts are reduced to 1 or 2 repetitions, while ancillary or assistance exercises are performed with 3 to 5 repetitions. The use of assistance exercises maintains muscle mass and conditioning, while the explosively performed 1 and 2 repetition exercises further sharpen the nervous system's ability to activate muscle fibers.

- Stage 5 Active Rest Stage – Shortly prior to competition the athlete could reduce the workload in their primary activities, but increase their general conditioning. This gave rise to the concept of "tapering" or reducing workload to maximize muscle recovery.

Block Periodization

In 1965 Leo Matveyev, building on previous ideas practiced by Boris Kotov, Lauri Pihkala and Lazlo Nadori,[8] offered a training concept which considered structured recovery being more important than linear progression training. [4,5,6,18] Russian Olympic success during the nineteen fifties and sixties advanced Matveyev's periodization concept throughout Europe. Eventually, the practice of out working one's opponent began being replaced with a strategic balance of work and proper recovery. Versions of his periodization model were soon adapted by all sports.

In the mid-1980s, Yuri Verkhoshansky began conceptualizing his "Supertraining" shock concepts. [17] Verkhoshansky proposed that shorter accumulative shock workouts could sustain longer periods of peak power and strength. This application was of great value to multiple competition sport athletes who found it difficult to train like Olympic weightlifters and powerlifters. Verhosshansky's Conjugated Successive System (CSS), is considered the origin of both "Plyometric" and "Block Periodization" concepts.

Block Periodization attempts to address team sports' issues with Matveyev's traditional periodization model. [5,6] Team sports athletes have many competitions during a sports season and must improve in areas other than overload strength and power. Simultaneously distributing training focus on multiple areas results in high training volumes. These high volumes can reduce peak effectiveness in all focus areas. [14] Blocks are shorter periods (3 to 6 weeks) structured to produce short term peaks in power output. Support for these shorter periodized blocks came from Iñigo Mujika in his 2009 book *Tapering and Peaking for Optimal Performance*, [13] where he suggested that peak power could only be maintained for a maximum of three weeks. Block Periodization attempts to extend maximum output by shortening the workout stage and diversifying the exercise choices into complementary adjuncts.

Define the Work

You must weigh the impact of any planned work if you expect to recover from it. It is therefore important to clearly define what you are really working for. If you are a powerlifter, your recovery requirements will be vastly different from an Olympic weightlifter, football player, body builder or spartan racer. Proper recovery from the work depends on clearly understanding what physical work is required for your objectives.

Before you can properly plan the work, you should understand what effect the work will have on the body, particularly the muscles involved. It has been said that every system of the body is designed to support the brain and muscular system. Nothing happens without brain function, and without muscle function, life cannot be sustained or duplicated. Muscles are metabolic engines, demanding and utilizing food energy. A variety of muscle fibers exists to help the body perform different types of work. (11) Whether work defines a muscle's chemical structure or a muscle's chemical structure defines a muscle's best work are both likely true. Observe the work to determine the most involved muscle fibers. Work differences place demands on different muscle fiber types. To achieve overall performance improvement, the athlete must make improvements to the muscle fibers best suited for the performance.

Muscle Fiber Types

Only the average internal muscles and those responsible for less voluntary work have a higher endurance capacity. Primary movers are chemically divided evenly for both power and endurance work. Work concentrations can shift the chemical profiles of chemically intermediate muscle fibers to benefit either endurance or power concentrations. Based on Myosin ATPase staining studies, there are seven skeletal muscle fiber types in humans. However only three fiber types are most often referenced in exercise studies: Type I (Slow Oxidative [SO]), Type IIa (Fast Oxidative Glycolytic [FOG]) and Type IIb or Type IIx (Fast Glycolytic [FG]). [11]

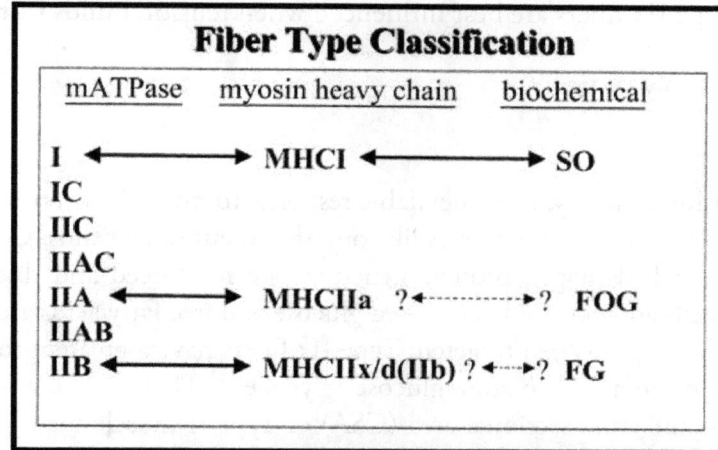

Fiber Type Classification

Type I fibers are used primarily during endurance activities and Type IIx fibers are used when power is required. The Type IIa fibers can be influenced by either endurance or power work and are thought to shift their chemical profiles to aid in the type of work being performed. Considering fiber types is important in exercise program design, because if you are a power athlete it will be counterproductive to reduce Type IIx power producing work for Type I and Type IIa endurance work volumes.

Fiber Recruitment

Researchers have examined how power and endurance activities can influence muscle fibers types, and simply, the more repetitions performed, the more Type I fibers improve their function and size. While quickly moved, heavier loads influence the size and function of Type IIx fibers.

Nerve Influences Fiber

Each muscle fiber is activated by a nerve fiber, and the speed at which that nerve delivers impulse influences the fiber's type. Impulses from slow motor neurons chemically influence Type I fibers. Intermediate impulse speeds influence Type IIa fibers and Type IIx fibers are influenced by the larger fast motor neurons' impulse speeds. Organelles in the muscle and tendons signal for the required muscle tension to handle the workload. The necessary speed of impulse is then delivered. More Type I fibers begin the work if the workload is lighter requiring less initial muscle tension.

Muscle Fiber Recruitment Order

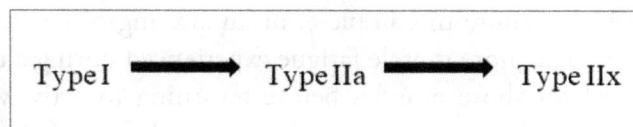

However, as tension builds with fatigue, more Type IIa and IIx fibers are recruited. Near exhaustion, the athlete is forced to alter form and speed the movement to complete the final repetitions, thus charging Type IIx fibers with the final work. If only one powerful movement is required, there is a similar recruitment pattern from Type I through Type IIx fibers (although much faster). Although Type IIx fibers are eventually recruited with exhaustive activities, the slower buildup of tension reduces their maximal effect. Type IIx fibers are best influenced when tension builds instantly with little to no exhaustion. [9,11]

Muscle Fiber Size

Muscle size increases, or hypertrophy, is an inevitable response to muscular exertion. After being stressed, muscle fibers attempt to restructure themselves like our aforementioned callus. Cell bodies are increased in the cytoplasm of the cell, damaged protein structures are reinforced and thickened, pathways and receptors in and on the cells are increased and stored glucose and free fatty acids are multiplied. This happens regardless of the fiber type. When targeted, Type IIx fibers have a greater growth potential because of their affinity to both protein and to store glucose (glycogen). Therefore, low volume, heavily explosive exercise can increase the cross-sectional area (CSA) of Type II muscle mass. [21] Increases in muscle mass can help to stabilize, cushion and increase leverage potential around the body's joints. Therefore, suitable increases in muscle mass can benefit the power athlete. However, not all muscle mass is the same. Increases in Type I fiber mass can also provide leverage, cushion and stability; however, these fibers receive slower nerve impulses which may diffuse nerve impulse speeds preferred by Type IIx fibers. [11,12]

Think of the path of water. Water trying to find its path will seek larger openings before smaller ones. A path of least resistance is its choice. The large openings take the impulse of water while simultaneously reducing pressure on the smaller openings. If reversed, and small pathways are made more accessible then the larger pathways will suffer a reduced surge of water. Neural drive is much the same.

Bodybuilders are not as powerful as Olympic weightlifters because their higher volume routines result in Type I fiber hypertrophy. The enlarged Type I neural pathways have reduced Type II pathway impulse. Alternatively, an Olympic weightlifter's focus on Type IIx fibers can limit Type I benefits. Type I fibers provide advantages to bodybuilders trying to control body composition. Type I fibers with higher mitochondria content are more efficient in reducing body fat potential because they are continuously removing glucose from the blood. Type IIx fibers have more limited glucose uptake potential because they release glycogen more sparingly. With nowhere to provide immediate energy, excessive serum glucose seeks a storage site. Neither training intention here is right nor wrong if the work objectives and desired outcomes are understood.

General Rules of Recovery

1. Schedule both heavy workout days and light workout days, preferably with the heavier days occurring after off days, and lighter workouts occurring later in the work week. This reduction of intensity improves recovery time and helps to prevent fatigue-related injuries.

2. Muscle exhaustion or momentary muscular failure (not advised when seeking maximal explosive power) [15] is defined as a failure to complete, or an altering of technique/form to successfully complete a movement. The more muscle fatigue experienced during a training session, the more rest should be allowed for those muscles before returning to activity. This recovery can vary based on the age, muscle fiber type, sleep and nutrition habits of the client. As a rule, during

a workout, if the athlete experiences a moment of complete muscle exhaustion for one repetition during any exercise, then 24 hours of recovery should be planned for that muscle group. If multiple incidents of failure occur, then consider at least 48 hours of recovery before exercising that muscle group again. If the workout intensity is set extremely high and muscle failure is the primary objective during every set of exercise during the workout, then 72 hours of recovery is highly suggested.

3. Neurological fatigue is more subtle and harder to recognize compared to muscle exhaustion. Strength and power athletes often avoid a complete loss of movement speed to avoid fatigue related reductions in nerve impulse. Much of strength and power depends on the nervous system being able to deliver a strong and clear message to its associated muscle fibers. As the nerve fatigues, the neurotransmitters (calcium, sodium, magnesium, potassium) decline, causing subsequent reductions in motor units (nerve and muscle fibers) recruitment. This minimized muscle fiber recruitment lowers leverage potential and thus strength and power output. After lighter load days (below 90% of the 1 repetition max 1RM), an athlete should consider allowing at least 48 hours before the same movement pattern is revisited. After heavy load days (above 90% of the 1RM) the athlete should allow at least 72 hours before the movement pattern is repeated. Also, higher repetition activities (endurance work, muscle exhaustion work) can negatively impact nerve recovery. Either avoid training for power and endurance simultaneously on the training calendar or at least avoid training both activity types on the same day.

4. Adequate sleep, well-balanced nutrition and proper hydration must be emphasized to optimize the post exercise recovery. After all, the workout is just a stimulus that causes the body to protect itself. The body's cells cannot reinforce against physical stress without these essentials of recovery.

The Team Sports Athlete

Although athletes like to appear fit and want to be generally healthy, athlete's bodies are primarily built for an athletic advantage over an opponent and at a sport's position. Therefore, athletes must stay focused on improvements in power, speed and strength at a much higher level than the general fitness client. Competition against team members vying for starting roles and against their opponents drives athletes to constantly consider methods of increasing peak performance. One of the traditional methods for helping athletes reach peak strength and power has been to track workloads across a variety of focus areas and then manage each area's recovery through periodization. In field and court sports there are over a dozen fitness characteristics or focus areas that should be addressed and improved upon to help athletes increase their overall performance advantage.

Athletic Focus Areas

1. Overload Strength
2. Overload Power
3. Speed Power
4. Functional Strength
5. Agility/Rhythm/Tempo
6. Flexibility
7. Balance
8. Movement Transitions
9. Linear Speed
10. Cardiorespiratory Conditioning
11. Visual Acuity
12. Body Composition Control
13. Restoration Therapy

With so many focus areas, how can an athlete expect to reach peak performance in any one of them? A large amount of physical energy is required to address all these areas and dividing this energy limits peak maximum effectiveness in each area. All athletes experience this, but it is just an expected part of their preparation for competition. The athlete and coach gain a competitive advantage when they creatively figure out how to capitalize on a specific area where an opponent might be deficient. Maybe the only thing separating two similar athletes is better balance, and an improved plan of work and recovery in that area might make the difference between winning or losing. During the preparatory period, sometimes referred to as the macrocycle (e.g., the time period of training toward a long term goal which could be one training year, or four years for a college athlete.), an athlete's focus areas will be individually periodized if added to the plan. The total training plan must examine total daily workloads, including team practices and factor in appropriate recovery to optimize all focus areas. Program success often depends on how creatively the training variables are arranged during the training cycle. This arrangement of the variables can be referred to as "Specificity of Training." Specificity can be unique to a particular sport, sport position or to an individual athlete, and is best managed when coaches create individual plans that address the issue of recovery.

Due to training facility schedule restraints and the numbers of athletes training at any given time, team workout plans cannot address individual specificity as effectively. Coaches can at best manage team weekly workloads by checking off whether assigned repetitions are achieved and then adjusting one repetition maximums. Coaches can also manipulate volume, frequency, duration, cadence and technique, through the use of pre-season, in-season and off-season calendars (European counterparts: preparation, first transition, competition and second transition). Although the training variables are broadly applied in these types of programs, they work effectively, especially with younger athletes needing basic strength development. However, as the athletes move into their professional careers or if the athlete performs an individual skill activity as in track and field or strength and power events, specialized training is essential to address specific needs. Many highly specialized athletes therefore shop the world for knowledgeable coaches and training environments that produce champions.

Overlapping focus areas make training and performance analysis very difficult. Although strength and conditioning and sports coaches desperately want to quantify excellence and address failures and successes numerically, it's a slippery slope because training numbers too often do not explain why the Chicago Bulls dominated the NBA of the 1990s, or why Brazil has won so many World Cup soccer championships.

It is certain that each focus area is individually measurable, but quantifying a combination of these areas is more difficult, and measuring the "psychology" of heart, friendships, happiness or mental stability is far from being a numerical quantity. The most sensible approach toward analyzing your athletic programs may be to improve the numbers when possible and avoid crediting wins based on biometric statistics. After all it's what happens on the field or court during the competition that is the ultimate proof of success.

The Power and Strength Athlete

Unlike team sports which have more movement variability, power and strength activities are often performed individually and in a single direction. It is easier to examine how maximum power and strength gains are made in single directional activities. However, even power and strength sports range in movement complexity. One might consider sprints, long jump and triple jump being considerably more movement complex than high jumps, discus, shot put, javelin, Olympic weightlifting, baseball pitching and softball pitching. And even less complex are vertical jumps, broad jumps and powerlifting.

To avoid reductions in power and strength from poor postures and forms, great sports coaching is essential when movement complexity is higher. Complex activities cannot rely exclusively on great strength and conditioning. But the combination of great strength and conditioning, and great technique and great ability enhanced through coaching can produce great outcomes.

Programming and Periodization Considerations

- Programming - Applies changes to various training variables at a particular time in the training.
- Periodization - Establishes the total arch of time for training, and the divisions of that arch to best optimize recovery.
- Before you can periodize any program of training you need to understand the training variables.

Intensity and the Strength Training Variables

Intensity, frequency and duration have long been considered the standard variables of exercise design. But it is probably more revealing to consider intensity or perceived difficulty as a measure that can be intensified or lessened by manipulating a wider array of exercise training variables which include workload, volume, frequency, duration, cadence and technique. When training for strength, each training variable–although influential on training results–cannot be considered alone. Correctly combined and considering recovery, the training variables can create championship performances.

Training Variables Affecting Workout Intensity

Workload	Volume	Duration	Frequency	Cadence	Technique
▶	▶	▶	▶	▶	▶
Resistance, incline, drag etc.	More repetitions, sets, exercises, distance, less rest	Time	When movement is repeated during the week	Tempo continuous, movement slow	Contractions, isometric, bands

Workload

Using workload as the primary training object is a clear numerical method of evaluating work intensity. Alternatively, influences on exercise intensity involving volume, frequency, duration, cadence and technique are more difficult to quantify, and those training variables require more consideration and planning to avoid potential overtraining.

One essential consideration when using workload as the primary training object is how it relates to the training variable of cadence or movement speed. As previously discussed, the muscular system of humans is chemically designed for a variety of different types of work. Human bodies can both sprint and run a long distance, throw or carry a load to its destination, jump or climb to a point of elevation.

Jumping with the entire body's weight relies heavily on Type IIx muscle fibers, while the act of climbing requires efficient Type I fibers.

Heavier workloads therefore influence greater changes in Type II nervous system pathways, while lower workloads influence greater changes in Type I nerve pathways. Recruitment speed is often associated with the terms "movement speed" or cadence. This is often confusing and will be discussed ahead. However, regardless of terminology, when considering the perceived intensity of exercise, workload and the pace at which load is moved are inseparable.

The success of power and strength sports depend primarily on heavy loads requiring fast muscle fiber recruitment speeds. Power and strength athletes clearly understand the objective of an ever-increasing workload, but physical limitations make continuous progression nearly impossible. Coaches and athletes must therefore creatively manage all the training variables to gradually manipulate the body into accepting greater workloads. Even if this means periodically reducing workloads to assure muscle tissue growth, nervous system adaptations and recovery.

Often working on their own and experimenting with their training programs, strength and power athletes have gained individual successes. Historically observant coaches have compared those athlete's training rituals for similarities and differences and formulated models of best strength training practices.

Famed Russian Olympic Lifting Coach Alexandre Prilepin, after being guided by Metveye's periodization research, used percentages of his athlete's one repetition max (1RM) to control workload intensities. The percent workloads were then applied at various stages of his periodized programs.

Prilepen's Table

Intensity (% 1RM)	Reps Per Set	Optimal Total of Reps	Total Range of Reps
Below 70%	3 - 6	24	18 -30
70 – 79%	3 - 6	18	12 – 24
80 – 89%	2 - 4	15	10 – 20
90% and above	1 - 2	7	4 - 10

Prilepen's Table would eventually be used and argued over by both Olympic and powerlifting communities. However, regardless of its exact specificity to either sport, the table's true value is in the concept of graduated workloads - how to elicit a specific training effect and manage recovery using graduated workloads.

Volume

Volume considers the total number of achieved repetitions during a workout. A repetition is a single movement of a particular exercise and a set is a group of repetitions. Considering volume alone, it is easy to see that a marathon is a high-volume activity, while a high jump is a low-volume activity. It would be a disadvantage for a marathoner to engage exclusively in low-volume work and the opposite would hold true for the high jumper. It is essential to choose work volumes that match the energy requirement of an athlete's sport. To quantify work volume, multiply the number of repetitions performed by the total number of sets.

a)   4 sets x 10 reps = **40 repetitions (More Volume)**
b)   (1 set x 10 reps) + (1 set x 8 reps) + (1 set x 6 reps) = **24 repetitions (Less Volume)**

Forty repetitions in example a) above would be considered a greater volume than the twenty-four repetitions in example b), and volume considered alone as a measure of intensity would mean more repetitions would require more planned recovery.

Considering volume and workload together is the basis of periodization because volume and workload multiplied can quantify the total work performed and indicate daily overall intensity. Numerically knowing the rise and fall of daily and weekly intensity levels helps plan better recovery.

a)   4 sets x 10 reps x 100 lbs = 40 x 100 = 4,000 lbs/moved
b)   1 set x 10 reps x 150 lbs = 1,500 lbs/moved
   1 set x 8 reps x 175 lbs = 1,750 lbs/moved
   1 set x 6 reps x 200 lbs = 2,000 lbs/moved
   1,500 + 1,750 + 2,000 = 5,250 lbs/moved

Considering workload and volume together gives a more complete measurement of the intensity of the work performed. In the example above, a greater volume of forty repetitions was still performed to accomplish the 4,000 pounds/moved, but if intensity were strictly being measured by the amount of total weight moved, the heavier total weight moved in example b) would require more recovery.

Frequency

Frequency of work considers the amount of rest allowed between sets (b/s) of an exercise. Longer rests between sets generally are considered less intense workouts compared to a workout with less rest between exercise sets.

a)   20 sets (45 seconds rest b/s) = **More Intense**
b)   20 sets (1 minute and 15 seconds b/s) = **Less Intense**

What if more rest is allowed for moving more workload during the overall workout? Then the sets with the longer rest may be considered more intense.

a)   20 sets during the workout using 5 exercise movements (45 seconds rest b/s) total weight moved **7,000 pounds**
b)   20 sets during the workout using 5 exercise movements(1 minute and 15 seconds b/s) total weight moved **9,000 pounds**

However, intensity of exercise sets based on frequency is often more nuanced and should be determined by the workout's objective. If the workout's purpose is to challenge the muscle tissue and increase exercise intensity through muscle fatigue, then less rest between exercise sets may be just as intense and require similar recovery considerations as the workout with longer rest periods but heavier workloads. A more impacting consideration of frequency is the time needed between exercise sessions or how often an exercise or body area is used. Optimal recovery often hinges on this critical component of the workout plan. Here again is where the "General Rules of Recovery" previously mentioned in this chapter should be considered and applied.

Duration

Changes in workout duration can affect an exercise session's intensity. Workouts that last longer accompanied by increased workload and volumes will require more recovery than shorter workouts involving less overall work. A one-hour workout with 30 sets moving 10,000 pounds is more intense than a 45-minute workout with 20 sets moving 7,000 pounds.

Studies have shown optimal strength training workout durations should fall into a forty-five minute period. Intense workouts lasting longer than forty-five minutes have been demonstrated to lower testosterone levels. Lowered hormone levels post workout might increase the time needed for tissue healing and regeneration. [22]

Cadence

Cadence or movement speed was touched upon when we discussed workload, and we associated both with the concept of speed of muscle fiber recruitment. Because of its profound effects on the perceived exercise intensity, movement speed and cadence should always be considered in planning recovery. As previously mentioned, workloads usually dictate the cadence of an exercise or movement. As loads increase, muscle fiber recruitment speeds must generally increase to move the load. However, heavy loads often force cadences to be disrupted by pauses, and slows external movement speeds to a grind. Powerlifters refer to the "grind" as an essential part of their training protocols. Grinding to a near halt may seem counterintuitive, but grinding induces a reflexive response from the involved motor units, driving the nervous system to increase muscle fiber recruitment speed. Although the movement externally is slow, internally nerve impulses are fast.

In contrast to maximum tension created by extreme loads moved quickly, a slow and controlled movement speed paired with a continuous cadence can increase the muscle's time under tension. Slower and continuous cadences incrementally build tension through accumulative muscle fiber fatigue. As more and more fresh muscle fibers come to the aid of their exhausted counterparts, tension is accumulated. Fiber exhaustion stresses the structural protein matrix and depletes cellular chemical stores, fatty acids and glycogen. Post workout, recovered muscle fibers replenish and reinforce their stores and structures. Over time through this enlarged capacity, muscle fibers add tension into their combined structure which builds strength.

- Slower movement speeds with constant cadence = **time under tension of muscle fiber**
- Faster movement speeds with irregular cadence = **maximum tension via nerve impulse**

If we just consider cadence alone, 4 sets x 10 repetitions performed to complete exhaustion with slow, constant movement can be considered more intense than 4 sets x 10 repetitions performed with faster movement speeds and an irregular cadence allowing for momentary respites.

a) 4 sets x 10 reps x 100 lbs with Constant Cadence = **More Intense**
b) 4 sets x 10 reps x 100 lbs with Irregular Cadence = **Less Intense**
c) 4 sets x 6 reps x 200 lbs with Irregular Cadence **= More Intense**

Athletes can certainly move lighter objects with faster movement speeds, and they often do when using throw-and-release objects like medicine balls, bags, hammers, blocks, etc. But this is considered Speed Power and not advised for extreme overload settings using barbells and dumbbells. Releasing or swinging a lighter overloaded object reduces injury potential and increases athleticism and neuro-muscular control. The explosive athletic power required in throwing, punching, kicking, jumping and sprinting are greatly benefited by using single cadence, lighter overloaded movements.

Technique

Technique considers the details of an exercise movement. Subtle changes in posture, hand positions, focused muscle contractions, variations in movement ranges and the addition of equipment can all change the intensity of the exercise to produce a greater result.

Hartzell's Strength Curve Revelation and Louie Simmons

Before Coach Dick Hartzell, athletes had randomly used the concept of accommodating or variable resistance, using cables, springs, manual resistance and rubber bands. But Hartzell had an idea in the early 1980s when he invented Flexbands®. Hartzell recounts he began using bands with his younger high school athletes to reduce resistance training injuries. [3] As he expected, injuries declined, but unexpectedly, according to Hartzell, his athlete's strength gains increased. Hartzell anecdotally attributed these gains to an ever-increasing resistance along the exercise's range of motion. Where the exercise was normally easy due to an athlete's mechanical strength advantage over the resistance, the bands made the movement more difficult. Challenging the strength curve was not a new concept. During the 1970s, the manufacturer of exercise equipment, Arthur Jones, had invented a patented cam-altered pulley system for his Nautilus® exercise machines. The shell shaped cam attempted to counter the exercise's strength curve by positioning the cam to move the cabled resistance further from the direction of linear force, thus pulling harder on the cable where the exercise should have been easiest and normalizing the resistance where the exercise was predicted to be most difficult. However, rather than buying costly machines, Coach Hartzell's hack applied a simple low-cost industrial rubber band directly to an athlete's actual training movements and accomplished very similar strength curve results.

Like most coaching success stories, Louie Simmons' is built on the expertise of many, but Simmons experienced a breakthrough of his own. Simmons willingness to experiment was one of his most fortunate attributes, and in the early 1990s he saw Dick Hartzell's rubber bands and decided to bring them into his Westside Barbell club and apply their simple strength curve demands directly to powerlifting's big three lifts: bench press, squat and deadlift.

Applied technique, as in the previous example, can sometimes change the entire outcome of an exercise session. Technique is often nuanced and can be highly influential on physical outcomes, but more importantly, techniques can provide positive mental adaptations as well. The mere suggestion of something new and secretive being added to the workout can positively impact confidence and participation. It can make all the difference toward successful outcomes if an athlete sincerely believes in the training and participates at a higher level.

Programming Training Variables

To succeed, a well-constructed exercise plan requires an understanding of the athlete's physical demands. This understanding combined with a variable use, a coaching philosophy of training, can challenge the body to improve. Because both understanding and philosophical ideas are subjective, one coach or athlete's programming may be vastly different from their competitors. Very much like the endless possibilities of musical chords, the blend of training variables can make something harmonious or something discordant. Proper exercise variable programming should dovetail for maximal recovery with the proper use of periodized time.

Periodization

Matveyev's periodization model evolved over time. His original construct had three training periods: Preparatory, Transition and Competition. The Preparatory period consists of a higher volume work performed with lower resistance. The stages that followed had lower and lower volumes accompanied with ever increasing resistance. Finally, as the athlete entered the performance/strength stages of training, volume decreased even further, with added focus on improving performance technique. Matveyev later added a fourth transitional period of Active Rest.

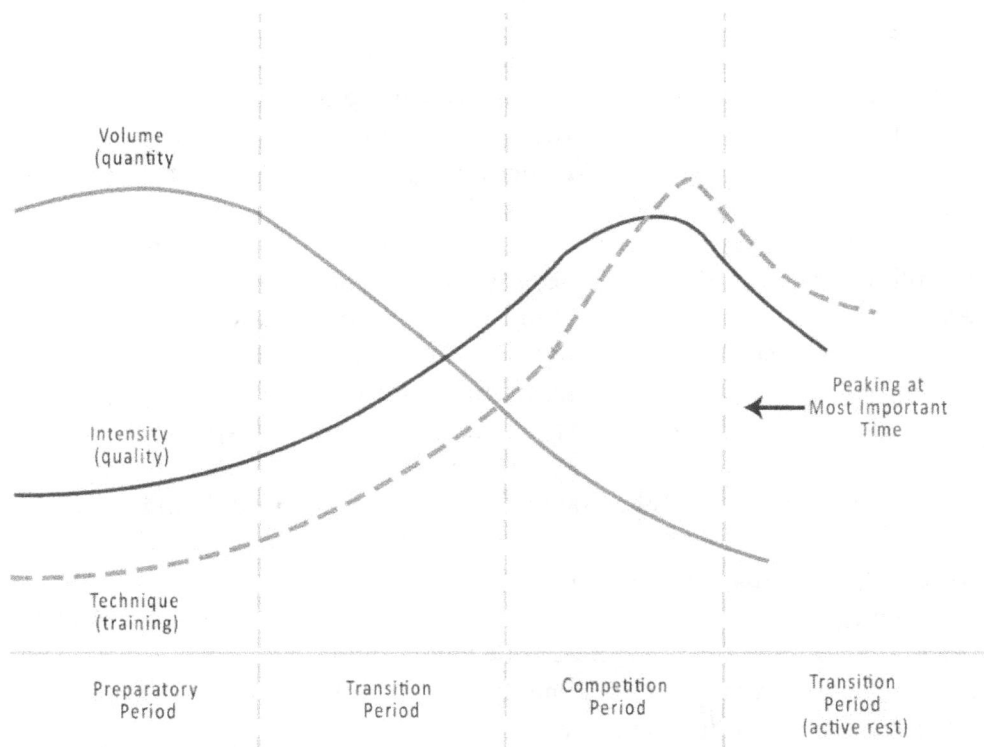

Matveyev's original program used a four-year Olympic calendar. This was the time required for an athlete to reach their peak power output for the next Olympic games. The calendar was divided into manageable cycles where goals could be set and gradually approached. Peak performances were planned for the height of the competitive cycle.

The entire training calendar was referred to as the **macro**cycle and depending on the competition dates, further divisions of three-to-four month **meso**cycles were marked. Each mesocycle was further divided into weekly **micro**cycles, and each microcycle was constructed of daily training sessions.

Macrocycle –	Year(s)
Mesocycle –	Block of Months
Microcycle –	Block of Weeks

2021			
Macrocycle			
3 Month Mesocycle	3 Month Mesocycle	3 Month Mesocycle	3 Month Mesocycle
12x 1 week microcycles	12x 1 week microcycles	12x 1 week microcycles	12x 1 week microcycles

Matveyev established the basic rules of Periodization:

1. Start with low intensity work, and gradually increase the difficulty of the workouts.
2. Be progressive, but not overly aggressive when increasing workout intensity. Working to complete exhaustion is neurologically counterproductive.
3. Plan both heavy and lighter days during the weekly microcycles.
4. Recovery is critical, so divide the work into manageable goal setting periods.
5. As the athlete progresses toward the competition period, exercise should become more specific to the athlete's competition requirements.

Traditional versus Block Periodization

Although periodization is limited by the constraints of time and how a calendar can be divided, more recent periodization protocols for team sports athletes have revealed positive results. The classical or traditional model of periodization was designed for athletes on Olympic trajectories. Team sports seasons are only a few months long rather than years long, resulting in the need for mesocycle management that more accurately accommodates team sport athletes' schedules.

Block Periodization advocates suggest that the traditional model attempted to improve too many athletic focus areas simultaneously within the sports calendar. The magnitude of the work volume would certainly be detrimental to recovery and reduce strength and power outcomes. High volumes of work are always problematic for recovery. There are only so many hours in each day and academics, occupations, team practice, athletic training and family weigh on available time for strength and conditioning workouts. Good programming, regardless of periodization format, should always consider the sports season calendar and concentrate only on focus areas appropriate for that time of the training calendar. Plotting a yearly sport Activity Concentration Chart can help visualize what focus areas need to be concentrated on and when.

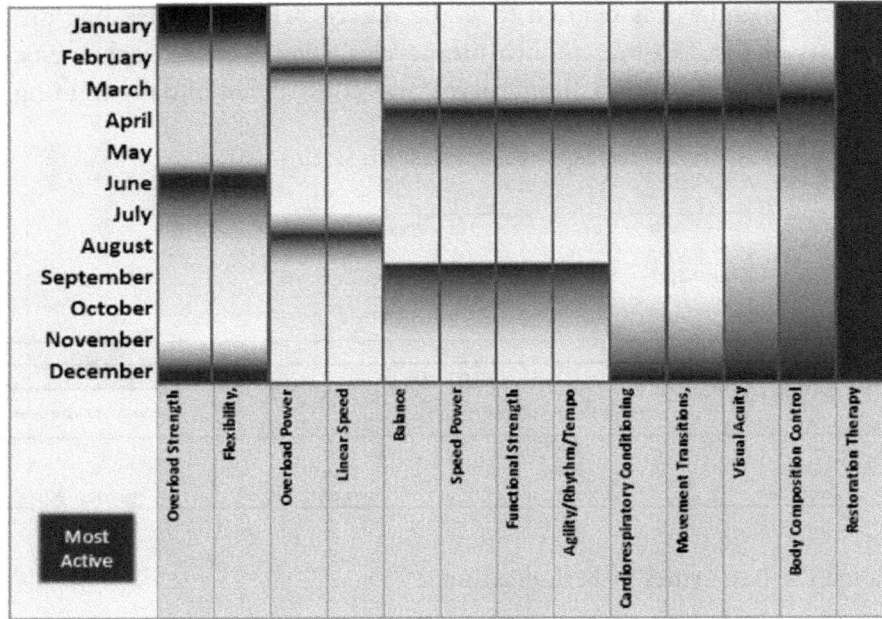

In the figure above, we get a visual idea of how focus area concentrations can be distributed. A traditional periodization trajectory for "Overload Strength" might have an American football athlete training from the start of the off-season in November until just before the start of spring practice in mid-February. Incremental increases in intensity can be planned for 16 weeks or for two eight-week cycles. In his traditional plan, Matveyev considered the GAS principle of stress adaptation, and managed intensity by increasing it gradually over three stages he called Preparatory, Transition and Competition. Even though stress is mitigated using these stages, Matveyev's Preparatory stage would have been too long for a team sport like American football. Dividing the "Preparatory Phase" into more manageable blocks aids recovery by restructuring the volume of work required.

The value of Block Periodization appears to be further condensing intensity into even shorter periods. Like Metveyev, Verkhoshansky also managed intensity in stages. Each Block of time was further divided into its own three stages called, Accumulation, Transmutation and Realization. In 2006, Verkhoshansky outlined his first Block Periodization concepts using a three-block model consisting of two 6 to 12 week periods of strength, power and speed transition, followed by one 3 to 5 week period of sports specific technique training with a taper.

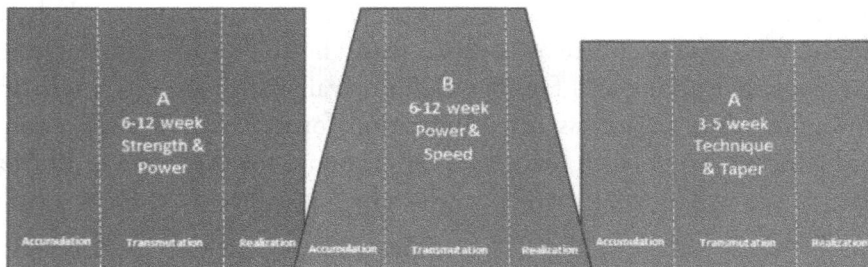

The Football Activity Concentration Chart, can still be used when applying Block Periodization principles (see table below). Using 5-week blocks and pairing compatible focus areas helps to concentrate intensity into even more manageable windows of time. In Blocks 1-3 Flexibility pairs well with Overload Strength's tendency to eccentrically load. This combination can improve muscle sarcomere length, improving strength with this muscle growth potential.

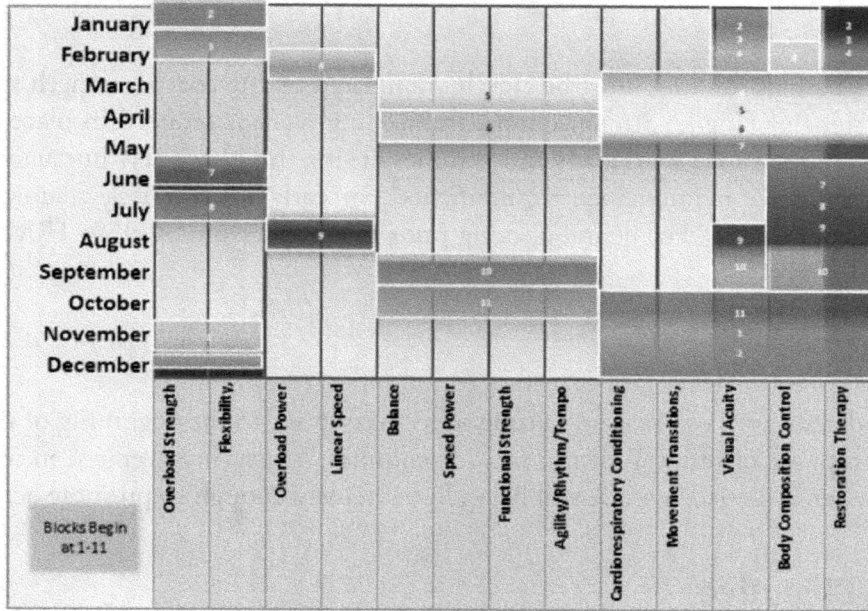

Current Periodization Model

Although terminology has changed slightly, current periodization theory mirrors the historical models by creating a framework of work intensity over time which is designed to promote recovery. A model promoted by the National Strength and Conditioning Association instructs that a period should be divided again into four phases of training: "Preparation Phase," "First Transition," "Competition Phase" and "Second Transition."

Preparation Phase

This training phase is considered an "Off-Season" period for team sport athletes. It is a protracted period of strength and condition improvement, introducing incremental increases in load and intensity. The phase begins with lower intensity (50-75% of 1RM) and higher volume (3-6 sets 8-20 reps) to higher intensity (85-95% 1RM) lower volume (2-6 sets 2-6 reps) over the course of the period. Because there are no competitions in this phase, more emphasis is directed toward less specific sports movements and instead toward the improvement of total strength, speed, power and physical conditioning.

First Transition

This phase of training, considered "Pre-Season," aims to transition the base strength and conditioning gained during "Preparation" toward a more explosive speed and power outcome. This is achieved by increasing workload during overload resistance training (85-95% 1RM) and lowering work volume (2-5 reps). Overload work is paired with over-speed work in the form of plyometric training involving lower workloads (30-50% 1RM) with low volumes (2-5 reps). This combination of applications during this phase focuses more on neural drive improvements over that of muscle tissue improvements.

Competition Phase

This "In-Season" phase of training must be closely monitored by the coach, strength staff, and athletic training staff for signs of fatigue. Strength and conditioning work is reduced in place of added sports team practice and competition. Workloads and volumes during this phase may fluctuate to address both muscular and neural drive maintenance requirements. For early week muscle maintenance: 85-95% 1RM with 2-5 sets of 3-6 reps. For neural peaking prior to competition: 50-95% 1RM with 1-3 sets of 1-3 reps.

Second Transition

This can be considered the "Post-Season," a time of recovery prior to the beginning of the next Preparation or Off-Season phase of training. It can include complete rest or involvement in other recreational activities that broaden athleticism while still being low intensity enough to promote activity recovery.

The Training Objective

Focus areas, programming training variables and proper periodization of the sports calendar have been covered. But what is it you are training to achieve? Neither Traditional, Block or Current periodization models have wanted to stray from Hans Selye's General Adaptation Syndrome (GAS) theory. All seem to consider that managed stages of workout intensity are required to help the athlete adapt to workout stress and avoid the harm resulting from exhaustion.

Management of Exercise Stress	General Preparation	Strength /Power	Peaking	Active Rest
	This includes muscle tissue improvements (hypertrophy) via protein synthesis and improved enzymatic delivery. Training that results in muscle strength, size, stability, blood flow and work capacity.	For safety and best outcomes, strength must be established before increasing power. Then a transitioning of training to faster movement speeds for increased neural adaptations.	Workouts become increasingly more technique driven and specific to the actual competitive event. Intensity is pared prior to the event to maximize recovery.	A period of rest involving multi-joint activity with reduced intensity. It is a period of transition prior to beginning the next General Preparation.
Traditional Periodization Metveyev	**Preparatory**	**Transition**	**Competition /Taper**	**Active Rest**
Block Periodization Verhosshansky, Issurin, Kaverin Bondarchuk's	**Accumulation**	**Transmutation**	**Realization**	**Active Rest**
Current Periodization Terminology	**Preparation Phase**	**First Transition**	**Competition**	**Second Transition**
Sports Season Periods	**Off-Season**	**Pre-Season**	**In-Season**	**Post- Season**

Periodization Conclusion

There will always be conversations about best practices related to athletic strength and conditioning. During these discussions, it is important to understand the difference between Programming and Periodization. Regarding programming, understanding about Focus Areas Concentrations and that Training Variables pairing is endless, but critical. Regarding Periodization, once the basic considerations for proper recovery are factored in, it is important to understand there are limited ways to divide a sport's calendar. Periodization has proven to be a sound management method of both time and stress load. Everyone understands the value of goal setting. Periodization is time set to incrementally achieve goals while avoiding overwork, and it appears the shorter these blocks of time the more achievable the goals.

See Appendix B for additional resources on Periodization

- image of Annual Plan (Macrocycle)
- Volume & Periodization 2019 Slide
- Video: Periodization of Exercise

References: Chapter 14

1. Bompa, T.O. *Theory and Methodology of Training: The key to athletic performance*. Dubuque, IA: Kendall/Hunt, 1994.

2. Selye, H. *Stress without distress*. New York: J.B. Lippincott, 1974.

3. Haff, G. G., Triplett, N. T. *Essentials of Strength Training and Conditioning-NSCA, 4th ed*. Human Kinetics: Champaign, IL, 2016.

4. Hatzell, D. Interview by Jim Evans. *Armstrong Neighborhood Channel: Loose Change*. 9 Sep 2016. Accessed 8 January 2021.http://youtube.com/watch?v=MGK19Y2j6wg

5. Issurin, V. "Block Periodization: Scientific Concept and Implementation." Presentation at Rowing Coaches' Clinic, October 15, 2010. doi: members.ehf.eu/1530

6. Issurin, V.B. "New horizons for the methodology and physiology of training periodization." *Sports Med*. 40, no. 3 (March, 2010): 189-206. doi: 10.2165/11319770

7. Issurin, V. "Block periodization *versus* traditional training theory: a review." *The Journal of Sports Medicine and Physical Fitness*. 48 no. 1 (March, 2008): 65-75. doi: 18212712

8. Issurin, V. Interviewed by Yosef Johnson. *Otivation Sports Performance*, 17 June, 2012. Accessed 29 January 2021. Available at: otivation6.17/otivation.2012.Issurin.

9. Issurin, B.V. "Periodization Training from Ancient Precursors to Structures Block Models." *Kinesiology* 46 (September, 2014): 3-9. doi: 279325049

10. Komi, P.V., Tesch, P. "EMG frequency spectrum, muscle structure, and fatigue during dynamic contractions in man." *Eur J Appl Physiol Occup Physiol* 42, no. 1 (September, 1979): 41–50. doi: 10.1007/BF00421103

11. Kraemer, W.J., et al. "Physiological changes with periodized resistance training in women tennis players." *Med Sci Sports Exerc* 35, no. 1 (January, 2003): 157-168. doi: 10.1097/00005768-200301000-00024

12. Lievens, E., Klass. M., Bex. T., Derave, W. "Muscle fiber typology substantially influences time to recover from high-intensity exercise." *J Appl Physiol* 128, no. 3 (March, 2020): 648–659. doi: org/10.1152/japplphysiol.00636.2019

13. Matveyev L. *Fundamentals of Sports Training*. Moscow: Progress, 1981.

14. Metzger JM, Moss RL. "Effects of tension and stiffness due to reduced pH in mammalian fast- and slow-twitch skinned skeletal muscle fibers." *J Physiol* 428 (September, 1990): 737–750. doi:10.1113/jphysiol.1990.sp018238

15. Mujika, I. *Tapering and Peaking for Optimal Performance*. Chicago: Human Kinetics, 2009.

16. Painter, K.B., Haff, G.G., Ramsey, M.W., et al. "Strength gains: block versus daily undulating periodization weight training among track and field athletes." *Int J Physiol Perform* 7, no. 2 (June, 2012): 161-169. doi: 10.1123/ijspp.7.2.161

17. Plisk, S.S., Stone, M.H. "Periodization strategies." *Strength Cond J*. 25, no. 6 (December, 2003): 19-37. doi: 2003/12000

18. Sale, D.G. *Medicine and Science in Sports and Exercise*. 20, no. 5, Suppl. (October, 1988): S135–S145. doi: 10.1249/00005768-198810001-00009

19. Siff, M.C., Verkhoshan, Y.V. *Supertraining, 4th ed*. Denver, CO: Supertraining International, 1999.

20. Stone, M.H., O'Bryant, H.S. *Weight Training: A Scientific Approach*. Minneapolis: Burgess, 1987.

21. Stone, M., O'Bryant, H., Garhammer, J. "A hypothetical model for strength training." *Journal of Sports Medicine and Physical Fitness* 21, no. 4 (December, 1981): 342–351. doi: 7339218

22. Stone, M.H., Keith, R.E., Kearney, J.T., Fleck, S.J., Wilson, G.D., Triplett, N.T. "Overtraining: a review of the signs, symptoms and possible causes." *Journal of Applied Sports Science Research* 5, no. 1 (February, 1991): 35–50. doi: 1991/02000

23. Travis, K.S., Ishida, A., Taber C.B., Fry, A.C., Stone M.H. "Emphasizing Task-Specific Hypertrophy to Enhance Sequential Strength and Power Performance." *J Funct Morphol Kinesiol* 5, no. 4 (December, 2020): 76. doi: 10.3390/jfmk5040076.

24. Villanueva, M.G., Lane, C.J., Schroeder, E.T. "Influence of Rest Interval Length on Acute Testosterone and Cortisol Responses to Volume-Load Equated Total Body Hypertrophic and Strength Protocols." *J Strength Cond Res* 26, no. 10 (October, 2012): 2755–2764. doi: 10.1519/JSC.0b013e3182651fbe

SECTION 4

RECOVERY & NUTRITION

15
RECOVERY FROM TRAINING

By: Philip Bishop, Ed. D.
Professor Emeritus of Exercise Science, University of Alabama

OF ALL THE things that coaches and trainers can do for their athletes, the most neglected may be the area of recovery. As a long-time researcher in the area of sport performance, I noticed that there were hundreds, maybe thousands now, of research papers investigating training techniques, but almost nothing investigating recovery from training. But think about it, an elite athlete might train four hours a day for six days per week, making 24 hours per week of training, but a week has 168 hours, so what about those other 144 hours, shouldn't we pay attention to those too?

In fact, for high-level sportsmen, they train so intensely that a major challenge for them is adequately recovering between workouts, such that they are capable of maximizing the benefits of the next workout. In my younger days, I was a very successful ultra-distance runner. In the height of my competitive era, I ran 20 miles (32Km) on Monday, and again on Tuesday. On Wednesday, I'd cut back a bit to about 15 miles (24 KM) but Thursday, I ran 20 miles again. Friday I'd do another 15, then Saturday about 15 or 16 miles more. That gave me a bit over 100 miles (160Km) per week of training. The sad part is that I was so ignorant that almost ALL of it was done at the same long-slow-distance pace, with the only variety provided by the hilly terrain of western Virginia where I trained. I paid NO attention to my recovery, and likely ran even my winning races in a fatigued state.

As coaches and trainers, our temptation is to make sure our athletes are "well trained" as a result of plenty of hard work. Frequently coaches and trainers will proudly make comments such as, "They may beat us, but they won't out-work us!" Unfortunately, in our desire to get the best from our team, we are failing them when they don't get sufficient recovery. Again, for high-level competitors, they likely are working so hard that it is difficult for them to recover for the next workout.

What needs recovery?

Our body's highest priority is maintaining homeostasis of all systems. Workouts vary greatly in which systems they impact and each individually will vary widely in their responses to the same workout. In

293

most cases, generally speaking, our muscles need time to recover from high-intensity or long-duration stressors. As good coaches, we seek to be specific in our training, trying to stress and train the systems most important for success in the sport for which we are training.

In most cases, fuel will need to be replenished. The best research at this time suggests that providing carbohydrates and protein within 30-60 mins after a workout provides the most benefit. Although a few people have claimed benefits from low-carbohydrate diets, this would NOT be recommended for most. Again, humans vary greatly, so short off-season experiments with carbohydrates or other diet changes might yield contrary findings on an individual basis.

The key is making sure sportsmen are getting adequate fuel of a high quality. We don't know enough about micro-nutrients to be able to say which ones are crucial to recovery—and again this is likely highly individual anyway. That is why a nutrient-rich diet with sufficient carbohydrates is our best overall option. Individuals with deficiencies will need more attention. Many female competitors are low in red blood cells, which are crucial in carrying oxygen for oxidative metabolism, and may need supplements to try to maximize red blood cell production.

Fatigue is multifactorial depending on the training stressor and the individual, therefore it can be difficult to pinpoint what is causing the fatigue to each body system. So instead of being concerned with exactly what may be fatiguing our athletes, we should instead experiment with different treatments for speeding recovery.

Speeding Up Recovery

There are a lot of treatments which have been tested for speeding recovery between training bouts. The simplest of these is passive rest. Athletes should rotate heavy/high intensity workouts with lower intensity workouts. But, again we need to remember that a recovery schedule/modality that works for one individual, may be totally ineffective for another. Monitoring individuals and treating them as individuals is the KEY.

Ice-baths and hot-and-cold baths are popular. Sports teams that implement cold-water immersion after training sessions perceive it to be beneficial, but our research suggests that some individuals do worse after cold-water exposure in recovery. So studying individuals is essential. Although we haven't tested contrast therapy (hot-and-cold baths), I would expect similar results, in that some will benefit, and others can be negatively affected.

Let's take a moment and examine how we might conduct such a study on our own team. Sports with clear objective performance criteria are the easiest to study. So, for our first example, let's look at 10Km runners.

- Monday: A very tough workout after a weekend off. After the workout everyone has a 30-min session of leg immersion in cold water.
- Tuesday: Start the practice with a 5Km or 10 Km time trial for these runners. We compare their run time to their personal record (PR) to see how well they have recovered from Monday's workout. Those who are running closest to PR would appear to have benefited and those running further from their PR would seem to be negative responders to the ice bath. But one time is not enough for conclusive results, so you must repeat this.
- Thursday and Friday we repeat this procedure, or the next week we do it again. Those who show consistent benefits will get this treatment, whilst those who got worse consistently will try a DIFFERENT treatment for recovery.

- If we find consistent improvement or consistent worsening over the course of 6 or 8 workout comparisons, we make a decision as to what works for that person.

An alternative to cold water, which is much more pleasant, is massage. The key disadvantage of massage is that it is labor-intensive to administer to a large group. One variation is to use foam rollers so that individuals can vary the nature of the treatment, and also so that the labor requirements are mostly eliminated. Similar to the ice water baths and hot-cold baths, some will benefit and some will worsen with this treatment.

Both your tradition and experience may suggest other recovery techniques to test, but the key principle in my mind is that few treatments will work for everyone, so experimentation is a requirement to discover what works best for each individual person.

Some sportsmen seem to ignore the value of sleep in recovery. Although we do not know of research specifically on sleep and sport performance, it should be obvious that sportsmen in heavy training will need to get plenty of high-quality sleep. Again, how much sleep is vital to optimal performance, and how this sleep is obtained is likely highly variable among sportsmen.

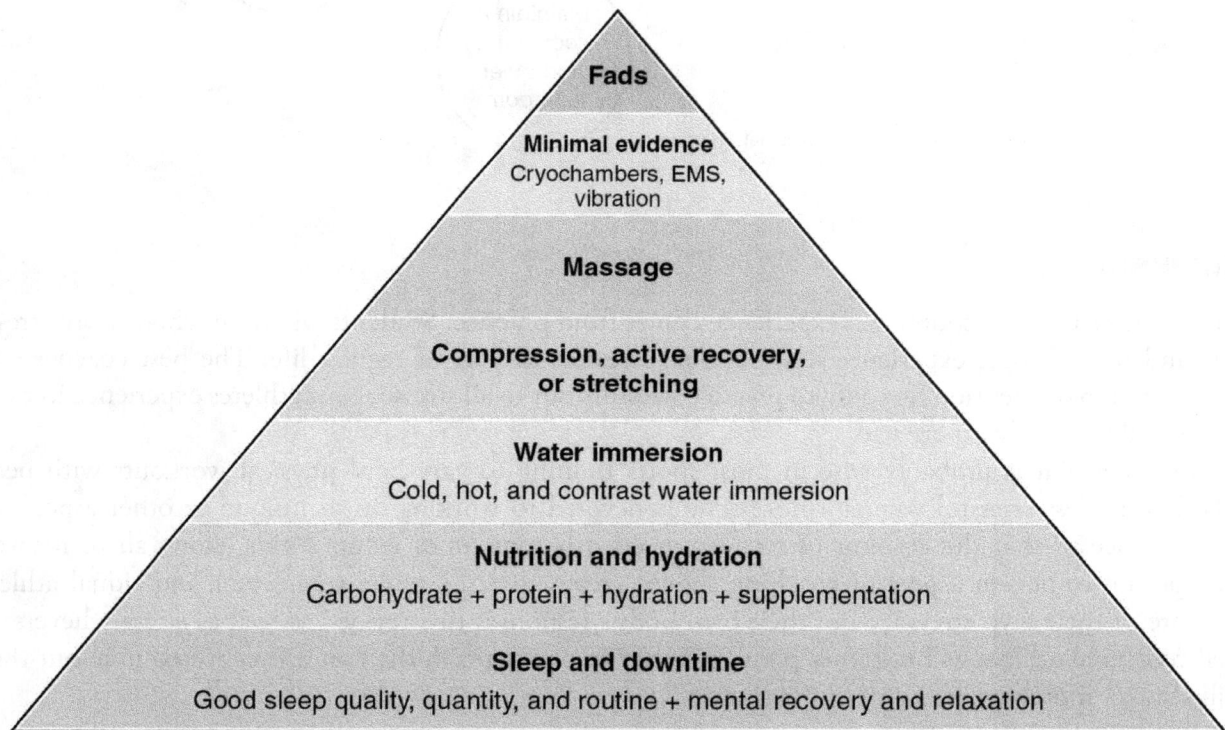

Fads

Minimal evidence
Cryochambers, EMS, vibration

Massage

Compression, active recovery, or stretching

Water immersion
Cold, hot, and contrast water immersion

Nutrition and hydration
Carbohydrate + protein + hydration + supplementation

Sleep and downtime
Good sleep quality, quantity, and routine + mental recovery and relaxation

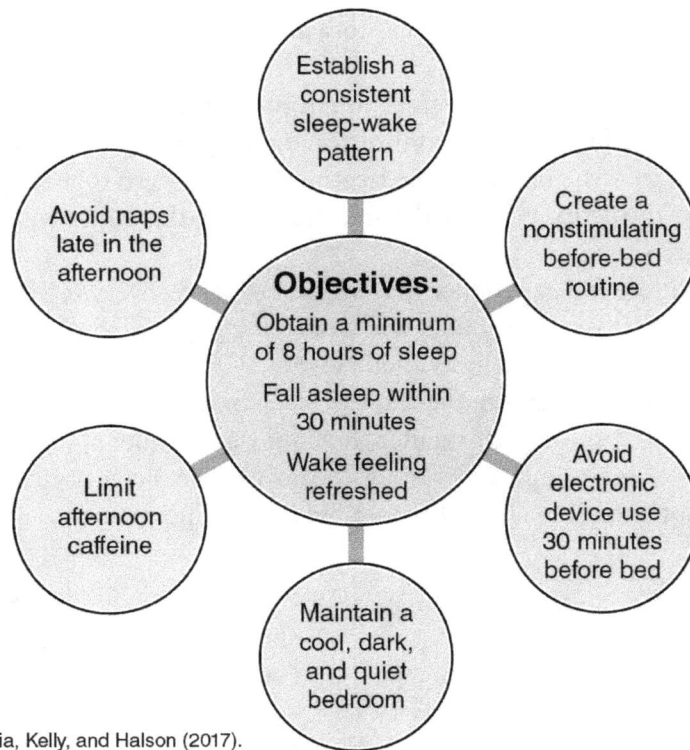

Adapted from Caia, Kelly, and Halson (2017).

Stressors

Not all stress that our sportsmen experience comes from practice. Students will have school work stressors, and most people experience interpersonal stressors as part of regular life. The best coaches and trainers will pay attention not only to practice stressors but to all stressors our athletes experience in their whole realm of daily experience.

In general, it is probably wise in most sports training to vary hard physical workouts with periods that are less stressful wherein more time is devoted to working on technique or other aspects of performance so that the amount of recovery needed is sometimes reduced–this allows all to recover. The person-to-person aspect of coaching should create an atmosphere where each individual athlete is aware of their own stressors and their own body's responses to stressors, as well as stress-relievers. A well-recovered athlete will not only perform better in competition than an un-recovered one, but they will also get more out of each training session.

Heart Rate Variability Monitoring

Monitoring heart rate and heart rate variability has become an extremely popular research area. New technologies have made monitoring heart-rate variability (HRv) feasible for coaches and sportsmen. Typically, HRv measurements are made first thing upon rising in the morning. The variability can be expressed several ways, but log-transformed root mean square of successive R-R intervals, or the standard deviation of the normal-to-normal R-R intervals seems the most useful for monitoring athletes. Portable devices are sold which can make these measurements for the athlete.

Although this might seem a bit counter-intuitive, a decrease in variability is typically associated with a poorer status for an individual. It would not be too difficult to set up a system wherein sportsmen check their own HRv status at specific times each day and give these numbers to their coaches before training each day. The coaches and trainers decide on how much stress the sportsmen can handle depending on the variability the athlete has experienced that specific day. If the variability is high, meaning the heart rate has changed a lot throughout the day, then the athlete can handle more stressors during the workout. An even simpler approach, which has not been as closely examined, is to look at the resting heart-rate upon first arising. It could be for many people that HR is also effective as an indicator of work capacity.

Monitoring and providing adequate recovery time between workouts, as well as implementing tactics that help speed up recovery will be a significant way to get major improvements in elite sportsmen. Focusing on the whole athlete, including their recovery, is key in helping them reach their fullest potential.

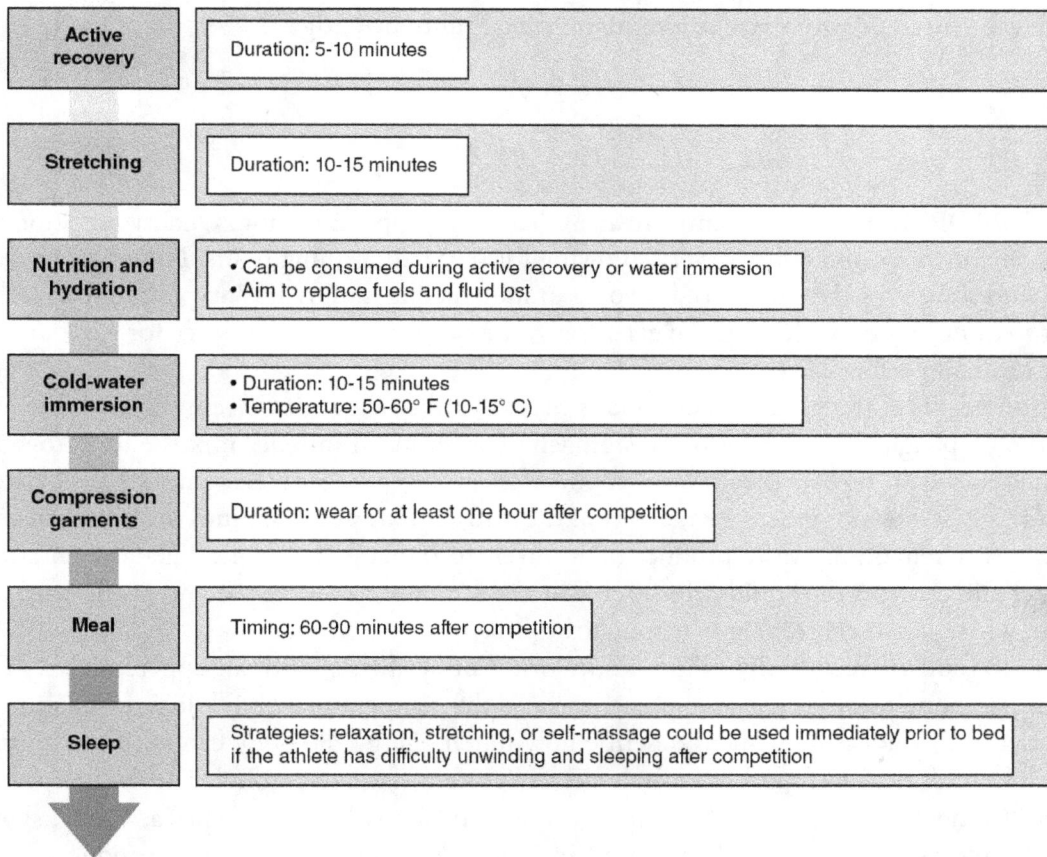

Active recovery	Duration: 5-10 minutes
Stretching	Duration: 10-15 minutes
Nutrition and hydration	• Can be consumed during active recovery or water immersion • Aim to replace fuels and fluid lost
Cold-water immersion	• Duration: 10-15 minutes • Temperature: 50-60° F (10-15° C)
Compression garments	Duration: wear for at least one hour after competition
Meal	Timing: 60-90 minutes after competition
Sleep	Strategies: relaxation, stretching, or self-massage could be used immediately prior to bed if the athlete has difficulty unwinding and sleeping after competition

References: Chapter 15

1.   French, D. N., and Torres, R. L. *NSCA's Essentials of Sport Science.* Champaign, IL: Human Kinetics. 2022.

CHAPTER 16
SPORT NUTRITION & HYDRATION

By: Chris Newport MS, RDN, LDN, EP-C, CISSN
Founder, Head Coach & Performance Dietitian at the Endurance Edge

JUST LIKE PROPER training is essential to an athlete, so is proper nutrition. Quality nutrition improves health and performance and aids recovery, allowing for repeated training bouts. Nutrition needs vary by sport, age, and sex, so it's important to develop a unique fueling and hydration plan for each athlete. It's important to understand the demands of each sport, the types of energy necessary for work and nutrient timing for optimal performance.

Digestion begins in the mouth when food is chewed and swallowed. Once swallowed, the food travels down the esophagus and goes into the stomach. The stomach muscles mix the food together with digestive juices to help further break down food. After mixing, the stomach empties the broken down food into the small intestine where a large part of the nutrients are absorbed into the bloodstream for the body to use. Any remaining waste product then travels to the large intestine. The large intestine helps absorb water and changes the liquid into stool. The stool is then moved to the end of the large intestine, the rectum, where it can exit the body through the anus.[1,2]

Calories in food are technically called "kilocalories" or "Calories" with an uppercase "C." This term refers to the amount of heat that is required to raise the temperature of 1 kilogram of water by one degree. It is a unit of measurement to describe how much energy the body can get from consuming a food or drink.[2] Calories are found in carbohydrates, protein, fat and alcohol. For the purposes of this chapter, we'll ignore alcohol. Carbohydrates are found in items like bread, pasta, beans, sugar, fruit, sports drinks and vegetables.[3] Protein is found in items like animal meats, dairy products, soy, beans, nuts and eggs.[4] Fats are found in items like avocado, olives, oils, nuts, seeds, nut butters and butter.[5]

Macronutrient & Micronutrient Needs for Athletes

Carbohydrates

Carbohydrates are broken down into glucose, which is the body's main source of fuel. Cells, tissues and organs all require glucose in order to function properly. Glucose can either be used immediately by the body, or it can be stored in the liver and muscles for later use.[3]

Simple carbohydrates are the most basic form of a carbohydrate. This means that these carbohydrates can be quickly broken down to use as energy. Fruits, cow's milk, white bread, white rice and table sugar are all examples of foods that contain simple carbohydrates.[3] It's recommended to limit added sugar intake to less than 10% of total caloric intake. Complex carbohydrates are made of many simple carbohydrates that are strung together. This means that it will take the body longer to break them down in order to use them for energy. Examples of complex carbohydrates are peas, beans, whole grains and vegetables.[3]

Protein

All cells contain protein, which is why the consumption of protein is so important. In order to help the body repair cells and make new ones, enough protein must be consumed. Protein can be remembered as the building block of life, and it is essential for growth and development.[4]

In other words, protein is necessary for building and supporting muscle tissue. It's also critical in creating antibodies for immunity. Proteins are made of smaller units called amino acids. There are 20 amino acids, of which humans can produce 10 of them. The essential amino acids (EAAs) are arginine, leucine, histidine, isoleucine, lysine, methionine, phenylalanine, threonine, tryptophan and valine. These amino acids are required in the diet.

Fats

Like carbohydrates, fats can also provide energy for the body. Fats are needed to help the body absorb certain vitamins and keep skin and hair healthy. Other essential functions of fats include brain development, controlling inflammation and blood clotting. It is important to remember that not all fats provide the same benefits. Healthier fats, such as nuts, seeds, avocado, and olives provide more health benefits than fats from butter, coconut oil or full-fat dairy products.[5]

Unsaturated fats are needed to provide many health benefits for the body and should be prioritized for consumption. These types of fats can help decrease the risk of heart disease, aid with brain development, and help the body grow and develop properly. Unsaturated fats are found in olives and olive oil, avocados and avocado oil, nuts, nut butters, seeds, and fatty types of fish like salmon.[5] Unsaturated fats tend to be liquid at room temperature while saturated fats tend to be solid at room temperature. Saturated fats do not provide the same health benefits that unsaturated fats provide. Overconsumption of these fats can lead to health problems, so consumption of these fats should be limited to less than 10% of total daily caloric consumption. Saturated fats are found in butter, coconut oil, fatty cuts of animal meats, like beef and full-fat dairy products, like whole milk, ice cream and cheese.[5,6]

Healthy Sources of Macronutrients

Carbohydrates	Proteins	Fats
Whole grains • Brown rice • Quinoa • Corn • Barley • Buckwheat • Millet • Oats • Popcorn Whole grain products • Whole wheat bread • Whole wheat pasta • Brown rice flour noodles or pasta Fruits • Apples • Berries • Bananas • Oranges • Cherries • Mango • Pineapples • Pears • Kiwi Vegetables • Broccoli • Spinach • Kale • Brussels sprouts • Asparagus • Okra • Cauliflower • Bok choy • Peppers • Lettuce • Mushrooms	Animal products • Clams • Crab • Lobster • Fish • Mussels • Shrimp • Beef • Chicken • Turkey • Duck • Eggs • Egg whites Protein powders • Whey • Egg white • Plant protein blends • Pea • Rice Low-fat dairy products: • Cow's milk • Greek or regular yogurt • Cheese • Kefir Soy products • Tofu • Tempeh • Soymilk • Edamame • Soybean spread Legumes • Chickpeas • Lentils • Peas • Kidney beans • Black beans	Fatty omega-3 fish • Salmon • Trout • Sardines • Albacore tuna Plant-based fats: • Coconut • Avocado • Olives Oils • Olive • Avocado • Canola • Peanut • Sesame • Sunflower • Safflower Seeds or seed butters • Chia • Flax • Pumpkin • Hemp • Sesame or tahini • Sunflower Nuts or nut butters • Almonds • Brazil nuts • Cashews • Macadamia • Hazelnuts • Pecans • Pistachios • Walnuts • Peanuts

Carbohydrates	Proteins	Fats
Dairy • Cow's milk • Yogurt Root vegetables • Yams • Beets • Potatoes • Onions • Carrots • Turnips Soy products • Tofu • Tempeh • Soymilk • Edamame • Soybean spread Legumes • Chickpeas • Lentils • Peas • Kidney beans • Black beans Sweeteners (<10% of total calories): • Honey • Maple syrup • Sugar		Animal-based fats (<10% of total calories) • Low-fat cheese • Ghee or butter • Mayonnaise • Egg yolk

Caloric needs for athletes

It's important for athletes to have enough calories, or energy intake. Inadequate caloric intake can cause short stature, delayed puberty, menstrual dysfunction, loss of muscle mass, and increased susceptibility for fatigue, injury, or illness.[7] Insufficient protein intake in athletes can result in the use of muscle protein being used as a source of energy. To avoid muscle loss, it is crucial to consume adequate protein every day. Athletes, especially growing adolescents, will need proper protein intake to grow, develop, and continue to perform well athletically.[8]

Consuming enough carbohydrates is necessary for athletes. Glycogen, which is stored in the liver and muscle, is the body's stored form of carbohydrates. It's the primary source of energy used during moderate to high intensity exercise. Glycogen is broken down into glucose, which is the brain and body's preferred fuel source. Inadequate carbohydrate intake can result in fatigue, decreased exercise performance, and the inability to properly recover after exercising.[9]

Undernutrition is the most common cause of growth retardation. Studies have shown that teenage athletes who regularly participate in vigorous sport training may need up to 5000 calories per day, so it is important to ensure adolescents are maintaining adequate daily caloric intake. Poverty, self-induced food restriction, malabsorption, and chronic systemic diseases are all main causes of inadequate intake, which can lead to malnutrition, impaired growth, osteopenia, anemia and different syndromes caused by micronutrient deficiencies.[34] Low energy availability (EA) is the result of a combination of high exercise energy expenditure and low energy intake. It is common in adolescents undertaking heavy training, especially females.[35] Low EA can lead to delayed puberty, menstrual irregularities, poor bone health, short stature, disordered eating and an increased risk of injury.[35]

Caloric needs for active adolescent male and females[6]

	Female			Male			
Age	12-13	14-22	22+	12-13	14-18	19-22	22+
Calories/day	2200	2400	25-35 kcal/kg	2400-2600	2800-3200	3000	30-40 kcal/kg

General carbohydrate, protein, and fat intake for adolescent age ranges.[6]

	Female				Male			
Age	12-13	14-18	19-22	22+	12-13	14-18	19-22	22+
Carb (% kcal)	45-65	45-65	45-65	45-65	45-65	45-65	45-65	45-65
Protein (% kcal)	10-30	10-30	10-35	10-35	10-30	10-30	10-35	10-35
Fat (% kcal)	25-35	25-35	20-35	20-35	25-35	25-35	20-35	20-35

	Female			Male		
Age	12-13	14-18	19-22	12-13	14-18	19-22
Carb (g/day)	248-358	270-390	270-390	270-423	315-520	338-488
Protein (g/day)	55-165	60-180	60-210	60-195	70-240	75-263
Fat (g/day)	61-86	67-93	53-93	67-101	78-124	67-117

In order to maintain adequate blood sugar and energy levels for energy and performance, athletes should eat several times throughout the day.[10] It is difficult to consume enough energy when consuming only one meal per day, so meals and snacks should be consumed roughly every 3-4 hours. Adequate daily consumption will allow for athletes to have enough energy to perform well at practice and during athletic events.[10] Furthermore, nutrient timing is the practice of timing the consumption of food and supplements around exercise to enhance athletic performance and recovery.[10]

If an athlete needs or wants to lose weight, but is not at risk for disordered eating patterns, ideally time the weight loss to not coincide with their peak season. A low-energy dense diet high in fruits, vegetables, whole grains, low-fat dairy, legumes/beans, lean meats and fish should be prioritized. Reducing the energy density of the diet can be more effective at lowering energy intake rather than reducing portion size. Ensuring adequate protein is being consumed will help with satiety and maintenance of muscle. Energy intake may need to be recalculated. Eating approximately 300-500 calories less per day than the athlete normally eats will result in a healthy rate of weight loss.[52] Weight loss of .5-2lbs per week is a healthy rate of weight loss. When it is greater than 2lb, it often is the result of lean body mass loss instead of fat mass, especially if the diet is lacking adequate protein intake. Furthermore, faster weight loss may lead to regaining lost pounds rather quickly.

Athletes in certain sports such as ski jumping, wrestling and cycling may want to gain weight in the offseason because it may be unrealistic or unhealthy to maintain such a low body weight all year round.[52] Athletes in certain sports like weightlifting or team positions that require size and strength, like football, the ideal weight gain is about .5-2 lbs per week. When weight gain is more than 1-2 lbs per week, this often leads to increases in fat rather than lean mass. By increasing intake to 300-500 calories more than what the athlete was originally consuming each day, this will allow for healthy weight gain. Eating every 2-3 hours or 5-9 meals per day can help increase caloric intake.[53]

Micronutrient Needs for Athletes

Vitamins and minerals, also referred to as micronutrients, are used by the body to help it perform its basic functions. Some of these functions that vitamins and minerals help with are growth, maturation, immunity, repairing cell damage and keeping nerves, bones, muscles and skin functioning properly.[9] Whole foods will be the best sources of vitamins and minerals. Fruits, vegetables, whole grains, cuts of meat and dairy are all very high in a variety of vitamins and minerals. Eating a variety of different foods throughout the day and week can help ensure that the body is getting different nutrients that it needs. Without adequate vitamin and mineral intake, a deficiency can occur. This is when the body does not receive enough of a particular micronutrient. When this happens, there can be adverse health implications.[9]

Micronutrients that are commonly insufficient in athletes include calcium, vitamin D and iron. Calcium is important for bone health, normal enzyme activity and muscle contraction. Calcium needs are high for adolescents to accommodate for the need for increased bone and muscle mass due to growth. Without enough calcium, bone or muscle growth can be affected. Consistent inadequate calcium intake also poses problems for bone health as humans age, especially females due to the reduction of estrogen. Bone breakdown can occur when calcium is low as the body uses the stored calcium to maintain normal biological functions.[11] Foods that are rich in calcium include low-fat cow's milk, yogurt, sardines, salmon, broccoli, spinach, and calcium-fortified products, such as plant milks (including soy and almond milk), orange juice and cereals.[6,7]

Vitamin D is needed for bone health and the absorption of calcium. Vitamin D also has an essential role in skeletal muscle growth, muscle function, immune and cardiopulmonary functions, and inflammatory modulation which influence athletic performance. Vitamin D can also interact with extraskeletal tissues to help regulate injury recovery and infection risk.[56] When not enough vitamin D is absorbed by the body, this also negatively affects calcium absorption and bone health. Vitamin D deficiencies are most common in those who have milk allergies, who are lactose intolerant or who follow a vegan diet.[12] A combination of vitamin D deficiency and elevated parathyroid hormone (PTH) levels can cause a decrease in bone mineral density. Athletes should ensure that vitamin D levels are adequate to optimize bone mineral density and avoid injuries such as stress fractures.[56] Few foods contain vitamin D, but it can be found in egg yolk, mushrooms, fatty fishes, such as salmon or tuna and vitamin D-fortified products such as milk, soy milk or almond milk. Vitamin D is best absorbed through the skin via sunlight.[7]

Iron is necessary for oxygen delivery to tissues in the body. Adolescents need more iron than adults to help with growth and increases in blood volume and lean muscle mass.[7] At around 14 years of age, females will need a higher consumption of iron due to menstrual losses. [6] Inadequate iron intake can lead to depletion of iron stores and iron-deficiency anemia. This can negatively affect athletic performance, especially in sports with higher aerobic demands. Fatigue, body temperature regulation and immunity can all be affected when not enough iron is consumed.[7,9] Food sources iron include lean red meats, beans, eggs, leafy green vegetables, and iron-fortified whole grains.[7,9]

Daily recommended intake of calcium, vitamin D, and iron for differing age ranges (chart)

a) Calcium: Ages 12-18: 1300mg, Ages 19-22: 1000 mg, Ages 22-50: 1000mg, Females ages 51-70: 1200mg, Males ages 51-70: 1000mg, <70+: 1200mg
b) Iron:
   i. Males and females ages 12-13: 8 mg,
   ii. Females ages 14-18: 15mg, Females 19-22: 18mg
   iii. Males 14-18: 11 mg, males 19-22: 8 mg
   iv. Female 19-50: 18mg, males 19-50: 8mg
   v. Males and females 51+: 8mg
f) Vitamin D: All ages: 600 IU.[6]

Hydration for Athletes

Water is essential to the human body for a variety of reasons, such as regulation of body temperature, keeping the eyes, nose and mouth tissues moist, protecting organs, carrying nutrients and oxygen to cells, keeping joints lubricated and helping flush out waste products.[13]

During exercise, water intake, or hydration, minimizes body mass losses associated with dehydration while ensuring fluid ingestion does not exceed sweat losses.[9]

Dehydration occurs when fluid intake is insufficient to replace fluid loss, such as sweat. It can impair cognition, technical skills and physical performance especially at higher levels of body mass or when heat stress is involved.[16] Even moderate levels of dehydration can increase physiological strain such as heart rate elevation and decreased cardiac output which make it more difficult for the body to dissipate heat.[14] Water losses ≥ 2% of total body weight impair exercise, skill, and endurance performance.[14,16]

Sweat

Respiration and sweat contribute to fluid losses during exercise, with sweating being the largest contributor. Sweating is the body's most effective physiological method of cooling itself. Evaporation of sweat is the primary cause of heat loss during exercise. This accounts for the importance of replacing fluids lost during exercise.[16]

Sweat contains water, electrolytes, urea and more. Electrolytes are defined as the minerals in the body that have an electrical charge. The most notable electrolytes found in sweat are sodium, potassium and chloride. These electrolytes are needed for water and pH balance, moving nutrients into cells, moving waste out of cells and making sure the nerves, muscles, heart and brain function properly.[18]

The rate of sweat loss is directly related to the exercise intensity. Lower intensity exercise results in lower sweat losses while higher intensity exercise generates a greater rise in core body temperature, resulting in larger sweat losses. Intermittent and endurance sports can cause heavy sweat loss over prolonged periods of time. Adolescents have diminished sweat rates compared to adults. This is beneficial to protect hydration status but can be disadvantageous due to the reduced ability to dissipate heat.[9] Larger individuals are at greater risk of excess sweating due to the larger surface area of skin that will generate more heat and produce more sweat. As skin increases in temperature, blood flow is sent to the skin to aid in cooling. Heart rate also increases to accommodate this and will continue to rise with increased sweating due to lower blood volume.

High temperatures and high humidity levels increase sweat rates as a function of environmental heat load. Skin temperatures rise with increased environmental temperature. Conversely, skin temperatures lower with higher air motion, which assists in sweat evaporation. Furthermore, the ground surface can play a role in an athlete's ability to stay cool. The rubber in turf retains more heat than grass, so athletes playing on turf will likely have an increased body temperature. Athletes playing on dark colored pavement surfaces or without shade will have core temperatures increase faster, larger sweat rates and increased risk for dehydration.

The sport plays a role in sweat rate as well. For example, due to the occurrence of convection in cycling, cyclists will have a lower sweat rate. Water sport athletes, such as swimmers or water polo athletes, will have a lower sweat rate because the body stays cooler in the presence of water. Soccer players and long-distance runners will have higher sweat rates because they are continuously moving, which generates more heat and increases their sweat rates. Football players often have larger sweat rates due to the protective clothing. Protective clothing and dark colored apparel insulates exposure to solar radiation, which then increases skin temperature and sweat rate.[16,57]

Monitoring Hydration Status

There are several ways of monitoring hydration. Thirst is a useful symptom that can be used to show that dehydration is present. Changes in body weight during practice may be a practical way of observing hydration status.[14] Athletes can measure body weight immediately prior to and immediately following activity. Changes in hydration are calculated as the difference between pre-and post-exercise body mass. The technique implies that for every 1g of body mass lost this correlates to 1 mL of water lost. Increases in body mass can inform the athlete that fluid ingestion was too much, and can increase the risk of hyponatremia. An excessive decrease in body mass can inform the athlete that fluid ingestion was not enough.[9] Ideally, body weight losses should not exceed 2% of starting body weight.

Another method of measuring hydration are urinary markers, including reduced urine volume, a high urine specific gravity, a high urine osmolality or a dark urine color. Urine color is a common and simple way to assess hydration status, with a lighter color correlating with hydration and a darker color correlating with dehydration. Urine specific gravity can be measured with a refractometer and is not as practical or easily accessible. Bioelectrical impedance is another noninvasive technique used to estimate total body water (TBW) by using a low amperage current passed between skin electrodes. However, this may not be a valid technique when electrolyte concentrations change, as they often do with sweating.

In order to stay hydrated, athletes should keep fluids readily available and easily accessible during training sessions and events. Coaches, athletic trainers and events should promote water breaks and ingestion of fluids during exercise regardless of thirst level.[14] During activities, it is recommended that athletes consume 150 mL to 300 mL of fluid every 15 min to 20 min. Taking water breaks will help meet the recommendation.[7]

Sports Drinks

Sports drinks can be a convenient way of delivering energy from carbohydrates as well as replacing lost fluid and electrolytes. Proper replacement of electrolytes during exercise will help with the avoidance of muscle cramps. Muscle cramps are more likely to occur with the loss of sodium through sweat, so by keeping electrolyte levels high, this helps the body avoid cramping.[20]

Before exercise, a sports drink may be optimal to choose over water due to its carbohydrate content for energy. In addition, the sodium content may reduce urine loss before exercise.[19] Sports drinks should generally be prioritized during and after exercise after heavy fluid loss through sweat has occurred.[7, 20]

For events lasting longer than 60-90 minutes, sports drinks containing 6% carbohydrates and 20 mEq/L to 30 mEq/L of sodium chloride are recommended to replace energy stores, fluid loss and electrolyte loss.[7] Most sports drinks contain about 6-8% carbohydrate (6-8g/L). When concentrations are above this, it can impair gastric emptying and lead to gut upset during exercise.[19] The sports drink will help replace fluids and electrolytes that were lost during sweat while helping with recovery.[19]

Sodium and potassium should be included in the sports drink. The sodium content in the sports drink will help drive the thirst mechanism and increase absorption and fluid retention for the athlete to remain hydrated.[19, 20] Low sodium drinks may not always be optimal for athletes that need quick rehydration. The presence of potassium in sports drinks will also help maintain electrolyte balance and assists with muscle contraction during exercise.[19]

Fluid recommendations for exercise:

Pre-exercise	During exercise	Post-exercise
• 5-7 ml/kg of body weight 4 hours prior • Another 3-5 ml/kg 2 hours prior if urine is dark or the athlete cannot urinate	• Based on individual sweat rate • Consume amount of fluid to minimize body weight loss of <2% • For events >60-90 minutes or for hot or high intensity exercise, choose a sports drink containing carbohydrates and electrolytes that is well tolerated	• 1-1.5 L/kg body weight lost of fluid with sodium

Heat-related illness

Heat-related illness refers to heat cramps, heat exhaustion and heat stroke. These conditions occur when the body is not able to cool itself off properly, and body temperature rises faster than it can cool down.

Heat cramps are muscle pains or spasms that commonly occur in the abdomen, arms or legs. Heavy sweating during activity makes heat cramps more likely to occur. The high sweat rate depletes the body's salt and moisture, which causes muscle cramps. Heat cramps may also be a symptom of heat exhaustion. If heat cramps occur, stop all activity and sit in a cool place, drink clear fluids or a sports drink, and do not return to strenuous activity for a few hours after the cramps subside. If the heat cramps do not subside within one hour, seek medical attention.

After several days of exposure to high temperature with inadequate or unbalanced fluid replacement, heat exhaustion can develop. If left untreated, heat exhaustion may progress to heat stroke. If symptoms worsen or last longer than one hour, seek medical attention. Signs and symptoms of heat exhaustion including heavy sweating, cold, pale, clammy skin, fast, weak pulse, nausea and vomiting, muscle cramps, fatigue, dizziness, headache, or fainting.

Out of all heat-related illnesses, heat stroke is the most dangerous. Heat stroke occurs when the body cannot control its temperature. Body temperature rises quickly, sweating mechanisms fail and the body becomes unable to cool down. Within 10-15 minutes, body temperature can rise to 41°C (105°F) or higher. Unlike heat cramps or heat exhaustion, if an individual shows signs and symptoms of heat stroke, do not give the individual anything to drink. Signs and symptoms of heat stroke are hot, red, dry, or damp skin, headache, fast and strong pulse, dizziness, nausea, confusion, or loss of consciousness.[17]

Heat related illness or deaths are preventable. It is important to monitor athletes to make sure they are not exhibiting any signs or symptoms of heat illness. Most importantly, stay hydrated and replace electrolytes. Take breaks in air conditioned, cool, or shaded areas. Monitor athletes' paces during practices where temperatures are higher than normal. Schedule practices and events during lower temperatures. Wear light-weight, light-colored and loose-fitting technical fabrics when possible. Also, apply sunscreen 30 minutes prior to going outdoors for all skin colors. Sunburned skin negatively affects the body's ability to cool itself.[17]

Physiological differences between sport types and nutrient needs

Aerobic exercise is any activity using large muscle groups that can be maintained continuously and is rhythmic in nature. Activities that are primarily aerobic are cycling, dancing, hiking, long-distance running, long-distance swimming and walking.[1] Aerobic exercises use the cardiorespiratory system, which is the heart and lungs, in order to supply oxygen and help muscles use oxygen during exercise.

Aerobic metabolism involves the creation of energy known as adenosine triphosphate or ATP through the combustion of carbohydrates, fat and amino acids in the presence of oxygen. As the duration of exercise increases beyond 3 minutes and intensity decreases, energy from aerobic metabolism is prioritized.[22] The majority of ATP is obtained from carbohydrates or triglycerides depending upon the exercise intensity and duration. As exercise intensity increases, there is a gradual switch from triglycerides as the main fuel source for energy production to the use of carbohydrates for energy production.[22]

Anaerobic exercise is intense physical activity of very short duration that is fueled by energy sources within contracting muscles.[21] Activities that are primarily anaerobic are sprinting, short-distance swimming, high-intensity interval training and weightlifting.[21] Anaerobic exercise is fueled by energy sources within contracting muscles. It is independent of the use of inhaled oxygen as a source of energy.

Anaerobic metabolism involves the creation of energy (ATP) through the combustion of carbohydrates in the absence of oxygen. The adenosine triphosphate phosphocreatine (ATP-PC) energy system is important as an energy source in physical activities that need a lot of energy per second (about 3 seconds or less). Exercises that are very short-term and high-intensity, such as sprinting or weightlifting, require the ATP-PC system. This energy is provided for only a short period of time. For slightly longer durations, aerobic glycolysis can occur to produce lactic acid to generate ATP for energy. Glucose from the bloodstream or from glycogen in glycolysis will be used as a fuel source for intramuscular ATP and PC stores. Proteins and triglycerides can not be metabolized to provide ATP during anaerobic exercise.

Although each energy system can be looked at individually, this does not mean that only one energy system can function during exercise. No energy source of ATP is ever turned "off." All sources will supply some ATP at all times. Anaerobic energy sources provide the majority of ATP needed to perform high-intensity and short-duration maximal physical activity. Sports like weightlifting, shot-putting, high-jumping and diving rely mainly on ATP and PC as an energy source due to their high intensity and short nature. Events requiring maximal power will also need ATP from other metabolic sources.

Aerobic metabolism provides the majority of ATP to perform long-duration, low-intensity physical activity. Cross-country skiing, cycling, mid-long distance swimming, skating, pentathlon, rowing and triathlon rely on aerobic metabolism.[23] Intermittent sports, such as basketball, football, ice hockey, field hockey, rugby, soccer, tennis, boxing and volleyball will vary between the use of aerobic and anaerobic metabolism.[22]

Due to the longer exercise duration of intermittent and endurance sports compared to skill and power sports, it is important to remember to schedule refueling breaks when necessary for athletes. For example, many endurance athletes find it difficult to continue to hydrate throughout an event. If the difficulty of staying hydrated repeatedly occurs during an endurance event, hyperhydration (drinking more water than needed) may be an option prior to exercise. The downsides of this are potentially having to urinate during exercise.[26] Hyponatremia is also a concern when fluids are ingested at excessive levels. As duration of an activity increases along with fluid ingestion, especially in warm-hot conditions, the risk of hyponatremia increases. The ingestion of sodium containing beverages will reduce the risk of hyponatremia.[9]

When training is over one hour, 30-60 grams per hour of carbohydrate-electrolyte sports drinks are recommended for improved performance. For endurance sports and intermittent sports that last longer than 90 minutes, 60-90 grams of carbohydrates-electrolyte solution may have advantages such as extending running time, preserving sprint speed, and preserving sport-specific skill. Daily carbohydrate intake varies between 5-12 g/kg/day depending on intensity and needs of the athlete.[24] Endurance sports are completed over a longer time without breaks, so athletes in this field are most likely to need refueling during practice or an event.[26] For heavy daily training (4+ hours per day), higher carbohydrate intake closer to 9-10 g/kg/day may be needed to restore performance.[24, 25]

Many skill sports will require a high level of focus, yet are not as demanding on the aerobic or anaerobic exercise systems. Archery, curling, equestrian, golf and shooting are primarily skill-based sports. To ensure that mental performance is at its best, it is important to continue to consume balanced meals throughout the day to ensure that blood sugar levels remain stable and provide the brain and body necessary nutrients to perform well. A low carbohydrate diet is not recommended because it will disrupt cognitive function. Caffeine may not be recommended for skill sports either due to possible side effects such as shakiness, dizziness, and increased heart rate. After caffeine consumption, the mental tempo will increase first and speeds of association increases, but a noticeable decrease in the quality of work being done has been shown.[58]

Anthropometrics, gender and nutritional needs

Anthropometrics are quantitative measurements of the muscle, bone and adipose tissue that are used to assess the composition of the body. Body composition, along with sex, age and activity level help to to give guardrails for energy and macronutrient consumption. The main measurements of anthropometry for nutritional status are height, weight, body mass index (BMI), body circumferences (waist, hip, and limbs) and estimated body fat.

The two main components that make up total daily energy expenditure (TDEE) are resting metabolic rate (RMR) and activity level. Normally, RMR makes up approximately 60-70% of total daily energy expenditure. This can be multiplied by a physical activity (PA) factor that correlates to the activity level of an individual in order to estimate the TDEE. The TDEE can then be used to estimate how much energy should be consumed every day.[27]

Resting metabolic rate (RMR) is the total number of calories required to keep your body functioning at rest. These functions include breathing, circulating blood, organ functions and basic neurological functions.[27] Resting metabolic rate can be calculated using direct or indirect calorimetry. Since those methods are often costly and impractical, several metabolic equations have been developed to calculate the RMR of an athlete. One method is the Mifflin-St Jeor equation, that factors in gender, height, body weight and age.

Men = (9.99 x body weight) + (6.26 x height) - (4.92 x age) + 5
Women = (9.99 x body weight) + (6.26 x height) - (4.92 x age) - 161
Weight = kilograms, height = centimeters, age = years

Factors that influence RMR include age, genetics and gender. After peak growth has been achieved, RMR decreases about 2% per decade of life. Some people are genetically predisposed to have faster or slower metabolisms. On average, males have greater muscle mass and lower body-fat percentage than females do. Because of this, males will generally have a higher RMR. Those with more mass will have a higher RMR, particularly those with lean body mass (more muscle).[9] Athletes that are the same weight with a higher body-fat percentage will generally have a lower RMR than those with a lower-body fat percentage.[27]

The PA coefficient is the number correlating to the activity level of an individual that can be multiplied by RMR to calculate total daily energy expenditure.

Physical activity multipliers to calculate total energy expenditure:

Sedentary — little to no exercise (multiply by 1.2)
Lightly Active — light exercise 1–3 days/week (multiply by 1.375)
Moderately Active — moderate exercise 3–5 days/week (multiply by 1.55)
Very Active — hard exercise 6–7 days/week (multiply by 1.725)
Extremely Active — hard daily exercise and training (multiply by 1.9)[27]

After calculating the RMR, multiply that number by the PA coefficient that correlates to the athlete to get the estimated caloric needs of the athlete.

Example: A 17 year old male who is 175 cm tall and weighs 68 kg who plays tennis 6-7 days per week.

(9.99 x 68kg) + (6.26 x 175cm) - (4.92 x 17) + 5 = 1696
1696 x 1.725 = 2926

For weight maintenance, growth and proper athletic performance, this 17 year old male should be consuming approximately 2900 calories per day.

Once caloric needs are determined, estimate the macronutrient needs, beginning by estimating the protein needs. One gram of protein equals approximately 4 calories.

Athletes should be consuming a minimum of 1.2-1.8g/kg/day.[9] It's important to consider the total percentage of protein intake should be no less than 10-15% of total caloric intake. The maximum amount of protein intake per day can be upwards of 2.2-3.0g/kg/day. However, the total percentage of protein intake should allow for adequate amounts of carbohydrates and fat as described previously. For the purposes of gaining muscle and strength, 25-30% of total calories should come from protein.

Example: A 17-year-old male who is 175 cm tall and weighs 68 kg.

- Minimum needs are 1.2-1.8g/kg:
  o 1.2gx68kg = 82g/day
  o 1.8gx68g = 122g/day
  o The athlete should be consuming at least 82-122g of protein per day.
    ▪ 82*4 calories per gram = 328 calories
      • 328/2900 = 11% of total calories from protein
    ▪ 122*4 = 488 calories
      • 488/2900 = 17% of total calories from protein
  o Since he is a tennis player looking to maintain muscle mass and still growing, he may need closer to 20% of total calories from protein, or 2900*.20 = 580 calories = 145 grams or 2.1 grams/kg body weight

For reference, approximately one ounce of cooked weight of a lean protein source like chicken, fish, pork or beef contains approximately 7 grams of protein.

35g protein = 1 cup whole shrimps
33g protein = 1 cup extra firmed cooked tofu
25g protein = 1 cup nonfat, plain greek yogurt
20g protein = 1 cup edamame
18g protein = 1 cup lentils

Next, calculate carbohydrate needs, which are crucial for exercise performance, which should be 3-8g/kg/day.[9] Similar to protein, one gram of carbohydrate equals approximately 4 calories. Generally, carbohydrates should make up 35-60% of total caloric intake, allowing for adequate protein and fat intake.

Example: A 17-year-old male who is 175 cm tall and weighs 68 kg.

- Using 3-8g/kg:
  o 3gx68kg = 204g/day
  o 8gx68g = 544g/day
  o The athlete should be consuming at least 204-544g of carbohydrate per day.
    ▪ 204*4 calories per gram = 816 calories
    ▪ 544*4 = 2176 calories
    ▪ Since the athlete's total recommended caloric intake is 2900, as an active tennis player, a more appropriate range is 50% of total calories, or 2900*.50 = 1450 calories

- 1450/4 calories per gram = ~362 grams
- 362/68kg = ~5g of carbohydrates per day.

For reference, here are some common foods and their grams of carbohydrates (CHO).

1 cup cooked brown rice = 52g CHO
1 mango = 50g CHO
1 cup cooked rice noodles = 42 g CHO
1 cup cooked lentils = 40g CHO
1 medium sweet potato = 35g CHO
1 cup edamame = 18g CHO
1 small apple = 15g CHO

Finally, calculate the fat needs for the athlete. One gram of fat equals 9 calories. Ensure that the percentage of total fat intake doesn't drop below 12-15% of total energy intake. A diet adequate in healthy fats is crucial for adolescents to help with the synthesis of hormones, to assist in normal bodily functioning, and to promote healthy growth and maturation. Adolescents have been found to have improved aerobic efficiency related to an increased dependency on fats for energy production, so adequate fat intake for adolescent athletes is crucial. In general, children depend more rapidly on lipids in comparison to adults, so a diet too low in fat should not be recommended.[9]

Similarly, diets high in fat may lead to excessive weight gain. Fat provides more than twice the calories than carbohydrates or protein provides, so it can become easy to over consume on a high-fat diet. A high-fat diet can also impair metabolic functioning and lead to cardiovascular disease. Coronary heart disease is a chronic, progressive disease with origins beginning early in life, so it is crucial for adolescents to adopt healthy, balanced eating patterns to decrease disease risk.[9]

Example: A 17 year old male who is 175 cm tall and weighs 68 kg.

- As calculated above, this athlete needs 2900 calories per day, with about 20% of calories from protein and 50% of calories from carbohydrates.
  - 50% + 20% = 70%
  - Subtract total energy needs from protein and carbohydrate needs to determine fat. Ensure it is above minimum needs.
    - 100%-70% = 30% of total calories from fat
      - 2900 * .30 = 870 calories per day.
      - 870/9 calories per gram = ~97 grams per day.

For reference, here are some common foods containing fat.

Almonds: 16g fat = ¼ cup whole almonds
Olive oil: 15g fat = 1 tbsp oil
Cashews: 14g fat = ¼ cup whole cashews
Salmon: 11g fat = 6 oz. filet of salmon.
Egg: 5g fat = 1 egg

Pre, During & Post Workout Nutrition

Proper sports nutrition for athletes ensures adequate energy production related to exercise and recovery. By consuming enough energy throughout the day with proper macronutrient distribution ranges, athletes will have enough energy from carbohydrates to perform well, can recover properly with adequate protein and carbohydrate intake and can function properly during exercise with healthy fat consumption.[9]

Consuming a **pre-workout** meal or snack replenishes glycogen stores and can have positive effects on athletic performance. One to four hours pre-workout, athletes should consume 1-4 g/kg of carbohydrates.[25] These foods should be familiar and well-tolerated foods for the athlete to deliver quick energy. The closer to practice or competition time the snack is consumed, the smaller in size it should be. Also, the snack should be higher in simple carbohydrates to deliver quick energy. They may include fruit, dried fruit (i.e., raisins, apricots, or cranberries), pretzels, crackers or fruit juice. Athletes can consume a larger mixed meal or snack when there is a greater amount of time between eating and competition, which allows for more digestion to take place. Include more complex carbohydrates for sustained energy like brown rice, sweet potatoes or legumes.

Carbohydrate ingestion **during** exercise has been shown to improve exercise performance even when the exercise is high intensity (>75% VO_2max) and short duration (~60 minutes).[26] In this case, sports drinks may be the best tolerated. For exercise lasting longer than 60 minutes, carbohydrate consumption in the form of simple carbohydrates should be consumed.[9, 25] Food options with simple carbohydrates that can be tried include bananas, dry cereals, crackers, granola bars, fig bars, carbohydrate gels, gummies or pretzels. All food and drinks that will be used during competition should be used in training first to ensure adequate tolerance and enjoyment.

Post exercise, 1-1.5g/kg of carbohydrate should be consumed within 30 minutes of the cessation of prolonged exercise.[9, 25] This is when the body is more likely to store exogenous carbohydrates as glycogen for the next training session. Also, consume at least 20-25g protein within 2 hours post workout for ideal muscle protein synthesis, which helps maintain and build muscle.[9, 25] By consuming both carbohydrates and protein together, this may help reduce delayed onset muscle soreness after exercise.[25] Food choices should be well tolerated and enjoyed and can include edamame, Greek yogurt and fruit, smoothies, store bought protein shakes or bars, jerky and crackers.

Potential foods and drinks to avoid pre, during and post workout will vary for each athlete. However, any known foods that the athlete is allergic to or intolerant to should be avoided. Gastrointestinal (GI) issues such as nausea, vomiting, abdominal angina and bloody diarrhea are very common in athletes, especially in endurance athletes. During exercise, blood flow to the GI tract is impaired which is likely the main cause of developing GI symptoms. This can impair both athletic performance and recovery.[29] Research suggests that athletes who are not accustomed to fluid and food ingestion during exercise have a two-fold risk of developing GI issues. The gut is highly adaptable, so endurance athletes should incorporate nutritional training into their exercise plans as well.[29]

Some athletes tolerate certain foods differently during exercise. Milk products and foods that are high in fiber or fat may commonly increase the risk of developing GI distress during exercise.[7, 29] This is why it is important to test the consumption of different foods on practice days rather than event or game days to know if a food can be tolerated or not. Fiber is not digestible, so the fiber will pass through the intestinal tract. This will increase bowel movements, which is not ideal for exercise or maintaining hydration status. It is recommended to consume a low-fiber diet before an event if GI symptoms are likely. Legumes, high-fiber cereals, and many fruits and vegetables contain a high fiber content.[29]

High-fat meals should be avoided prior to exercise because they can delay gastric-emptying, make athletes feel lethargic and ultimately negatively affect athletic performance.[7] Depending upon sport type, some athletes will need fat prior to exercise to create a well-balanced meal. Because long distance athletes will continuously be exercising for long periods of time, having adequate consumption of both carbohydrates and fat as a fuel source is important. In anaerobic sports, fat intake is less likely needed.[29]

The intake of fructose, especially in isolated form (as in certain sports drinks and sodas) or as high fructose corn syrup, may also be associated with an increased risk of developing GI symptoms. When fructose is consumed in combination with glucose, research suggests that GI symptoms may not develop and are better tolerated. Foods high in fructose that may need to be avoided include sodas, fruit juices, dried fruit, apples, agave, and honey. The combination of fructose and glucose are found in table sugar and whole fruits, which is why fruit may still be an ideal pre-workout food choice.[29]

Exercise causes both physical and psychological stress. Stress during exercise activates the autonomic nervous system which increases the release of neurotransmitters in the GI tract. The gut is directly connected to the brain through the vagus nerve, which is why stress may be the cause of GI symptoms prior to exercise, especially on competition or game days.[59] If all food items seem to have been eliminated, be sure to rule out any potential medical condition. Furthermore, consider mental training from a certified sports psychologist to manage stress prior to competition.

Ergogenic Aids

Ergogenic aids are any training technique, mechanical device, nutritional ingredient, pharmacological method or psychological technique that can improve exercise performance.[36] Dietary supplements are considered nutritional ergogenic aids. Dietary supplements intended for improvement of athletic performance and faster recovery are known as sports supplements.[37] Whey protein, creatine, amino acids, caffeine, vitamin and mineral complexes, beta-alanine and glutamine are commonly used.[37]

Common supplements used by athletes and their potential exercise effects:

- Branched-chain amino acids (BCAAs): Can be metabolized in the skeletal muscle to provide energy during exercise. Research shows a possibility of greater gains in muscle mass and strength during training.
- Caffeine: May enhance performance in intermittent and endurance activities when taken prior to exercise. Genetic differences in our ability to metabolize caffeine may affect how different athletes perform and feel using it.
- Creatine: Helps supply muscle with energy for short-term activities that are mainly anaerobic. May increase strength, power, and work from maximal effort muscle contraction. Can help the body adapt to training regimens, but has little value for endurance sports.
- Protein (powders, shakes, etc.): Builds, maintains, and repairs muscle. Optimizes muscle training responses during and after exercise.
- Beta-alanine: Helps reduce muscle fatigue and loss of force production. Research has shown inconsistent effects with high-intensity exercise for a short duration. Little to no benefits have been shown in activities longer than 10 minutes.
- Glutamine: May help with recovery of muscle strength and reduce muscle soreness after exercise.
- Vitamin and mineral complexes: Do not directly improve athletic performance, but can help minimize free-radical damage to skeletal muscle, inflammation, and soreness.[38]

The prevalence of sport supplements has greatly increased within the past decade, but athletes rarely seek information from educated resources. Many supplements can be properly utilized for increased athletic performance, but athletes must understand proper dosage and which supplements are allowed to optimize athletic performance and eliminate adverse health effects.[37] If athletes take supplementation without guidance, there is an increased risk of negative effects on the athlete's health, especially in adolescent athletes. Recent research has shown that there is a relatively low level of knowledge among adolescent athletes regarding supplementation with 12% of athletes stating they would use banned substances for an advancement in sports. Coaches and athletes can refer to the International Society of Sports Nutrition (ISSN), World Anti-Doping Agency (WADA), and NSF International for information about safe supplement use.

Supplements used to improve athletic performance can have side effects and could interact with medications that athletes may be taking. The active constituents of botanical or other ingredients that are commonly marketed as ergogenic aids are unknown or uncharacterized. Many products contain multiple ingredients that have not been adequately tested in combination with one another, which can cause adverse health effects.[38] A third-party certification should be an important consideration for athletes who want to protect themselves from quality control or banned substances. This certification ensures that an independent organization has reviewed a product and determined that it is safe for the user.[40]

Certain ingredients like caffeine and testosterone should be avoided. Caffeine in doses over 500mg can cause insomnia, nausea, vomiting, tachycardia and arrhythmia.[38] Testosterone boosters can cause polycythemia, increased blood viscosity, prostatic hyperplasia, hepatotoxic effects, hepatic neoplasia and dysfunction and sleep apnea.[39] The following are on the Banned Substance Control Group (BSCG) dietary supplement ingredient advisory list:[40]

- Selective Androgen Receptor modulators (SARMs): Andarine, cardarine, ostarine
- Growth Hormone Releasing Peptides (GHRPs) and other peptides: GHRP-1, GHRP-2, GHRP-6
- Synthetic stimulants. Common in pre-workout supplements or fat-burners. These are ingredients that are constituents, extracts, or concentrates or plants or herbs that can be considered as legal supplements.
  o Aegeline/bael tree extract, acacia, DEPEA, DMAA, geranium extract, DMBA, DMHA, kigelia africiana, DMPEA, higenamine, hordenine, isopropyloctopamine, NMPEA, orchilean, oxilofrine, phenylethylamine HCL
- Certain pharmaceutical nootropics: Phenibut, picamilon, piracetam, tianeptine

"The difference in how these products are regulated and the recommendations that are made about them across different countries raises the question of whether and how harmonization could be implementable since there exists a substantial difference in diet, historical knowledge and the consumer, across these countries." https://www.sciencedirect.com/science/article/pii/S0273230020300738#sec3

Not all supplements have been evaluated for efficacy or safety prior to entering the market. Supplements can be marketed at any concentration as long as the daily recommended value is on the label. If the daily recommended value is undetermined, supplements can be marketed without this information. Dietary supplements can be sold in any combination of ingredients, which may also pose health effects due to possible interactions between ingredients. Analyses have shown the presence of lead, arsenic, mercury, cadmium, or pesticides in 40 different dietary supplements in the United States. In addition, botanical supplements have been found to contain plant species that are not listed on the label. Supplement labels can fail to state the intended purpose of the supplement, fail to identify the active ingredient, not recognize any side effects or not include the maximum dosage.[41]

Manufacturers of products set their own standards, so the same products from a different manufacturer may be different in composition, strength, or bioavailability.[41] Many companies make claims about their product in order to increase sales, and not all of these claims may be true. The outcomes of studies of many performance-enhancing substances are often equivocal. This makes it confusing for the consumer on which supplement to purchase.[38] Claims can often be poorly understood.

Supplements containing herbal extracts have been seen to cause liver and kidney toxicity. The same has been shown with pure caffeine anhydrous ingestion.[37] Harm may be caused from heavy metal and other contaminants found within supplements. Larger doses of a supplement are associated with greater toxicity of any contaminants that may be present. This supports the need to ensure a supplement has been through third party testing.[41]

Supplement Considerations

- Identify important components when looking for a multivitamin.
- Most basic multivitamins contain vitamins and minerals at levels that do not exceed the daily value. Some individuals may need to pay attention to vitamin A or iron to avoid over consumption of these nutrients.
- Generally, adolescents should try to find a multivitamin tailored to their age and gender. Multivitamins for young males will contain less iron than multivitamins for young females since the need for iron is higher for younger females.[43]
- Look for products that have a third-party certification on the label.[42]
- Demonstrate how to read a supplement label.
  - The serving size is the manufacturer's recommended serving expressed in the appropriate unit. Example: 1 scoop.
  - Servings per container lets the consumer know how many servings of the supplement are provided.
  - Amount per serving provides the quantity of each dietary ingredient present in the supplement.
  - The % Daily Value (DV) tells what percentage of the recommended daily intake for each nutrient is present in the supplement.
  - If an ingredient has an asterisk or other symbol in place of the %DV, this means a DV has not been established for that specific ingredient.
  - Any foot notes on the label will provide explanations for symbols, such as asterisks, for further explanation.
  - The amount of dietary ingredients in each serving is declared in metric units. This is important to see how much of a specific ingredient is being ingested.
  - The list of all ingredients will be in decreasing order by weight.[44]
- Describe how a supplement can fit into a healthy diet.
  - For any adolescent to perform well, proper hydration and a nutritionally adequate diet should be prioritized. After a proper dietary foundation has been set, dietary supplements can be added to the diet to help meet athletic goals or increase athletic performance. A sport supplement should not be substituted for a healthy diet.[38]
  - To supplement something means to add an extra element. Dietary supplements can be thought of in the same sense. For example, adding protein powder to a smoothie can help enhance the smoothie to meet athletic goals. Whole foods are still being prioritized, while the protein powder helps enhance the smoothie.

Special Issues in Sports Nutrition

There are special issues with athletes that may affect their nutritional status and needs. Overreaching and overtraining is one of the most common. Overreaching is further accumulation of training volume or intensity combined with insufficient or impaired recovery. If one is not careful overreaching can be the precursor to overtraining. The recovery period can take days to weeks.[45, 47] Overtraining is persistent underperformance despite more than two months of recovery combined with changes in mood and the absence of symptoms or diagnoses of other possible causes of underperformance. The recovery period can take weeks to years.[46, 47]

Signs and symptoms of overtraining include increases in resting heart rate and arterial pressure, insomnia, amenorrhea, reduced appetite, weight loss or weight gain, and anorexia. Blood markers may reveal alterations in glutamine, iron, ferritin, hemoglobin and hematocrit.[48] There may also be changes in metabolic, immunologic, muscle, inflammatory, and hormonal responses.[47] Fatigue, excessive muscle pain, depression, mood change and decreased athletic performance can all occur when proper rest and recovery is not enforced.[48]

Common eating disorders include anorexia nervosa, bulimia nervosa, orthorexia nervosa and binge-eating. Risk factors for disordered eating patterns include having a close relative, such as a parent or sibling, with disordered eating or a mental health condition or having a history of anxiety disorders or dieting. Many individuals also report that disordered eating began in efforts to restrict food too much in order to lose weight. Other risk factors include type 1 diabetes, poor body image, bullying or continuously being exposed to the message that thinner is better through social media, television, the internet, etc.[51] Athletes involved in certain sports may also be at higher risk of disordered eating (ED). For example, sports like ballet, running, figure skating, gymnastics and diving that emphasize aesthetics or leanness or weight class sports like wrestling, martial arts and rowing are at increased risk.[22, 50] Participating in endurance sports where a low body weight is advantageous like in cycling, long-distance running or cross-country skiing are also at risk.[22] Finally, disordered eating may appear in sports where body contour-revealing clothing is worn like ballroom dancing, volleyball, swimming or diving.[22]

For adolescent females, strenuous athletic training, high exercise energy expenditure and low energy intake can all affect the normal menstrual cycle. This can result in a shortened luteal phase or amenorrhea. Training too much, not eating enough or a combination of the two can result in low energy availability which has a negative effect on the reproductive hormones in females. The menstrual cycle can also be disrupted by hormonal contraceptives which can decrease the amount of estrogen and progesterone produced in the body.[35] Strategies to promote healthy views of body image are to focus on health rather than weight. Focus on goals unrelated to body weight. For example, it may be better to focus on being injury-free and able to train or other non-weight related accomplishments. Call out bullying. Also, explain social media and teach adolescents that they do not need to look like a certain athlete in order to perform well.[55]

The female athlete triad is a syndrome consisting of three interrelated conditions of menstrual dysfunction, osteoporosis and disordered eating that can affect active females.[22, 50] Physical signs of female athlete triad include:

- Noticeable weight fluctuations
- Stomach cramps
- Menstrual irregularities
- Difficulty concentrating
- Dizziness and fainting

- Feeling cold all the time
- Fatigue/sleep problems
- Dry skin and hair, brittle nails
- Muscle weakness
- Impaired immune function
- Dental problems[51]

Disordered eating resources to contact if an athlete presents signs and symptoms:

- United States: National Eating Disorders Associations (NEDA) https://www.nationaleatingdisorders.org/help-support/contact-helpline (800) 931-2237
- United Kingdom: Beat Eating Disorders https://www.beateatingdisorders.org.uk/support-services/helplines
  - Helpline: 0808 801 0677
  - Students: 0808 801 0811
  - Youth: 0808 801 0711
- Southeast Asia Eating Disorder Treatment Information and Resources https://www.eatingdisorderhope.com/treatment-for-eating-disorders/international/southeast-asias-eating-disorder-resources
- Hong Kong Eating Disorders Association (HEDA) http://www.heda-hk.org
- Japan:
  - 摂食障害の自助・ピアサポートグループ NABA Tel: 03-3302-0710
  - Eating Disorders Community Peerful http://peerful.jp
  - Eating Disorder Hope Japan http://edrecoveryjapan.com
  - Japan Association for Eating Disorders (JAED) https://www.jafed.jp

References: Chapter 16

1. "Your Digestive System & How it Works." *National Institute of Diabetes and Digestive and Kidney Diseases*. Accessed February 5, 2021. https://www.niddk.nih.gov/health-information/digestive-diseases/digestive-system-how-it-works. Published December 1, 2017.

2. "Expert Questions and Answers." *Nutrition.gov*. Accessed February 5, 2021. https://www.nutrition.gov/expert-q-a.

3. "Carbohydrates." *MedlinePlus*. Published November 18, 2020. Accessed February 8, 2021. https://medlineplus.gov/carbohydrates.html.

4. "Protein in diet." *MedlinePlus*. Published January 5, 2021. Accessed February 8, 2021. https://medlineplus.gov/ency/article/002467.htm.

5. "Dietary fats explained." *MedlinePlus*. Published January 5, 2021. Accessed February 8, 2021. https://medlineplus.gov/ency/patientinstructions/000104.htm.

6. U.S. Department of Agriculture and U.S. Department of Health and Human Services. *Dietary Guidelines for Americans, 2020-2025, 9th Edition*. December, 2020. Available at DietaryGuidelines.gov.

7. Purcell, L.K., Canadian Paediatric Society, Paediatric Sports and Exercise Medicine Section. "Sport nutrition for young athletes." *Paediatr Child Health* 18, no. 4 (2013): 200-5 doi: 10.1093/pch/18.4.200

8. Webb D. "Athletes and Protein Intake." *Today's Dietitian*. Published June 2014. Accessed February 9, 2021. https://www.todaysdietitian.com/newarchives/060114p22.shtml.

9. Smith, J.W., Holmes, M.E., McAllister, M.J. "Nutritional Considerations for Performance in Young Athletes." *Journal of Sports Medicine* (August, 2015). doi:10.1155/2015/734649.

10. Kerksick, C.M., Arent, S., Schoenfeld, B.J., et al. "International society of sports nutrition position stand: nutrient timing." *J Int Soc Sports Nutr* 14, no. 33 (August, 2017). doi: 10.1186/s12970-017-0189-4

11. "Calcium: Fact Sheet for Health Professionals." NIH Office of Dietary Supplements. Published March 26, 2020. Accessed February 10, 2021. https://ods.od.nih.gov/factsheets/Calcium-HealthProfessional/.

12. "Vitamin D: Fact Sheet for Health Professionals". NIH Office of Dietary Supplements. Published October 9, 2020. Accessed February 10, 2021. https://ods.od.nih.gov/factsheets/VitaminD-HealthProfessional/.

13. "Water: Essential to your body." Mayo Clinic Health System. Published July 22, 2020. Accessed February 10, 2021. https://www.mayoclinichealthsystem.org/hometown-health/speaking-of-health/water-essential-to-your-body.

14. Arnaoutis, G., Kavouras, S.A., Angelopoulou, A., et al. "Fluid Balance During Training in Elite Young Athletes of Different Sports." *J Strength Cond Res* 29, no. 12 (Decmeber, 2015): 3447-52. doi: 10.1519/JSC.0000000000000400

15. "Hydration Assessment of Athletes." Gatorade Sports Science Institute Web. Published October 2006. Accessed February 10, 2021. https://www.gssiweb.org/sports-science-exchange/article/sse-97-hydration-assessment-of-athletes.

16. Nuccio, R.P., Barnes, K.A., Carter, J.M., Baker, L.B. "Fluid Balance in Team Sport Athletes and the Effect of Hypohydration on Cognitive, Technical, and Physical Performance." *Sports Med* 47, no. 10 (October, 2017): 1951-82. doi: 10.1007/s40279-017-0738-7

17. "Frequently Asked Questions (FAQ) About Extreme Heat." Centers for Disease Control and Prevention. Published June 1, 2012. Accessed February 15, 2021. https://www.cdc.gov/disasters/extremeheat/faq.html.

18. "Fluid and Electrolyte Balance." MedlinePlus. Accessed February 15, 2021. https://medlineplus.gov/fluidandelectrolytebalance.html. Published October 1, 2020.

19. "Sports Drinks." Sports Dietitians Australia. Accessed February 16, 2021. https://www.sportsdietitians.com.au/factsheets/fuelling-recovery/sports-drinks/. Published June 26, 2015.

20. Dolan S. "Electrolytes: Understanding Replacement Options." ACE Fitness. Accessed February 15, 2021. https://www.acefitness.org/certifiednewsarticle/715/electrolytes-understanding-replacement-options/.

21. Patel, H., Alkhawam, H., Madanieh, R., Shah, N., Kosmas, C.E., Vittorio, T.J. "Aerobic vs anaerobic exercise training effects on the cardiovascular system." *World J Cardiol* 9, no. 2 (February, 2017): 134-38. doi: 10.4330/wjc.v9.i2.134

22. Kraemer, W.J., Fleck, S.J., Deschenes, M.R. *Exercise physiology: integrated from theory to practical applications, 1st ed.* Philadelphia: Wolters Kluwer/Lippincott Williams & Wilkins Health, 2012.

23. Niebauer, J., Borjesson, M., Carre, F., et al. "Recommendations for participation in competitive sports of athletes with arterial hypertension: a position statement from the sports cardiology section of the European Association of Preventive Cardiology (EAPC)." *Eur Heart J* 39, no. 40 (October, 2018): 3664-71. doi: 10.1093/eurheartj/ehy511

24. "Materials for Practitioners." Gatorade Sports Science Institute. Accessed February 17, 2021. https://www.gssiweb.org/en-ca/for-practitioners.

25. Williams, C., Rollo, I. "Carbohydrate Nutrition and Team Sport Performance. Gatorade Sports Science Institute." Accessed February 17, 2021. https://www.gssiweb.org/sports-science-exchange/article/sse-140-carbohydrate-nutrition-and-team-sport-performance. Published February 2015.

26. Jeukendrup, A.E. "Nutrition for endurance sports: marathon, triathlon, and road cycling." *J Sports Sci* no. 29, suppl. 1 (September, 2011): S91-9. doi: 10.1080/02640414.2011.610348

27. Kelly, M.P. "Resting Metabolic Rate: Best Ways to Measure It-And Raise It, Too." ACE Fitness. Accessed February 17, 2021. https://www.acefitness.org/certifiednewsarticle/2882/resting-metabolic-rate-best-ways-to-measure-it-and-raise-it-too/.

28. *Nutrition Care Manual.* Academy of Nutrition and Dietetics. Accessed Feb. 17, 2021. https://www.nutritioncaremanual.org/.

29. "Nutritional Recommendations to Avoid Gastrointestinal Distress During Exercise." Gatorade Sports Science Institute. Accessed February 18, 2021. https://www.gssiweb.org/sports-science-exchange/article/sse-114-nutritional-recommendations-to-avoid-gastrointestinal-distress-during-exercise.

30. Spriet, L., Smith, H. "Practicing Sports Nutrition: Maintaining Hydration and Proper Fueling." Gatorade Sports Science Institute. Accessed February 18, 2021. https://www.gssiweb.org/docs/CanadaEnglishLibraries/sport-specific-materials/practical-sports-nutrition-maintaining-hydration-and-proper-fueling.pdf?sfvrsn=6.

31. Brown, K.A., Patel, D.R., Darmawan, D. "Participation in sports in relation to adolescent growth and development." *Transl Pediatr* 6, no. 3 (July, 2017): 150-59. doi: 10.21037/tp.2017.04.03

32. Allen, B., Waterman, H. "Stages of Adolescence." HealthyChildren.org. Published March 28, 2019. Accessed February 18, 2021. https://www.healthychildren.org/English/ages-stages/teen/Pages/Stages-of-Adolescence.aspx.

33. "Review: Introduction to the Reproductive System." National Cancer Institute. Accessed February 18, 2021. https://training.seer.cancer.gov/anatomy/reproductive/review.html.

34. Soliman, A., De Sanctis, V., Elalaily, R. "Nutrition and pubertal development." *Indian J Endocrinol Metab* 18, suppl. 1 (November, 2014): S39-47. doi: 10.4103/2230-8210.145073

35. Desbrow, B., Burd, N.A., Tarnopolsky, M., Moore, D.R., Elliott-Sale, K.J. "Nutrition for Special Populations: Young, Female, and Masters Athletes." *Int J Sport Nutr Exerc Metab* 29, no. 2 (March, 2019): 220-27. doi: 10.1123/ijsnem.2018-0269

36. Kerksick, C.M., Wilborn, C.D., Roberts, M.D., et al. "ISSN exercise & sports nutrition review update: research & recommendations." *J Int Soc Sports Nutr* 15, no. 1 (August, 2018): 38. doi: 10.1186/s12970-018-0242-y

37. Jovanov, P., Dordic, V., Obradovic, B., et al. "Prevalence, knowledge, and attitudes towards using sports supplements among young athletes." *J Int Soc Sports Nutr* 16 (July, 2019): 27. doi: 10.1186/s12970-019-0294-7

38. "Dietary Supplements for Exercise and Athletic Performance: Fact Sheet for Health Professionals." NIH Office of Dietary Supplements. Accessed February 21, 2021. https://ods.od.nih.gov/factsheets/ExerciseAndAthleticPerformance-HealthProfessional/ Published October 17, 2019.

39. Herriman, M., Fletcher, L., Tchaconas, A., Adesman, A., Milanaik, R. "Dietary Supplements and Young Teens: Misinformation and Access Provided by Retailers." *Pediatrics* 139, no. 2 (February, 2017). doi: 10.1542/peds.2016-1257

40. "Dietary Supplement Ingredient Advisory List." BSCG. Accessed February 22, 2021. https://www.bscg.org/dietary-supplement-ingredient-advisory-list/.

41. Starr, R.R. "Too little, too late: ineffective regulation of dietary supplements in the United States." *Am J Public Health* 105, no. 3 (February, 2015): 478-85. doi: 10.2105/AJPH.2014.302348

42. "Performance Enhancing Drugs." BSCG. Accessed February 23, 2021. https://www.bscg.org/performance-enhancing-drugs/.

43. "Multivitamin/mineral Supplements: Fact Sheet for Health Professionals." NIH Office of Dietary Supplements. Accessed February 23, 2021. https://ods.od.nih.gov/factsheets/MVMS-HealthProfessional/.

44. "How to Read a Supplement Label." Council for Responsible Nutrition. Accessed February 23, 2021. https://www.crnusa.org/resources/how-read-supplement-label.

45. Lastella, M., Vincent, G.E., Duffield, R., et al. "Can sleep be used as an indicator of overreaching and overtraining in athletes?" *Front Physiol* 9 (April, 2018): 436. doi 10.3389/fphys.2018.00436

46. Cheng, A.J., Jude, B., Lanner, J.T. "Intramuscular mechanisms of overtraining." *Redox Biol* 35 (August, 2020): 101480. doi: 10.1016/j.redox.2020.101480

47. Cadegiani, F.A., Kater, C.E. "Basal hormones and biochemical markers as predictors of overtraining syndrome in male athletes: the EROS-BASAL study." *J athl Train* 54, vol. 8 (August, 2019): 906-914. doi: 10.4085/1062-6050-148-18

48. Montesano, P., Di Silvestro, M., Cipriani, G., Mazzeo, F. "Overtraining syndrome, stress and nutrition in football amateur athletes." *J Hum Sport Exerc* 14, proc. 4 (2019): S957-S969. doi:https://doi.org/10.14198/jhse.2019.14.Proc4.58

49. "Downloadable Resources." CPSDA. Accessed February 24, 2021. https://sportsrd.org/downloadable-resources/.

50. Nazem, T.G., Ackerman, K.E. "The female athlete triad." *Sports Health* 4, vol. 4 (July, 2012): 302-11. doi: 10.1177/1941738112439685

51. National Eating Disorders Association (website). Published 2018. Accessed February 24, 2021. https://www.nationaleatingdisorders.org/.

52. Manore, M. "Weight Management for Athletes and Active Individuals." Gatorade Sports Science Institute. Published January 2018. Accessed February 24, 2021. https://www.gssiweb.org/sports-science-exchange/article/weight-management-for-athletes-and-active-individuals.

53. "Safe Weight Loss and Weight Gain for Young Athletes." HealthyChildren.org. Published February 3, 2012. Accessed February 24, 2021. https://www.healthychildren.org/English/healthy-living/sports/Pages/Safe-Weight-Loss-and-Weight-Gain-for-Young-Athletes.aspx.

54. Zamani Sani, S.H., Fathirezaie, Z., Brand, S., et al. "Physical activity and self-esteem: testing direct and indirect relationships associated with psychological and physical mechanisms." *Neuropsychiatr Dis Treat* 12 (October, 2016): 2617-25. doi: 10.2147/NDT.S116811

55. Hayes, D. "5 Ways to Promote a Positive Body Image for Kids." EatRight.org. Published February 24, 2021. Accessed February 24, 2021. https://www.eatright.org/health/weight-loss/your-health-and-your-weight/5-ways-to-promote-a-positive-body-image-for-kids.

56. de la Puente Yague, M., Collado Yurrita, L., Ciudad Cabanas, M.J., Cuadrado Cenzual, M.A. "Role of Vitamin D in Athletes and Their Performance: Current Concepts and New Trends." *Nutrients* 12, vol. 2 (February 2020): 579. Published 2020 Feb 23. doi:10.3390/nu12020579

57. Sawka, M.N., Cheuvront, S.N., Kenefick, R.W. "Hydration and Aerobic Performance: Impact of Environment." Gatorade Sports Science Institute. Published January 2016. Accessed March 2, 2021. https://www.gssiweb.org/sports-science-exchange/article/sse-152-hydration-and-aerobic-performance-impact-of-environment.

58. "Nutrition Information." USA Shooting. Published 2007. Accessed March 2, 2021. https://www.usashooting.org/11-resources/shootinginstruction/nutrition.

59. Clark, A., Mach, N. "Exercise-induced stress behavior, gut-microbiota-brain axis and diet: a systematic review for athletes." *J Int Soc Sports Nutr.* 13 (November, 2016): 43. doi:10.1186/s12970-016-0155-6

17
PRESSING REST: NEUROLOGICAL RECOVERY

By: Tim Anderson
Author, Co-Founder and Master Instructor Original Strength
&
Carson Molaro
MS, University of Louisville

Original Strength

Your body is awesomely and wonderfully made. It was designed to be strong and capable throughout your life at every stage in your life. In fact, you are meant to be "antifragile," or not easily injured. You were made to endure life and all of its challenges.

Yes, life happens. Accidents happen. Injuries happen. But the human body is designed to heal and even prevent injuries IF it is moving and operating properly. This means you are never limited by your current physical and mental condition, at least you don't have to be. If you move the way you were designed to move, you can restore your strength, mobility, speed, and power. Mobility that was once lost can return. Pain that has nagged you for years can go away. Your body knows how to handle these limitations. You can even restore or gain your ability to focus, remember, interpret, and analyze information quickly; all through moving the way you were designed to move.

Moving the way you were designed does indeed make you antifragile. It restores your health and vitality. We call this your Original Strength. This is the strength you were created to have throughout your lifetime. This is the strength that allows you to perform your job and live your life better, the way you want to. It's the strength that gives you the freedom to move and the ability to enjoy your life. This strength lives inside of you, and it is released when you move according to your design. We call this Pressing RESET.

In this chapter, we are going to show you how to press the reset button with yourself and your athletes, how to move the way bodies were designed, so you can restore the Original Strength you and your athletes were meant to have.

Why Reset: The science behind the resets

Humans were made to move, and they were made to move for a lifetime. In today's society, however, we seem to move less and less, and we start experiencing pain earlier in life. Can the key to maintaining efficient movement for a lifetime really be as easy as performing five simple movements? Original Strength believes just that. In their book *Pressing Reset: Original Strength Reloaded,* authors Tim Anderson and Geoff Neupert (2015) suggest that the more we move through our natural pattern of movement the more we develop our brain, and the more we develop our brain the more efficient we become at moving (p.22). This suggests the importance of both brain and body development through movement. Anderson and Neupert (2015) go on to elaborate that we strengthen this connection by building a "body map" with our proprioceptors found in our skin, joints, tendons and muscles that send signals to our brain that tell us where our body is and what it is doing (p. 23). The key to all of the resets is to have a strong core, or "x" as they call it at original strength. Anderson and Neupert (2015) state, "Your core is tied to everything, the body is interconnected and this interconnection solidifies our center" (p.32). In PR Resets: Understanding the Complexities behind the Simplicity, the way that we reset our bodies is by activating the nervous system (also known as the bodies operating system), and in doing that we restore our proper reflexive connection (Anderson 2018, p.5). Anderson and Neuport (2015) define reflexive control as a combination of reflexive stability, mobility, and strength, all of these also form the components of movement (p. 36). There are five essential movement patterns and engaging in these resets refreshes the central nervous system, creates efficient neural pathways in both the brain and body, and it restores/sharpens reflexive neuromuscular connections (Anderson and Neuport 2015, p. 38).

Original Strength has "5 Big Resets," and they are diaphragmatic breathing, head control, rolling, rocking and crawling/gait pattern (Anderson and Neuport 2015, p. 38). Diaphragmatic breathing helps to strengthen the core, and breathing with our chest weakens our core (Anderson and Neuport 2015, p. 41). Anderson and Neupert (2015) go on to add that because so many people often breathe with their accessory breathing muscles (the chest), we breathe in emergency mode which can lead to poor posture, early fatigue when exercising, high blood pressure, etc (p. 44).

Essentially, we are in a constant state of elevated stress when we breathe without our diaphragm. A study done in Italy looked at how important diaphragmatic breathing was in combating stress on the body. Exercise can increase the amount of cortisol and melatonin levels which can cause increased stress levels and may even lead to amenorrhea in female athletes who overtrain (Martarelli, Cocchioni, Sevri, and Pompei 2011). In the study, researchers took 16 endurance athletes and at the end of their workout took half of them and recovered for one hour, focusing on diaphragmatic breathing, while the other half just sat in a quiet space for an hour (Martarelli, Cocchioni, Sevri, and Pompei 2011). The findings of the study suggest that diaphragmatic breathing should be incorporated in all sports performance activities because it can increase performance and accelerate recovery (Martarelli, Cocchioni, Sevri, and Pompei 2011). *Original Strength Performance: The Next Level* by Tim Anderson, Chip Morton and Mark Shropshire (2018) talks about how the diaphragm is a spinal stabilizer and a stable spine leads to a more mobile and agile body (p.8). Anderson, Morton and Shropshire (2018) emphasize that a properly functioning diaphragm is essential for strength and helps to lay the foundation for optimal human performance and physical expression (p.10). Anderson and Neupert (2015) believe that real strength comes from being able to live in a state of peace, and diaphragmatic breathing can put us in a "peace mode" (p. 47). One of the fundamental components in diaphragmatic breathing is tongue placement. When we look at the tongue and diaphragmatic breathing, placing the tongue on the roof of the mouth encourages nasal breathing, and therefore diaphragmatic breathing (Anderson and Neuport 2015, p. 46). A study looking at tongue positioning during diaphragmatic breathing while doing isokinetic knee extension and flexion exercises were investigated, and the study found a 30% significant increase of knee flexion peak torque with the tongue on the upper roof of the mouth (di Vico, Ardigo, Salernitano, Chamari, and Padulo 2013)).

The second reset is head control, which is accomplished via head nods. Head control is important to your overall strength because your vestibular system (balance system) lives in your head (Anderson and Neuport 2015, p. 50). Why is it important to stimulate your vestibular system? The more you move, the more you stimulate your vestibular system the more neural connections you make in the brain and body (Anderson and Neuport 2015, p. 53). Anderson, Morton and Shropshire (2018) stress that optimal information into the vestibular system and then into the brain, leads to optimal action and reaction from the brain (p.10). The key to fine tuning this system is first through head movement and then body movement, this in turns keeps the body sharp because the nervous system is getting and giving good information (Anderson, Morton and Shropshire, 2018, p.10). Being able to incorporate diaphragmatic breathing with head nods along with the emphasis on proper tongue position can increase force production and endurance on flexion and extension (Anderson, Morton and Shropshire, 2018, p.11-12). Head nods not only restore posture, but optimize the function of your body's major systems (Anderson and Neuport 2015, p. 60).

The other resets are rolling, rocking and crawling or gait pattern movements. Rolling helps to activate your vestibular system and incorporates tying in your "x" or core when moving (Anderson and Neupert 2015, p. 67). Anderson and Neupert (2015) believe that rocking helps to build up both strength and coordination, because it is the primitive pattern that really starts to integrate the entire body (p.76). Similarly to rolling, rocking activates the vestibular system, but it goes a step further by connecting your shoulders to your hips (Anderson and Neupert 2015, p. 77). In an article written in the North American Journal of Sports Physical Therapy, rolling is suggested to be very beneficial for athletes who perform rotationally based sports such as tennis, golf, figure skating, etc. (Hoogenboom, Voight, Cook, and Gill 2009). The body relies on symmetry, and often athletes get stuck in movement patterns that do not promote symmetry (Hoogenboom, Voight, Cook, and Gill 2009). Hoogenboom, Voight, Cook, and Gill (2009) believe that the use of rolling, particularly for athletes, can address this dysfunction and enhance normal functional movement and provide adequate postural responses to motion. Crawling is the final component of the resets, and it ties everything together through motion. Anderson and Neupert (2015) suggest that crawling increases the communication between both hemispheres of the brain, therefore sharpening the neural pathways and their ability to send and receive signals (p.85-86). This only enhances your reflexes and makes them faster (Anderson and Neupert 2015, p. 86).

What happens when we engage in these movement patterns and just how does this impact our performance? Anderson, Morton, and Shropshire (2018) say that simply engaging in these activities will improve the performance of anyone because it helps them to live a better life (p.17). All of these activities stimulate the nervous system to be able to better send signals to motor neurons to produce movement. When you add a load or resistance the demand placed on the nervous system causes it to adapt, causing a greater neuromuscular response (Anderson, Morton, and Shropshire 2018, p. 17). Anderson, Morton, and Shropshire (2018) believe that by adding a load to the resets you will provide you with faster, more efficient neural pathways, which when talking about athletic performance is what we want (p. 17). It is important to note that we do not want to load our movements to the point that we compromise our bodies natural form, we want to be able to have our bodies move according to their designs (Anderson, Morton, and Shropshire 2018, p. 23). Anderson, Morton, and Shropshire (2018) have found that the best way to load the crawling progression is to have individuals drag or pull an object as they crawl (p. 23).

When an athlete has a healthy nervous system and a strong body deeply rooted in reflexive strength, they have the potential to express themselves in unlimited ways (Anderson, Morton, and Shropshire 2018, p. 65). If we can regularly engage in diaphragmatic breathing, we will experience all of the benefits mentioned earlier, but by relieving excessive muscle tension and guarding we lower tension, stress, anger and fear all of which can derail mental and physical performance (Anderson, Morton, and Shropshire 2018, p. 90). When we talk about the importance of rocking for performance, along with stimulating the vestibular system and relieving stress, this movement triggers the release of hormones that relieve pain and induce feelings of pleasure that can better our performance (Anderson, Morton, and Shropshire 2018, p. 90).

The human body is capable of amazing things. The human body was made to move, and to move for an entire lifetime. At Original Strength, they believe that the best way to enhance your body's movement is through stimulating the body's nervous system. The nervous system is our body's operating system, and if it is not functioning at optimal levels, then you will not be able to move as efficiently as you were made to move. In today's society, athletes are chasing after that special edge to give them a leg up on the competition. It is possible that performing these resets is one of the keys to increasing performance. Doing the resets under load can be even more beneficial for those looking for a performance edge because of the additional stimulus put on to the nervous system. The key to better movement and better performance could be regularly going through the 5 simple resets. As Leo Tolstoy once said "There is no greatness where there is not simplicity."

Pressing RESET

Your Original Strength is based on the Three Pillars of Human Movement. These are the pillars of movement we are designed to do each and every day. If we engage in these three things, we are Pressing RESET and strengthening the nervous system. These Three Pillars are:

1. Breathe deep with your diaphragm (belly breathe).
2. Activate your vestibular system (your balance and sensory integration system).
3. Engage in contra-lateral patterns (crawling, walking, marching) or midline crossing movements.

These three pillars are preprogrammed into each of our nervous systems. In fact, they are woven into the developmental sequence, the movements we moved through as children in order to become strong and antifragile.

A way to have efficient movement patterns, and ultimately greater performance, is to have a well-trained neuromuscular system, and just like everything else, it is important to train the neuromuscular system. To train this system, it is essential to take the body through a series of natural movement patterns that strengthen the neural connection between the brain and muscles. These movement patterns are referred to as RESETS. When moving through RESETS, connections are strengthened via the proprioceptors in the skin, joints, tendons and muscles. The idea behind a RESET is the movements are the most primitive human movements; they are the movements that humans are programmed to progress through. A baby first breathes with their diaphragm, then moves their heads around, followed by rolling around, rocking and finally, crawling. These basic human movements can unlock the key to enhanced performance.

It might seem strange, but the developmental sequence can actually *develop* us at any age and any stage of our lives. The Five developmental movements we are going to remember how to do are:

1. Belly Breathe
2. Learn to control the movement of our eyes and head
3. Roll on the ground
4. Rocking back and forth
5. Crawling

These simple movements are the key to restoring our Original Strength.

RESET #1: Belly Breathing, the very beginning of strength

Why?

- You were born a "belly breather."
- Your diaphragm (main breathing muscle) is a spinal stabilizer and it helps to protect your spine.
  - Proper diaphragmatic breathing allows you to move well.
- Diaphragmatic breathing helps to strengthen the core, and breathing with our chest weakens our core
  - Because so many people often breathe with their accessory breathing muscles (the chest), we breathe in emergency mode which can lead to poor posture, early fatigue when exercising, high blood pressure, etc
- Breathing is the "bridge" between your autonomic nervous system.
  - Proper breathing calms your nervous system and keeps you in the parasympathetic mode (rest and digest mode).
  - Breathing up in the neck and chest excites your nervous system and keeps you in the sympathetic mode (fight or flight mode).

How?

- Lie in this position.
- Place your tongue on the roof of your mouth and close your lips.*
- Breathe in and out of your nose and pull air deep down into your belly.

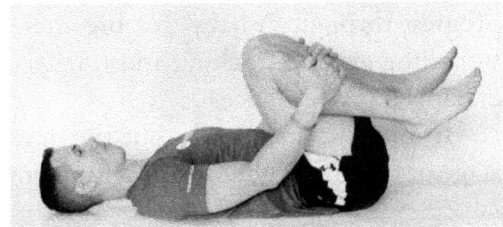

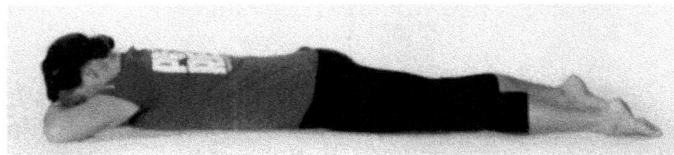

Position #1

It is super important that you learn to rest and keep your tongue on the roof of your mouth. This is where it belongs. It also helps your nervous system function optimally.

- Lie in this position.
- Place your tongue on the roof of your mouth and close your lips.
- Breathe in and out of your nose and pull air deep down into your belly.

Position #2

Don't make the mistake of dismissing how important breathing in your belly is. This is not just about getting air into your lungs. This is about building strength in your center. Your diaphragm is the chief stabilizing muscle in your inner core, it helps protect your spine

RESET #2: Head Control, the next layer of strength

Why?

- Controlling the movements of your head activates your vestibular system and improves its function.
  - o The VS is your balance system and your sensory information collection point.
  - o The more you move, the more you stimulate your vestibular system, the more neural connections you make in the brain and body
- Every muscle in your body is reflexively "wired" to the movements of your head.
- Head nods not only restore posture, but optimize the function of your body's major systems
- Head Control is <u>essential</u> to obtaining health and strength throughout your lifetime.

How?

Movement #1

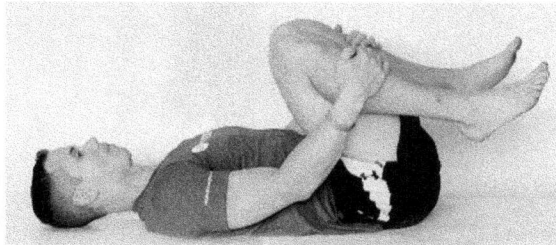

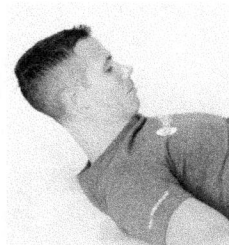

- Lie in this position.
- Place your tongue on the roof of your mouth and close your lips.
- Raise and lower your head by tucking your chin to your through and lifting your head off the ground as if to look through your knees.
- Lead the movement with your eyes.
- Do not hold your breath. Keep breathing through your nose.

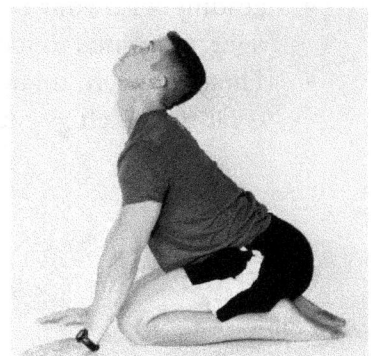

Movement #2

- Get into this position on your hands and knees.
- Place your tongue on the roof of your mouth and close your lips.
- Perform head nods by raising and lowering your head as far as your neck will allow you to move – PAIN-FREE.
- Lead the movement with your eyes.
- Do not hold your breath. Keep breathing through your nose.

Movement #3

- Get into this position on your hands and knees.
- Place your tongue on the roof of your mouth and close your lips.
- Rotate your head left and right as if you are trying to look at your "back pockets."
- Lead the movement with your eyes.
- Do not drop your head. Look over your shoulders.
- Do not hold your breath. Keep breathing through your nose.

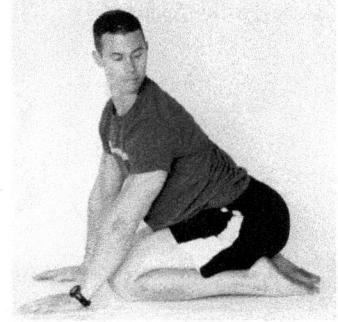

RESET #3: Rolling, connecting the shoulders to the hips

Why?

- Rolling further activates and strengthens the vestibular system.
- Rolling connects your shoulders to your hips, it connects your torso.
- Rolling nourishes the vertebrae of the spine.
- Rolling allows you to move fluidly and effortlessly.

How?

The Egg Roll

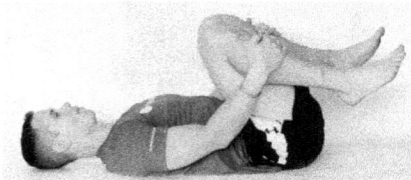

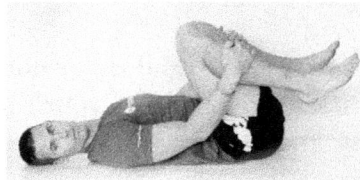

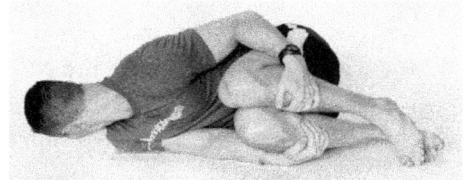

- Lie on your back and grab your shins.
- Place your tongue on the roof of your mouth and close your lips.
- Leading with your eyes, look right, rotate your head to the right, then rotate your body to the right. Continue to look as far to the right as your body will allow.
- Then, look left, rotate your head to the left, then rotate your body to the left. Continue to look as far to the left as your body will allow.

The Windshield Wiper

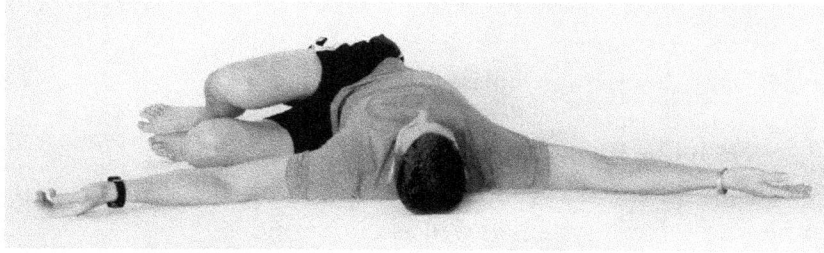

- Lie on your back and place your arms perpendicular to your torso.
- Bend your knees up towards your chest to lift your tailbone off the floor. Your feet will be in the air.
- Place your tongue on the roof of your mouth and close your lips.
- While keeping your shoulder blades in contact with the ground, rotate your legs from side to side.
- Keep your knees pulled up towards your chest even as you rotate your legs to the side. Do not let them drift away.

Upper-body Half Roll – from belly to back

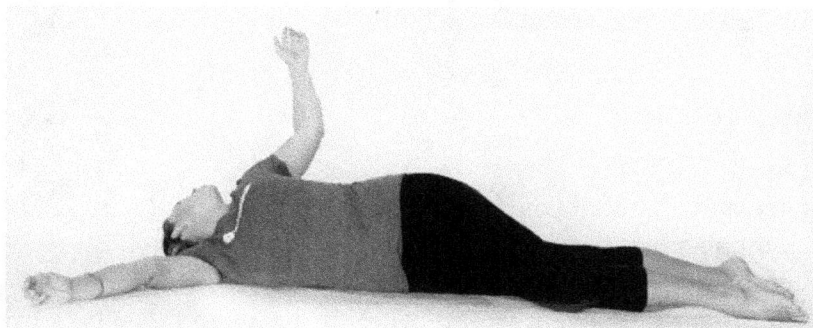

- Lie on your belly with your arms overhead.
- Place your tongue on the roof of your mouth.
- Bend your right elbow, look at it, and reach for the floor behind you. Try to touch the floor with your elbow.
- Then roll back to your belly.
- Repeat this on the left side.
- Keep your lower-body relaxed throughout the movement.

Reset #4: Rocking – total body integration

Why?

- Rocking further nourishes the vestibular system.
- Rocking integrates all the joints of the body into one whole body.
- Rocking helps to build up both strength and coordination
- Rocking coordinates the shoulders and the hips, preparing them for crawling and walking.
- Rocking soothes the nervous system as well as the emotions.

How?

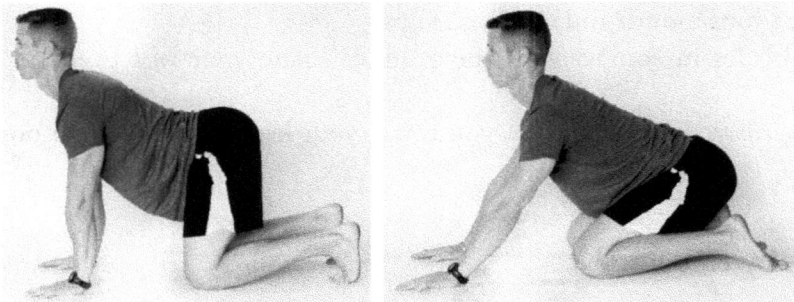

Feet can be in plantar flexion and/or dorsiflexion.

Rocking on hands and knees

- Get on your hands and knees.
- Put your tongue on the roof of your mouth.
- Hold your head up and keep your eyes on the horizon.
- Keep a tall sternum. Be "proud" and hold a big chest.
- Rock back and forth, shifting your weight over your hands and then back over your feet.
- Rock back as far as you can without losing your tall sternum.
- Keep your back flat. Do not let it round up or bow up.

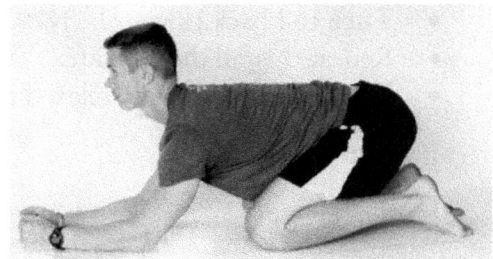

Commando Rocking

- Get on your forearms and knees.
- Put your tongue on the roof of your mouth.
- Hold your head up and keep your eyes on the horizon.
- Keep a tall sternum. Be "proud" and hold a big chest.
- Rock back and forth, shifting your weight over your forearms and then back over your feet.
- Rock back as far as you can without losing your tall sternum.
- Keep your back flat. Do not let it round up or bow up.

330

RESET #5: Crawling — Tying your X together

Why?

- Crawling connects both halves of the brain together, making it healthier and efficient.
- Crawling reflexively connects the body and ties it together.
  - It strengthens the nervous system.
  - It reflexively strengthens the body so that it can move efficiently, gracefully and powerfully.
- Crawling integrates other sensory systems with the vestibular system.

How?

Speed Skaters

- Get on your hands and knees.
- Put your tongue on the roof of your mouth.
- Hold your head up and keep your eyes on the horizon.
- Keep a tall sternum. Be "proud" and hold a big chest.
- Move your opposite arm and leg back together.

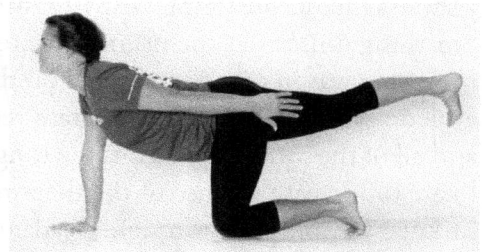

Hands and Knees Crawling

- Get on your hands and knees.
- Put your tongue on the roof of your mouth.
- Hold your head up and keep your eyes on the horizon.
- Keep a tall sternum. Be "proud" and hold a big chest.
- Move your opposite arms and together and crawl forward or backward.

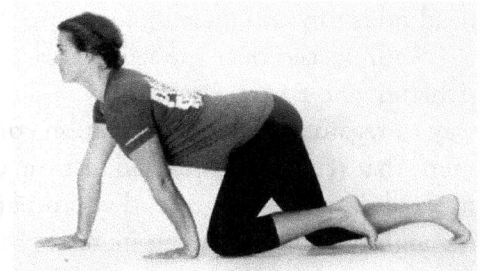

Leopard Crawling

- Put your tongue on the roof of your mouth.
- Hold your head up and keep your eyes on the horizon.
- Keep a tall sternum. Be "proud" and hold a big chest.
- Touch your opposite limbs together.
- Can touch hand to thigh, elbow to knees, etc...

Cross-Crawls

Do not dismiss the simplicity of this movement. This movement can be the easiest and most effective entry point that begins the restoration and strengthening of the nervous system. This movement can help rewire the brain, overcome learning disorders and set the body free to move and express itself.

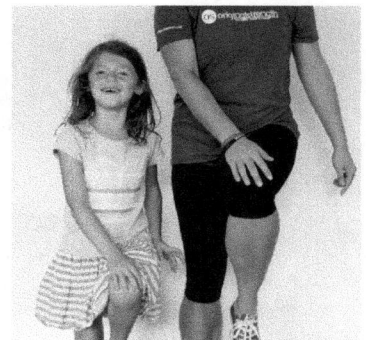

The Power in Your Design

The power of movement restoration, the hope of healing and the expression of strength all live inside your nervous system. All of these activities stimulate the nervous system to be able to better send signals to motor neurons to produce movement. Your very design contains the movement program intended to keep you strong, able and healthy. Spending just a few minutes every day relearning or remembering how to do these movements will enable you to live your life better, with strength and health.

Your body truly is awesomely and wonderfully made. It is designed to be strong and able, always. Everything you need to experience this is inside your nervous system waiting for you to move with it. In other words, your Original Strength is inside. It's your move...

Can RESETS Be Used To Provide a Performance Advantage?

Diaphragmatic breathing helps to strengthen the body's core and prevents the use of the accessory breathing muscles as the primary source. A study done in Italy looked at how important diaphragmatic breathing was in combating stress on the body. They found that diaphragmatic breathing could increase athletic performance and accelerate recovery. A fundamental component for diaphragmatic breathing and all of the other RESETS is the tongue position. Placing the tongue on the roof of the mouth is more likely to increase the use of the diaphragm and increase the amount of power produced (30% increase in knee flexion peak torque). Head nods are the next movement pattern. Head control is vital when building strength in the vestibular system. The more the vestibular system is activated the greater the neural connections between the brain and the body. Maintaining proper tongue position along with the head nods can also increase force production and endurance during flexion and extension movements.

Rolling, the next movement pattern helps to activate the core, and vestibular system even more. Athletes who participate in heavy rotational sports (swimming, tennis, baseball, etc.) can use rolling as a way to regain symmetry of rotation coming off of an injury. After rolling comes rocking, the first movement that truly begins to connect the upper and lower body in one fluid motion. Rocking is important for building up strength and coordination. The last RESET is crawling, which ties everything together through motion. Crawling increases the communication between both hemispheres of the brain, therefore sharpening the neural pathways and their ability to send and receive signals. All of these activities stimulate the nervous system, to better send signals to motor neurons to produce movement.

Loading Up the RESETS

The addition of a load to any kind of movement changes the type of stimulus put on the body, and therefore the outcome. Applying a load to any of the RESETS can have the capability of providing faster, more efficient neural pathways, which can increase athletic performance. It is critical that when applying a load to a movement that you apply the load properly, so that one does not compromise the body's natural form. All loaded RESETS, especially those done for the first time or with younger athletes, should be done with a supervisor who has been trained on RESETS.

Loading RESET 1: Belly Breathing

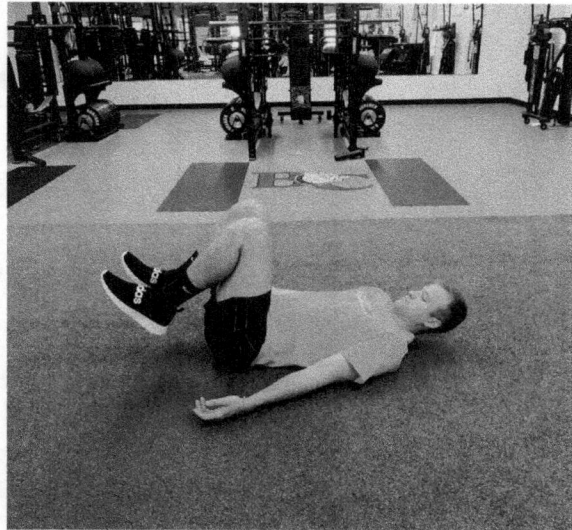

- Lie in this shortened position shown above
- Knees bent and pulled into the chest
- Neck in a flexed position
- Place your tongue on the roof of your mouth and close your lips.*
- Breathe in and out of your nose and pull air deep down into your belly.
- Perform 10 deep breaths

Loading RESET 2: Head Control

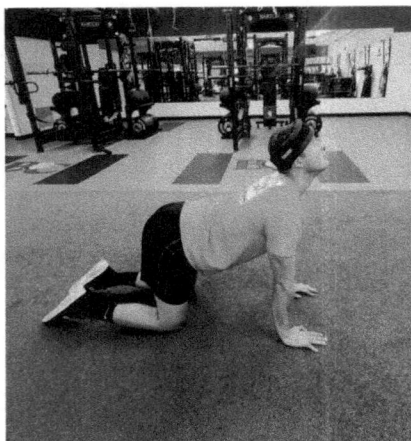

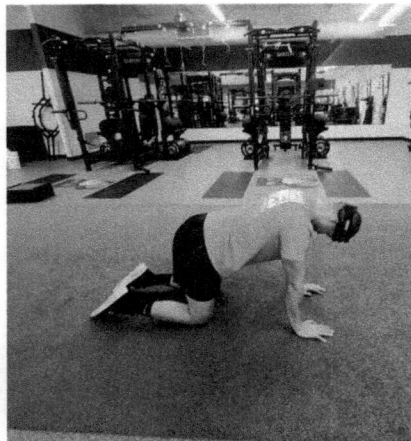

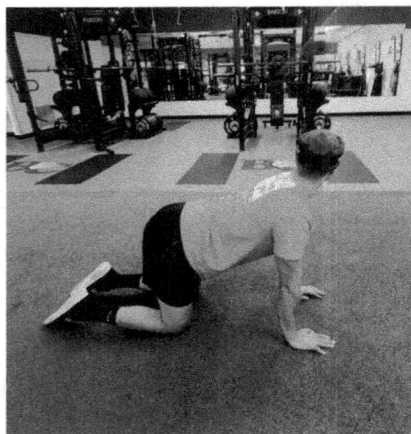

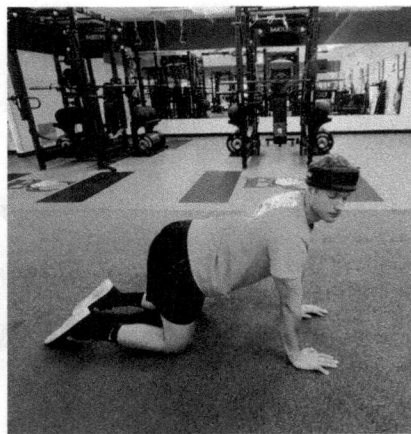

- Begin in a quadruped position (on your hands and knees as seen above)
- A 5 lb head weight is strapped around your head
- Make sure to continue to use your diaphragm when breathing, along with maintaining proper tongue placement
- Leading with your eyes perform 10 head nods up and down (yes's) followed by 10 side to side head nods (no's)

Loading RESET 3: Rolling

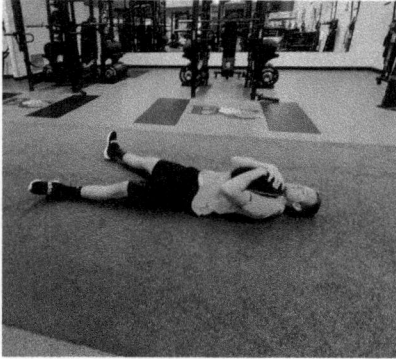

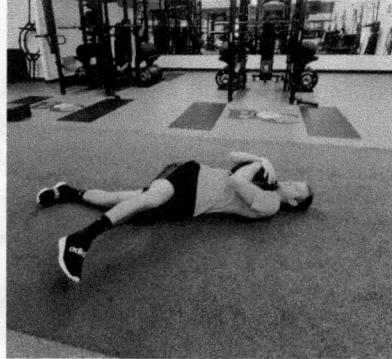

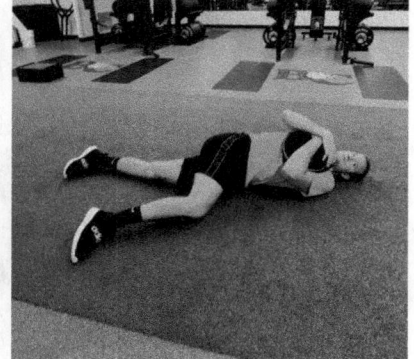

- Lie in this position to start
- Using a 25 lb sandbag, or whatever weight challenges you, without compromising good mechanics
- Roll over onto your stomach, leading with leg that is on the same side as weight

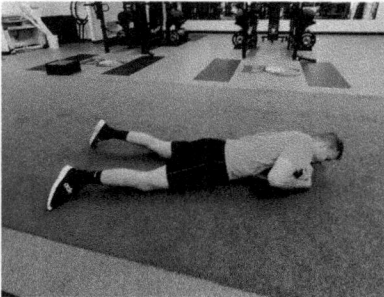

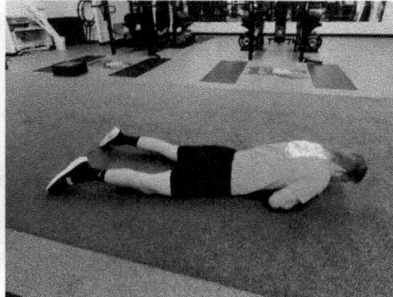

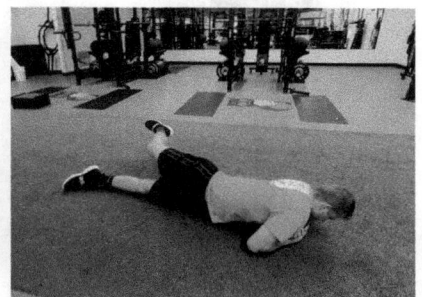

- Lift and swing your leg over to the opposite side of your body until finally you look like this

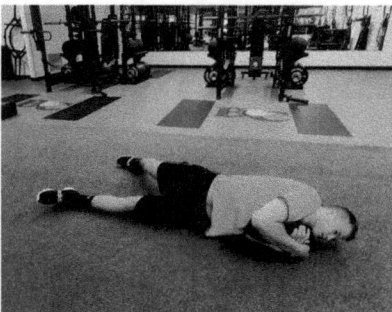

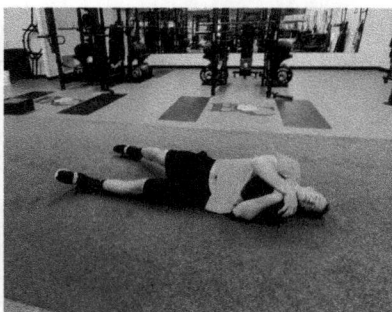

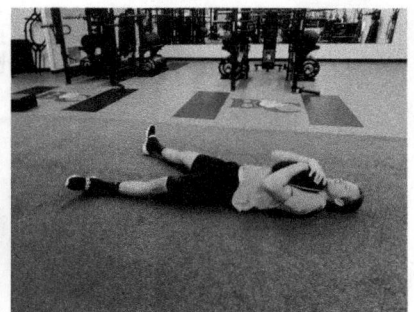

- Perform 5 rolls (rolling fully from your back to your stomach) then switch the side the weight is on and the leg you are using to lead with, and perform 5 more rolls

Loading RESET 4: Rocking

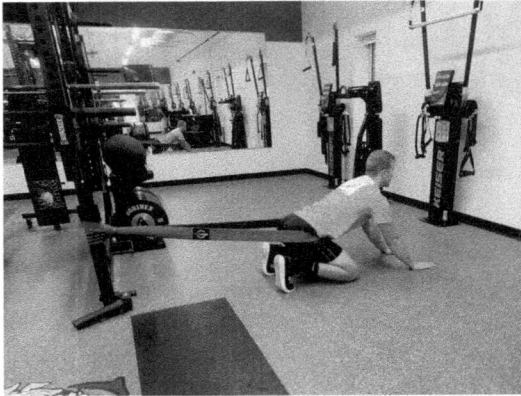

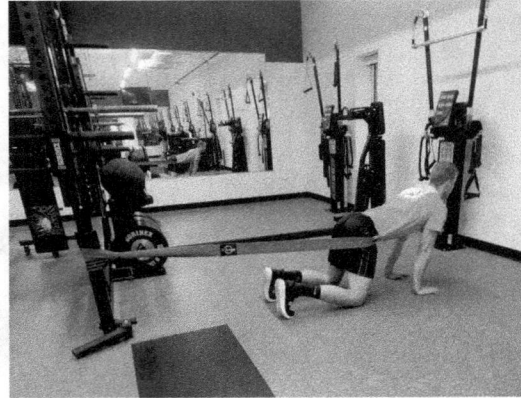

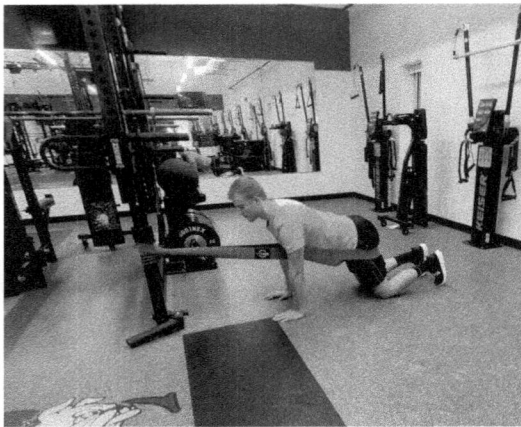

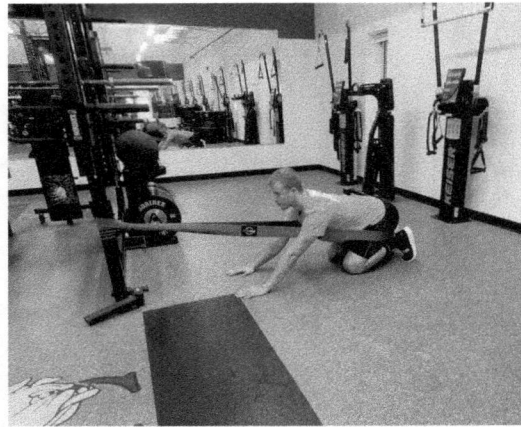

- Begin in a quadruped position (similar to the head nods) on your hands and knees
- Using a resistance band (light to moderate resistance) have the band wrapped around the upper hamstring
- Rock forwards and backwards at a controlled pace (2 secs forward, 2 secs backwards) 10 times
- Maintain a neutral head position
- Focus on diaphragmatic breathing and proper tongue placement (rough of the mouth)

Simple Daily RESET Restoration Plan

For whole body health and strength

This is one of many simple daily restoration plans to help you restore your body, become resilient and live your life with health and strength. Again, this is simple, but please don't underestimate how effective this can be. For best results, engage in the following routine daily, at least once:

Diaphragmatic breathing - While lying down in a comfortable position x 3 minutes - breathe in and out through your nose. Keep your tongue on the roof of your mouth. Focus on pulling air deep down into your belly. It may help to imagine trying to pull air down to your feet.

Why?

Because this is where strength starts. Breathing with your diaphragm makes you solid in your center and it helps your body work at optimum hormone levels. It keeps you in "peace and harmony" mode and out of "fight, flight and panic mode."

Head nods - While lying on your belly, prop yourself up on your forearms. Lift your head up and down x 20 repetitions, moving as far as your head will let you move. DO NOT move into pain. Simply move where your head will allow you to move. Oh, and lead with the eyes.

Why?

Because every muscle in your body is connected to the movements of your head. The body is designed to follow the head. Remembering how to move your head will, in a sense, sharpen and improve all the reflexive connections from your head to the rest of your body. This can help restore your reflexive strength!!

Rolling around on the floor - Roll anyway you want to roll: segmentally, egg rolls, backward rolls, frog rolls, or whatever for 3 minutes. Lead with your eyes and head when rolling. If you get dizzy, try slowing down, or reduce the range of motion of your rolls. OR, try a different roll altogether.

Why?

Rolling sharpens your balance and feeds your brain with rich nourishment; it makes your brain healthy. Rolling also connects your center, layering more strength on top of the solid foundation that diaphragmatic breathing started. Rolling prepares your body to coordinate complex movements like running!

Rocking back and forth on all fours - Keep your head up, stay "proud" in your chest and rock your butt back towards your feet for 3 minutes. Rock back as far as you can go while maintaining a strong chest (flat back). DO NOT move into pain. You can move to the edge of it, just don't move into it.

Why?

Because rocking integrates all the major moving joints of your body. It makes you whole and prepares your body to move like a gently flowing stream, like poetry. You were made to move with grace. Rocking also sets and restores your posture.

Cross-Crawling - Touch your opposite limbs together alternating for 3 minutes. They should move fluidly, together. That is, your right arm should move along with and at the same time as your left leg. Breathe in and out through your nose and keep your mouth closed.

Why?

Because cross-crawling is the simplest engagement of your gait pattern (walking). AND cross-crawling is the movement that can tie your brain together and connect your whole body. It can make you whole in both brain and body.

Get Up - Practice moving from the ground to standing for 3 minutes. Lie down on the floor and stand up. Repeat. Do this in as many ways as you can think of. Be creative.

Why?

Though not necessarily a Big 5 Reset, your ability to get up off the ground easily will improve your longevity and your quality of life. We must always master our bodies' movements and resist gravity with ease. When gravity starts to win the battle, we lose our resiliency.

That's it. It's about 15 minutes of gentle movement that will allow you to live your life with strength: the ability to live and do the things you want to do in life. It is simple. It is not fancy or complicated, but it works.

The 3 Minute Reset

Don't have 15 minutes to spare today? Do you have three? If you are pressed for time, have a hectic day, or you experience a particularly stressful situation, try the following three-minute reset. It will do your mind and body good.

- **Breathe with your diaphragm x 1 minute.** Stop wherever you are, in whatever position you may be in, place your tongue on the roof of your mouth and breathe deep down into your belly.
- **Rock back and forth x 1 minute.** Find a place to do this. It is worth it. Get on your hands and knees, hold your head up and your chest "proud," keep your tongue on the roof of your mouth, continue to breathe down into your belly, and rock back and forth.
- **Standing cross-crawls x 1 minute.** Touch your opposite limbs together, moving back and forth from side to side. Touch how you can, elbows to knees, forearms to thighs or hands to hips.

Wherever you can reach comfortably, touch your opposite arm to your opposite leg repeatedly for one minute. Do this and resume a less stressful or hectic and more energized day.

"... I am fearfully and wonderfully made..." Psalm 139:14

References: Chapter 17

1. Anderson, T. *Pressing Reset Understanding the Complexities Behind the Simplicity*. Fuquay Varina, NC: OS Press, 2018.

2. Anderson, T., Neupert, G. *Pressing Reset Original Strength Reloaded, 2nd ed.* Fuquay Varina, NC: OS Press, 2017.

3. Anderson, T., Morton, C., Shropshire, M. *Original Strength Performance—The Next Level, 1st ed.* Fuquay Varina, NC: OS Press, 2018.

4. di Vico, R., Ardigo, L. P., Salernitano, G., Chamari, K., Padulo, J. "The acute effect of the tongue position in the mouth on knee isokinetic test performance: a highly surprising pilot study." *Muscles, Ligaments and Tendons Journal* 3, no. 4 (October/December, 2013): 318-23.

5. Hoogenboom, B. J., Voight, M. L., Cook, G., Gill, L. "Using rolling to develop neuromuscular control and coordination of the core and extremities of athletes." *North American Journal of Sports Physical Therapy: NAJSPT* 4, no. 2 (May, 2009): 70-82.

6. Martarelli, D., Cocchioni, M., Scuri, S., Pompei, P. "Diaphragmatic breathing reduces exercise-induced oxidative stress." *Evidence - Based Complementary and Alternative Medicine* (February, 2011). doi:http://dx.doi.org/10.1093/ecam/nep169

SECTION 5

PROGRAM EVALUATION & TESTING

18
ATHLETIC PERFORMANCE EVALUATION

By: Philip Bishop, Ed. D.

Professor Emeritus of Exercise Science, University of Alabama

Why good measurement?

It is a well known saying in business, "If you can't measure it, you can't manage it." Likewise, the ONLY way we can know we are having a positive impact is by carefully measuring and monitoring our athletes. Measurement can be more complicated than it first appears. In order to use the results to the best of our ability to improve athletic performance, it is important to measure the right things, at the right times, in the right ways.

I once read a paper written by a very prominent medical school in the USA that featured several physicians and one statistical expert on their list of authors. The paper, which was peer-reviewed by scientific experts, was published in a very prominent research journal. The paper detailed how humans sense heat and cold and involved a pretty impressive design that allowed the doctors to manipulate skin and deep-body temperatures independently. When it came time to analyze their data, this highly-educated group, including an expert statistician, made a fundamental measurement error. They treated skin temperature and deep body temperature as if they were the SAME UNITS. After all, they were both in degrees Centigrade.

But why are the two measurements in Centigrade different? The difference can be illustrated with dollars. There are U.S. dollars, there are Australian dollars and there are Canadian dollars - but all have different values. You cannot add the three types of dollars because they each have a different value. The relative values change constantly. For example: if one US dollar equals 1.53 Canadian dollars and 1.33 Australian dollars, you'd be disappointed if you were given 100 Canadian dollars when expecting 100 Australian dollars, as the value of the Candian dollar is less.

But these well-educated scientists did not realize that one-degree Centigrade change of deep-body temperature was equal to about 3.6 degrees Centigrade change of skin temperature. That is, the whole range of human deep body temperature is from about 35C to about 40C, and above or below that is considered dangerous. The skin temperature is more variable, with lows of about 20C and highs of 38C.

When the scientists did their calculations, they neglected the measurement differences and naturally came to the wrong conclusion.

Careful measurement is very important. Fortunately, most sports measures are fairly simple.

Measuring Athletes

The most common measurement may be measurements of performance progress. To make this measurement well, we must start with an accurate baseline, or starting measurement. Because most performances are sensitive to fatigue, we need to measure the starting point when our athletes are at their very best. They need to be well rested, fed and hydrated. Because there is some variability in anyone's performance, to be very accurate we need to measure at least two or three times and either choose the average or the best.

This choice of average or best also requires knowledge of good measurement. Our average measurement will generally be more consistent than our "best" because "best" varies from day to day due to a lot of factors. The more measurements used in the average, the more stable the value will be. We can make a good decision to use either one, but we just need to understand that there are measurement trade-offs with each choice.

Once we have determined a baseline, we need to decide when to re-measure and how. Choosing the right time to re-measure can depend on multiple factors, and the coach/trainer's long range training plan will determine when and how often. For all re-testing however, the care to make accurate measurements is the same. For most sport performance, environmental factors, such as heat or altitude, will impact performance independently of actual improvements in capabilities. For example if a 10Km running baseline is measured in a cool environment, but the training progress measurements are made in a hot environment, then improvement will be masked by the added stress of the heat. Or if the progress measurement is made when the athletes are tired, the improvement will be underestimated.

Uses for a Good Measurement System

Only if we have a good measurement system used appropriately can we evaluate how our training program is working. It is important to do this for individuals as well as the whole team. Sometimes the top athletes will fail to show improvement, even though the lower-skilled performers show great improvement. In these cases, a coach/trainer must make a value-judgment to determine if that is a desirable outcome. But the only way to know is to make accurate measurements and keep good records.

In most cases, a good measurement program will help us evaluate our overall program. A detailed measurement system may most usefully identify strengths and weaknesses of our individuals and guide us in improving everyone's performance.

Hard Measurements

One of the fundamental facts of measurement is that all measurements have room for error. Our goal is simply to measure well enough that the errors are small enough not to mislead us. For some measurements, the error can be acknowledged and still be useful.

For example, if we want to estimate body fat, most systems of measurement such as Bioimpedance, give very large errors, and these errors may not be consistent. In contrast, a cheaper means of estimating body fatness is carefully measured skinfold thicknesses. If done correctly, the actual skinfold measurements can be very accurate and a good reflection changes in fatness. And, for a sport like body building, the skinfold thickness is the most important measurement, far more important than actual total body fatness. This is because lower skinfolds give better muscle definition, and intramuscular fat adds to the total muscle volume.

To use good measurement with skinfold, first learn to measure accurately. The sites can be found at https://www.exrx.net/Testing/BodyCompSites, and other places on the internet. Once good measurements are taken, I recommend measuring three sites in men: chest, abdomen and thigh; and three sites in women: triceps, suprailiac and thigh. Record these with the date and the name of the person measuring. Now, at subsequent dates, compare the simple sum of the three sites. If the sum is increasing, the person is getting fatter, regardless of what the scales may say (muscle weighs more than fat). If the sum is decreasing, the person is losing fatness, regardless of the scale readings. Because most of the body fat error comes in estimating fatness from skinfolds, this error is irrelevant when we ignore that conversion.

Performance and Physiological Testing

Fortunately, the most valuable measurements for athletes are the measurements related to their sport, such as race times, the amount of weight lifted, earned-run-average, on-base percentage, etc. matter the most. These measurements are specific to the sport and are the most relevant and easiest to measure.

But some more sophisticated testing may be helpful. For endurance athletes, we already mentioned that their ability to expend a lot of energy will depend on their ability to transport a lot of oxygen quickly to their muscles. The primary determinant of that capacity is the heart's ability to pump blood. A distance sportsman in training will experience a healthy enlargement of their left heart ventricle and an increase in the ability to pump blood with each beat. Their maximal heart rate may actually drop a couple of beats at maximum, but the maximal pumping ability will be higher for their size. A test of cardiac output is difficult to obtain, but a measure of maximal oxygen uptake is much more accessible and again is more useful than cardiac output, because maximal oxygen transport to the muscles is the goal. Expressing oxygen uptake relative to body weight is important for weight-supported sports, because the smaller the sportsman, the less total oxygen is needed.

Another useful measurement in many athletes is their so-called lactate threshold (it's not really a threshold because lactate is always in the blood). This is the point where lactic acid begins to accumulate rapidly in the blood. As we mentioned in the section on metabolism, the increase in lactic acid is not a bad thing in itself, but it does mark the point where the glycolytic system is beginning to store those H- ions temporarily whilst more ATP is produced without oxygen. The faster an athlete is moving when this happens, the faster or better they are likely to perform, with all other things being equal, to complete the race. It is also a useful marker in training because when athletes train at a level above this threshold speed, they are stressing the glycolytic system, and hopefully this stress will result in adaptations to the stress which improve performance.

Biomechanical measurements can also be useful in athletes, but these can be very hard to obtain. Essentially, biomechanical measurements involve filming the athlete in motion, then carefully analyzing their technique to improve performance, and sometimes lessen the chance of overuse injuries. To learn more about this go to https://www.nsca.com/education/articles/kinetic-select/biomechanical-analysis-in-practice/ which references a useful text.

One of the most difficult field measurements, but one of high value in many sports is assessment of individual hydration levels, especially for soccer or other sports of long duration. Currently there are three convenient means for roughly estimating hydration levels. Probably the best of these is changes in body weight over short time periods. A person sweating profusely will eventually become hypo-hydrated unless they drink an amount slightly greater than their losses. The measurement challenge with body weight is to make sure you are only weighing what you want to weigh. With weight as an estimate of hydration status, the athlete should wear minimum clothing and keep in mind that fluid in the gut or in the bladder will add to weight without contributing to true hydration.

Alternative measures such as urine color and urine specific gravity are helpful but can also be deceiving. They work well when a person is not sweating profusely and re-hydrating, but not so well in sports applications, where people are both losing sweat and also drinking. The urine measures are simply "averages" which represent what the kidney deposited in the bladder since the last void. So these measures are more useful before a workout. It is unfortunate that we do not have a good measure of hydration because dehydration puts people at greater risk for heat injury.

Sport Measurement

Measurement in sport is slowly but steadily improving. Automatic timing in swimming and running have made these measurements more accurate and free from bias of the person doing the measurement. Bias by measurers is problematic any time humans are involved, particularly in subjective sports measurement–where athletes are given a score or judged by a variety of techniques–such as in gymnastics, diving and some snow sports.

Having guidelines to minimize bias is helpful, like using rubrics such as those presented in several sources. For more on measurement issues see Bishop, P. *Measurement and Evaluation in Physical Activity Applications: Exercise Science, Physical Education, Coaching, Athletic Training, and Health*. 2nd edition. Textbook, Routledge Publishers. 2018.

Introduction to Basic Statistics

Being on the cutting edge of coaching/training requires that you keep up with the latest discoveries, which typically first appear in scientific journals. It is not recommended to take advice or research information from the internet. I have found much misinformation from that source in otherwise well-meaning people's posts.

To read and understand these science articles it helps to know a bit of basic statistics. First, most research on athletes will be repeated measures designs wherein a given group of skilled participants (skilled and trained athletes are different from those not training or training rarely, so beware of studies using untrained participants) undergo a treatment designed to improve performance and also undergo a control treatment that is known to have no effects, called a placebo. Most people vary slightly from measurement to measurement, so a small difference between the treatment and control conditions may be a fluke and not related to the treatment that is being tested. Because we can practically only test a sample of people, we will use inferential statistics to determine if any differences between treatments is real or just a fluke.

The simplest comparison in this situation is a paired-sample (1 group, or "dependent") Student's t-test. This is only a useful test for comparing two treatments. When we run our test, then the output is a "p" value. The "p" is simply the "probability" of a difference between the two treatments based on luck or fluke. Odds of a difference attributable to luck (as opposed to the effect of the treatment) should be very small, typically less than 5% ($p < .05$).

Common sense is important. If some treatment makes a major impact on an elite athlete's performance, perhaps be willing to use it even if there is only 90% confidence in the statistics. Observe the impact on the athlete or team, and if it's a positive outcome for most of them, then be open to using the new treatment.

Keep in mind that many useful treatments may have been accidentally dismissed. Take a simple hypothetical situation of testing a treatment that didn't statistically have a high mean of performance improvement. If 30% of the participants substantially improved their performance, but 30% of participants got worse by the same amount, then mathematically the mean would be unchanged. But those 30% who improved substantially–if the treatment is ethical, safe and not too expensive–should use it. Test it on all and see who consistently benefits and who gets worse. Those who benefit will use the treatment, but we will keep it far away from those who get worse.

If two different groups are tested over time, which scientists sometimes have to do because the treatment may take a long time or a major fraction of the training season, the two group means would be compared using an independent or 2-group t-test. Take note that t-tests of either type are only good to test two conditions or two groups. If we have more conditions or more groups, then we must do an Analysis of Variance (ANOVA). The principles of operation are the same and ANOVA gives you a p value just like a t-test.

Another very useful statistic for coaches/trainers is the Pearson Product-Moment Correlation. The correlation tells us the relationship between two independent variables. For example, we might be interested in the relationship between muscle cross-sectional area and strength. We would get a sample of people with a wide range of muscle sizes and strengths. We do not want to get all similar types of people, or it would distort the natural distribution of muscle size and strength and get an erroneous result.

If we gather a representative sample and get size and strength measurements from each person, we then can calculate the correlation between the two measurements. The maximal correlation is 1.0, and in this case, the worst possible correlation is -1.0, which would mean that the two measurements were perfectly inversely correlated, as one increased, the other decreased. This would also be useful data. So the actual worst situation in this case would be a correlation near 0–that is, there was NO relationship between the two measures. In general, the best correlation is + 1.0 or -1.0 and the worst is 0. Either a low (near zero) or a high correlation may be useful because these outcomes tell us the strength of relationship between the two characteristics–regardless of what they are.

Beware though, as scientists sometimes accidentally choose a sample that is NOT representative of the population of sportsmen. If they distort the distribution too badly they may present a falsely strong correlation. In a true story, some very good researchers measured the cross-sectional area of the muscles and the strength of a sample. Unfortunately, they measured both arms and legs and combined these data and then ran the correlation. Doing this resulted in two low correlations for legs and for arms, but when all were combined, the total correlation was high. The error resulted since the arms and legs are so drastically different in muscle size and strength. That is, the arms are typically much smaller and weaker than the legs, so the correlation was falsely inflated.

Running Your Own Statistics

The t-test and the correlation can be performed on most simple spreadsheets, so coaches could do their own statistics, if only two data sets were compared. If ANOVA or other statistical tests are needed, I recommend you visit your local college or university and seek their help. But now you know enough to read and understand most research.

19
ATHLETIC PERFORMANCE TESTING

By: Brian Edlbeck

Clinical Assistant Professor of Exercise Science Carroll University

Why Assess?

As a coach, it is important to put time and energy into assessing athletes. Assessment is simply quantifying performance variables. The question that presents itself is, what variables are you as a coach concerned with? To be able to answer that question, we need to answer why we assess athletes.

Assessment serves two primary purposes. The first is to hold athletes accountable for their training and development. If an athlete comes into a program understanding that coaches will quantify performance variables through assessment, this will promote compliance and desire to improve. The second purpose of assessment is to hold the coaches accountable. If you are writing a program designed to make an athlete jump higher and they do not jump higher after 12 weeks of training, are you doing what you've set out to do? The overall purpose of assessment is to hold both athletes and coaches accountable for their jobs and results.

It is a coach's responsibility to know the needs of each of their athletes and what will motivate them. While assessments hold coaches and athletes accountable to performance improvements, you want to ensure the assessments also motivate them, not hinder their performance or discourage them. Always be assessing athletes on metrics that can be used to truly help improve their performance, never losing sight of them as a whole person. The sample assessment categories and tests mentioned throughout this chapter are used to quantify specific variables for various athletes. Athletes will be looked at generally and not within individual sports.

General Motivation

If you put a record board or sign up on the wall to show who has the highest bench press, vertical jump or is the fastest, does that motivate athletes? Some athletes would be motivated by this. There will be athletes who will strive to see their name on the board or work extra hard to get their name on the wall. Knowing that they are the best of their peers and teammates can serve as a powerful tool to motivate them. The idea that if I work hard, I can see the benefits and quantify my improvements is a solid external reward tool. Others might view it differently; they might consider that they will not live up to their peers. They know they cannot beat someone, so why continue to try or put in the effort? They may think they are never going to be as good as their teammates. This could decrease motivation, and you may lose those athletes. You might have to look at other reward systems. All this to establish that we work with multiple personalities, drive and motivation factors within teams.

Motivate your athletes the best way you know how. As a strength and conditioning coach or a sports coach, develop a rapport with all your athletes. This will open up communication to determine the best way to motivate each athlete by highlighting them on the record board or giving them individual accolades for personal records and celebrating them in front of a team or individually. Ultimately, when looking into assessment, the main thing that needs to be considered is what is best for each athlete. When it comes down to it, we are working with people, not working with numbers. People matter—they are important. Many coaches lose focus on the people when too focussed on the numbers. Always prioritize the athlete and what is best for them.

Needs Analysis

To first determine what needs to be assessed, a coach needs to determine what is required to perform their chosen sport. For this, an overall look of the sport needs to be completed. For example, what does it take to be a great volleyball player or baseball player? Typically, an athlete does not need to be good at everything possible, but needs to be trained to make them successful for their sport. This will also be true of what assessments should be performed. As a coach, you will have strong athletes, quick athletes and fast athletes. Fueling a coach with this information may help a sports coach determine where each athlete can fit in to help the team. Further, by identifying the strengths and weaknesses of an athlete or team, a strength coach can best determine what training program is needed. This is typically how assessment can aid both the sports coach and strength coach to help each athlete or a team improve.

Moving forward, we will be looking at particular variables that are important in assessing all athletes regarding the sport they participate in. It would be up to the expertise of the sports coach and strength coach to prioritize which test may be more important than another in determining the needs of the athletes.

Assessment

Anthropometrics

Anthropometrics is one of the most utilized assessments throughout any health field. We generally look at the general stature of the body. Anthropometrics means measuring the size and proportions of the human body. The strength and conditioning coaches keep it straightforward by typically measuring two anthropometrics—height and weight. In addition, another anthropometric measurement, body composition, will be discussed later in this chapter. In addition to height, weight and body composition, you will see coaches measure girth measurements to know the actual size of the muscles or areas of the body. There are a lot of other anthropometrics used in various sports to measure an athlete for different reasons. American football uses hand width, which measures the tip of the thumb to the end of the pinky finger. This is supposed to identify a catch window for a wide receiver. Basketball coaches tend to look at wingspan versus height. Combat sports coaches will look at reach to determine how far an individual can reach with a strike. There are many forms of anthropometrics. Still, typically height and weight are utilized, along with body composition and body fat percentage.

A scale will be used to determine the weight, and a stadiometer is used to measure height. Typically, strength coaches will take this one step further than height and weight. They will report out what's referred to as a body mass index or BMI. BMI is a representation of comparison of height to weight. BMI is determined by taking an individual's weight in kilograms and dividing by their height in meters squared.

$$BMI = WT \div HT2 = kg/m2$$

By looking at the normative data, you can determine where individuals will fall when determining if they are a normal weight, overweight, underweight or obese. BMI is a good assessment for general populations. For individuals who carry excess muscle mass, BMI could be skewed. Some do not consider BMI to be a very valid measurement in two specific populations - the military and athletic populations. Too many people from those populations who are over 30 years old get classified as obese due to their muscle mass weight. When we look at their body fat percentage, we can see body fat is not an issue for these individuals, therefore they are not obese, or even overweight.

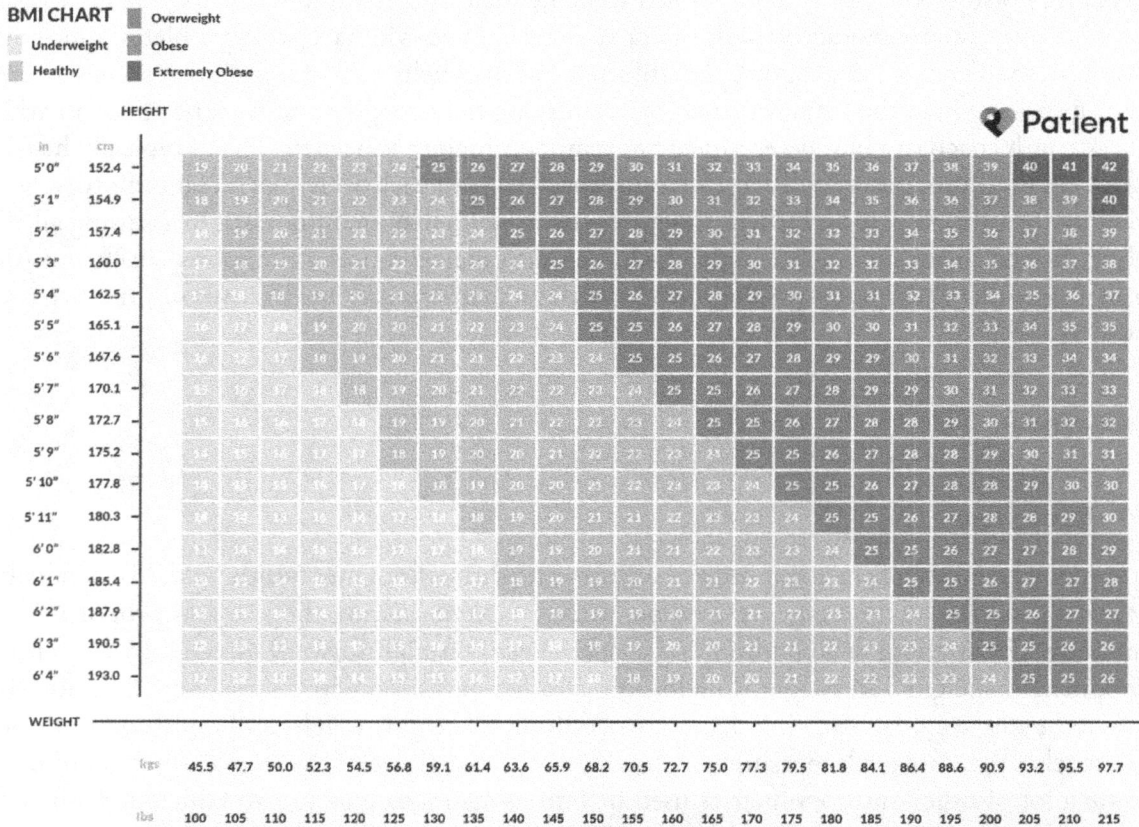

BMI CHART
Underweight · Healthy · Overweight · Obese · Extremely Obese

HEIGHT — ♥ Patient

in	cm																								
5'0"	152.4	19	20	21	22	23	24	25	26	27	28	29	30	31	32	33	34	35	36	37	38	39	40	41	42
5'1"	154.9	18	19	20	21	22	23	24	25	26	27	28	29	30	31	32	33	34	35	36	36	37	38	39	40
5'2"	157.4	18	19	20	21	22	22	23	24	25	26	27	28	29	30	31	32	32	33	34	35	36	37	38	39
5'3"	160.0	17	18	19	20	21	22	23	24	24	25	26	27	28	29	30	31	32	32	33	34	35	36	37	38
5'4"	162.5	17	18	18	19	20	21	22	23	24	24	25	26	27	28	29	30	31	31	32	33	34	35	36	37
5'5"	165.1	16	17	18	19	20	20	21	22	23	24	25	25	26	27	28	29	30	30	31	32	33	34	35	35
5'6"	167.6	16	16	17	18	19	20	21	21	22	23	24	25	25	26	27	28	29	29	30	31	32	33	34	34
5'7"	170.1	15	16	17	18	18	19	20	21	21	22	23	24	25	25	26	27	28	29	29	30	31	32	33	33
5'8"	172.7	15	16	16	17	18	19	19	20	21	22	22	23	24	25	25	26	27	28	28	29	30	31	32	32
5'9"	175.2	14	15	16	17	17	18	19	20	20	21	22	23	23	24	25	25	26	27	28	28	29	30	31	31
5'10"	177.8	14	15	15	16	17	18	18	19	20	20	21	22	23	23	24	25	25	26	27	28	28	29	30	30
5'11"	180.3	14	14	15	16	16	17	18	18	19	20	21	21	22	23	23	24	25	25	26	27	28	28	29	30
6'0"	182.8	13	14	15	15	16	17	17	18	19	20	20	21	21	22	23	23	24	25	25	26	27	27	28	29
6'1"	185.4	13	13	14	15	15	16	17	17	18	19	19	20	21	21	22	23	23	24	25	25	26	27	27	28
6'2"	187.9	12	13	14	14	15	16	16	17	18	18	19	19	20	21	21	22	23	23	24	25	25	26	27	27
6'3"	190.5	12	13	13	14	15	15	16	16	17	18	18	19	20	20	21	21	22	23	23	24	25	25	26	26
6'4"	193.0	12	12	13	14	14	15	15	16	17	17	18	18	19	20	20	21	21	22	23	23	24	25	25	26

WEIGHT

kgs	45.5	47.7	50.0	52.3	54.5	56.8	59.1	61.4	63.6	65.9	68.2	70.5	72.7	75.0	77.3	79.5	81.8	84.1	86.4	88.6	90.9	93.2	95.5	97.7
lbs	100	105	110	115	120	125	130	135	140	145	150	155	160	165	170	175	180	185	190	195	200	205	210	215

Aerobic Power

Aerobic power is looking at the body's ability to utilize oxygen for energy production. Oxygen comes into the body and is used to produce adenosine triphosphate (ATP). ATP is the body's number one energy currency and allows us to move our bodies. This is a variable that coaches typically want to assess. Aerobic power assesses an athlete's ability to bring oxygen into their bodies. Other terms that have been utilized for aerobic power are aerobic capacity, VO_2 max or oxygen capacity.

There are two ways to assess aerobic power. A coach can take an athlete's maximal effort and record or predict the amount of oxygen they bring into their bodies or utilize a sub-maximal effort then record or predict the amount of oxygen. If a coach wants to record the oxygen uptake, this uses specialized equipment.

The equipment is expensive and technical to use. I would not recommend for a sports coach or strength coach to record oxygen directly. This means the best way to assess aerobic power is to predict it using maximal or submaximal effort. Let's look at several potential assessment tools that can be utilized.

Pacer/Beep Test

The Pacer/Beep Test is a maximum effort test. To be able to utilize this test, you will need the following equipment:

- Tape measure
- 20 meters of linear space
- Audio device
- Beep recording (apps are available like on Top End Sports)
- Heart rate monitor (optional)

The Pacer/Beep Test is progressive. First, a coach needs to measure out 20 meters in a straight line. Next, an audio device plays instructions on performing the test and provides audio beeps when the individual must reach the 20-meter mark and then turn around. The test gets progressively faster until the athlete decides to stop. Once reaching maximal effort, a prediction equation or table is used.

Based on how long individuals could stay with the beeps, aerobic power (VO_2 max) is predicted.

Cooper's Test

The second test is not maximal, so the athlete does not have to go to the maximal effort, but needs more space for this test. Equipment required for this test includes:

- 400-meter track
- Stopwatch
- Cones
- Heart rate monitor (optional)

The space needed is a continuous loop. A track would work the best if it is flat with no elevation. Running on open roads, fields or trails may have too much elevation. This would impact the results of this test. The Cooper's test is submaximal, so the athlete should run at the highest pace they can while maintaining a constant velocity. The athlete will need to run continuously for 12 minutes. Once the 12 minutes are done, determine the distance accomplished and record it. A prediction equation is used to determine VO_2 max.

Queen's Step Test

A third test is the Queen's Step Test. This test requires no space, which makes it an excellent test to perform anywhere. The equipment needed includes:

- Stopwatch
- Aerobic step (16.25 in / 43.3 cm)
- Metronome
- Heart rate monitor (optional)

The athlete will need to step up and down onto the aerobic step at a specific rate. The cadence is set at 96 beats per minute for males and 88 beats per minute for females. Each time it beats, the athlete would take a step. This means it takes four beats for an athlete to get all the way up on the step and back down. For example, right foot up, left foot up, right foot down, left foot down. The test is performed for three minutes. After the three minutes, the heart rate is recorded and based on the individual's heart rate, VO_2 max can be determined.

There are pros and cons for each of the tests. The Pacer/Beep Test allows for smaller space to be used. It takes the individual to a maximal effort, which enables the coach to record a maximal heart rate, but audio equipment is needed. The Cooper's Test allows for everyone to start and stop at the same time and is a submaximal test. However a large area is required. The Queen's Step Test only needs minimal space to perform, but additional equipment is required and only one person can perform the test at a time.

When determining which test a coaching staff will perform, additional consideration of how much manpower is needed to run each test and how many athletes can be assessed simultaneously is needed. A coach can run people back and forth. The Pacer/Beep Test can be run with multiple athletes at a time, but needs multiple coaches to determine when each athlete finishes. If you are running 20 individuals, you have to know when each individual finishes and record the number of lengths run. It might be hard for one person to record all the data. The Coopers Test is relatively easy to run with one coach with multiple athletes running. This is because after 12 minutes, the athletes stop in place. Their distance run is then recorded before they leave the track. The Queen's Step Test is difficult to run in multiple groups due to the need for equipment.

Anaerobic Power

The next group of testing will look at an individual's ability to make energy without oxygen, otherwise termed anaerobic power, unlike aerobic power, which examines an individual's ability to produce energy with oxygen, thus looking at VO_2 max. Anaerobic power is assessing an individual's ability to make energy without oxygen. Again, three potential assessment tools will be looked at. Anaerobic power testing requires more equipment, but examples provided in this chapter will require less equipment than some of the other tests out there.

Running-Based Anaerobic Sprint Test (RAST)

The RAST does not require a lot of equipment or space. The equipment needed includes:

- Stopwatch
- 35 meters linear distance for sprinting
- 10 meters linear space to decelerate and rest
- Scale for body mass

The athlete runs a series of six sprints with 10 seconds of rest after each sprint. A coach will record the time it takes them to sprint the 35 meters at maximal velocity for each sprint. Two variables will be determined during this assessment tool. 1) Power output will be calculated for each of the six sprints. Power is measured in watts, and the following equation is utilized to determine that value.

The coach will determine maximum power out, minimum power output and average power output. 2) In addition to various power measurements, the coach will also calculate a fatigue index (FI).

In determining how much fatigue occurs throughout these six sprints, coaches will look at the fastest sprint, the slowest sprint and how much difference there is between the two. In theory, the athlete's fastest sprint should be one of the first couple. However, it might not be the first one, as they are getting used to the test. It could be the second one or potentially the third. The slowest sprint of six typically is either the fifth or sixth sprint as the athlete becomes fatigued. The FI indicates how quickly the athlete loses the anaerobic system. The RAST is a good test because not a lot of equipment is needed. It is hard to run multiple athletes at once because, typically, each athlete will require an individual timer. A downfall of these anaerobic capacity tests generally is they are very individual-based tests, unlike the aerobic power where we can test a lot of individuals at one time.

An advantage of the RAST is its ability to produce an FI value. For example, FI may inform a coach how quickly an athlete will fatigue during a task or sport—from a coach's standpoint. Using American football as an example, an average play in American football is typically six seconds. Therefore, the coach can determine how many plays an athlete should stay in before being rotated out.

Margaria-Kalamen Stair Climb Test

The second test is called the Margaria-Kalamen Stair Climb Test. Use this test only when you are sure it can be done safely. Equipment for this test is minimal:

- A flight of stairs with at least nine stairs
- At least 6 meters in front of the stairs
- Stopwatch
- Scale for body mass

The athlete is asked to stand 6 meters beyond the bottom step. The athlete then proceeds to sprint up to the ninth step as fast as possible. They only step on every third step: the third, sixth and ninth steps. You can see how safety comes into play as the coach asks the athlete to go as fast as they can ascending stairs but skipping stairs as they go up. The time is recorded once the athlete hits the ninth step. The athlete can run multiple trials. Power in watts is then calculated using the following equation:

Clock (to nearest 0.01 second)

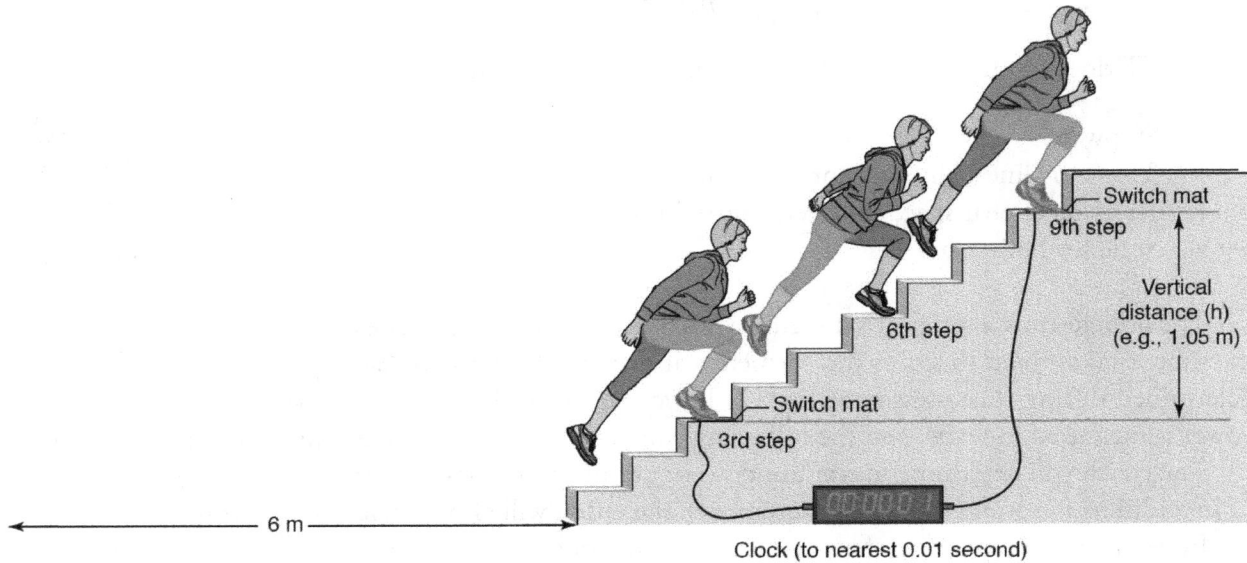

Reprinted by permission from Fox, Bowers, and Foss 1993.

Haff, G. G., and Triplett, N. T. *Essentials of Strength Training and Conditioning-NSCA* (4th ed). Champaign, IL: Human Kinetics, 2016.

Sargent Jump Test

Another test that is readily utilized to determine anaerobic power is the Sargent Jump Test. Again, it is a minimal equipment test. What is required to perform this test is:

- Wall
- Tape measure
- Step ladder
- Chalk or tape

The Sargent Jump Test asks the athlete to jump vertically as high as possible. It is not a difficult test to perform and thus is utilized by most sport and strength coaches. First, the athlete is asked to stand perpendicular to a wall and reach as high as possible with both feet remaining flat on the ground. Next, the athlete either marks the wall with chalk on their fingers or places a piece of tape. Then with more chalk on their fingertips or another piece of tape in hand, the athlete jumps as high as possible and marks the wall with the chalk or tape. A vertical jump height is determined by the distance between the two marks on the wall. The vertical jump height is then utilized to calculate the anaerobic power output of the athlete.

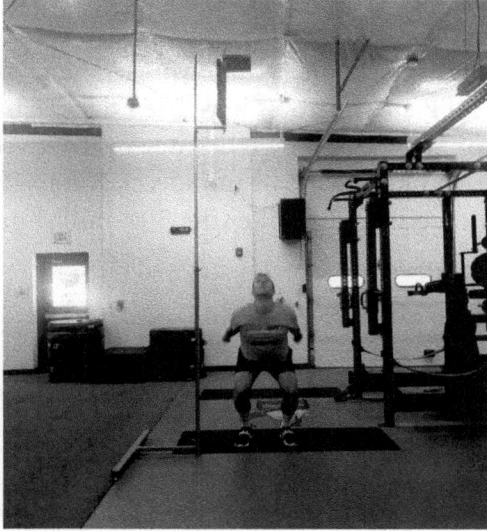

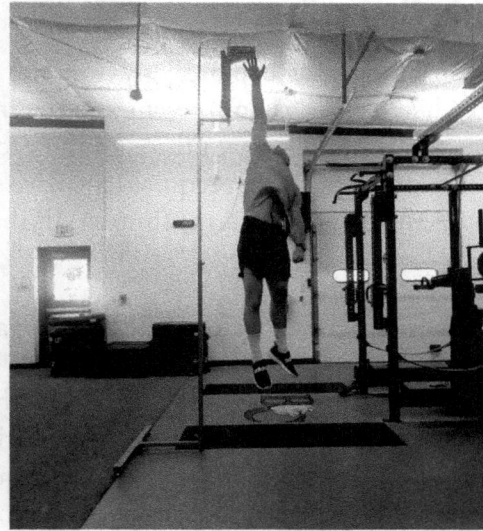

Haff, G. G., and Triplett, N. T. *Essentials of Strength Training and Conditioning-NSCA* (4th ed).
Champaign, IL: Human Kinetics, 2016.

Three different anaerobic power tests have been described within this section. All three will assess power output in watts. In addition to the power in watts, the RAST also will determine an athlete's FI. There are pros and cons to each of the three tests. RAST will assess maximal, minimal, and average power of the course of six sprints. The test will also evaluate the FI of the athlete, but a lot of manpower is needed if more than one athlete will be assessed at a time and a space of 45 meters is required to perform the test. Margaria-Kalamen Stair Climb Test only needs to be done once, so it goes very quickly. However, safety and the right stair set up needs to be taken into consideration. Sargent Jump Test is a quick test for athletes comfortable with jumping, but the right wall space is required.

Anaerobic power can be looked at by a coach in two different ways. First, it can be assessed as an absolute value that is measured in watts. Second, a coach could also look at the value as a relative term. That would be expressed in watts per kilogram. To determine that value, a coach takes the value obtained by the different assessment tools and divides it by the athlete's body mass in kilograms.

Anaerobic Capacity

Anaerobic capacity testing explores how well the anaerobic glycolytic system works. The glycolytic system is used when oxygen is not present and the initial ATP energy stores have been depleted. A glucose (sugar) molecule is broken down through the process of glycolysis. The efficiency of the glycolytic system is paramount in sports that require repetitive sprinting like basketball and soccer. A classic anaerobic capacity test is the 300-yd (274 m) shuttle. All that is needed to administer the 300-yard shuttle test is:

- Stopwatch
- Two lines spaced 25 yards (22.86 m) apart

The athlete runs down and back between the two lines six times as fast as possible. The time is recorded for the first 300-yd shuttle and the athlete is given five minutes to rest before the 300-yd shuttle is repeated. With the 300-yd shuttle requiring use of the glycolytic system to provide energy, the speed that each shuttle is run provides one indication of the strength of the glycolytic system. The similarity between the two times provides a strong indication of the athlete's anaerobic capacity with less difference between scores indicating a more efficient glycolytic system.

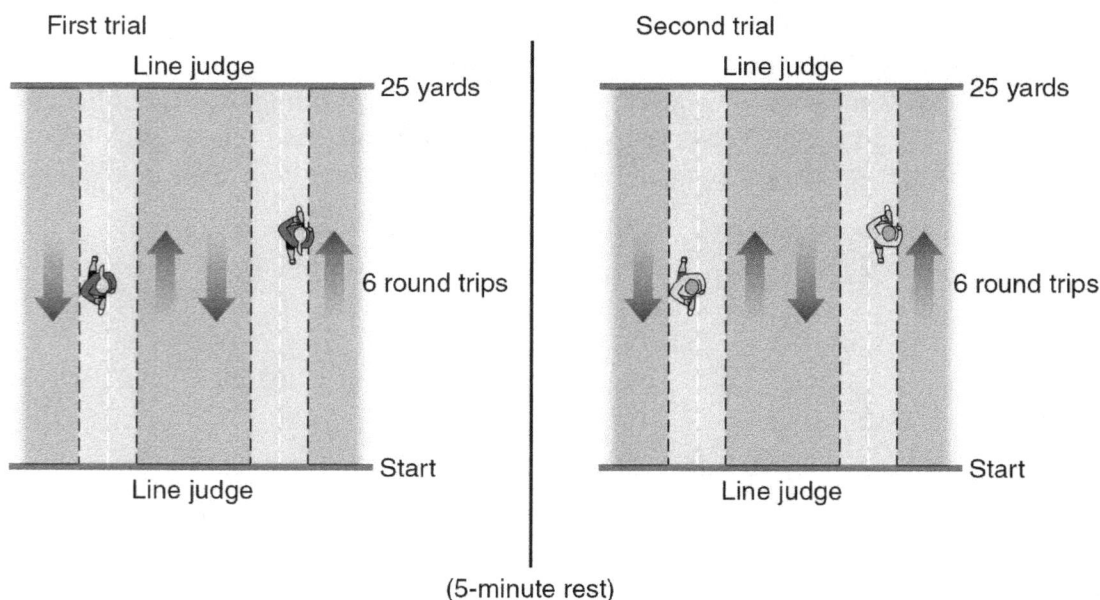

Adapted by permission from Gilliam 1983.

300-yard Shuttle

Muscle Endurance

Muscular endurance is something a little bit different than the first two categories of aerobic and anaerobic power. Muscular endurance is looking at the ability of a muscle to produce force over multiple repetitions. It looks at how many repetitions an athlete can perform before the muscle fatigues. The simplest way to do this is to use an individual's body mass. As a coach, you use the athlete's body mass to determine how many repetitions they can perform before they can't do any more. These are typically referred to as calisthenics assessments. Some assessments can be done in the weight room, but this section will focus on calisthenic-based assessment for muscular endurance.

The most typical calisthenics assessment is the push-up test and the sit-up test. At the end of this chapter are tables based on age and sex, showing how many the general population should perform.

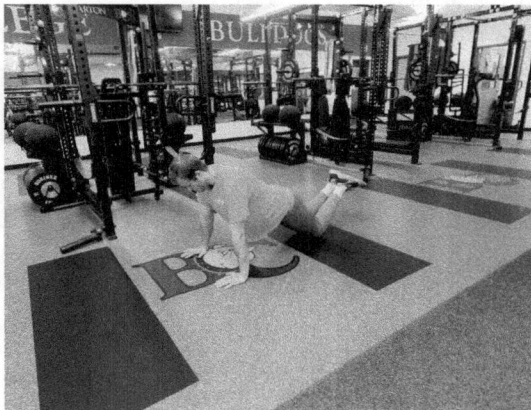

Modified Push Up Top Position

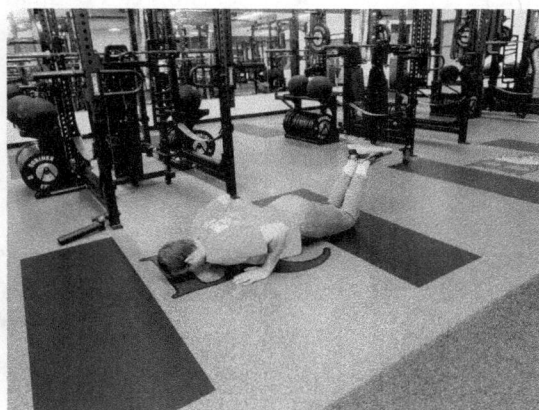

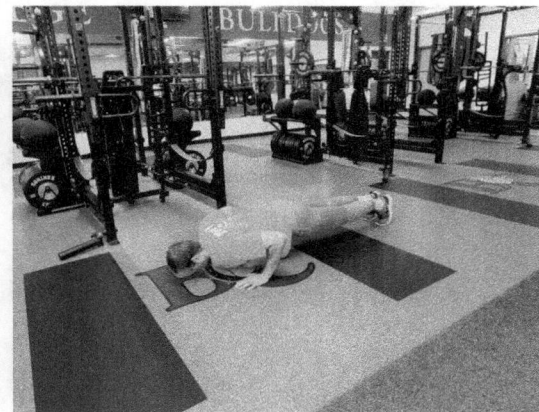

Modified Push Up Bottom Position

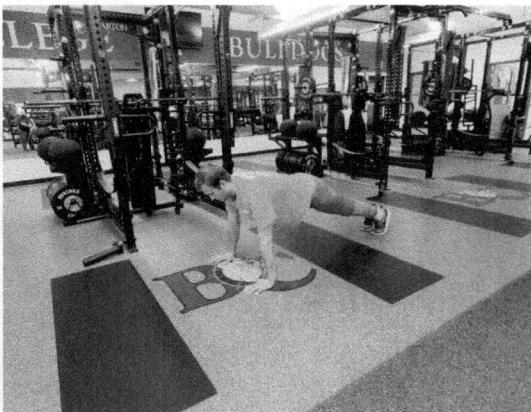

Push Up Top position

Push Up Bottom Position

In looking at the protocol of these, the most important thing is for a coach to stay consistent when having athletes perform the test. Calisthenic-based tests are very beneficial because multiple athletes can perform the test simultaneously, using a partner to count how many repetitions are being performed. Additionally, very minimal equipment is needed. The equipment includes:

- Partner
- Metronome
- Adequate floor space

The push-up test is a relatively standard test within the field. What needs to be paid attention to from a coaching standpoint is the pivot point of the movement. There are two options: 1) the standard push-up test uses the feet or the toes as the pivot point. 2) The modified push-up uses the knees as the pivot point. The pivot points typically have been associated with different sexes, with males performing the movement on the toes (standard) and females performing on the knees (modified). This is shown in the normative data above. If a female athlete wants to perform a standard push-up with the toes as the pivot point, they will fall into that normative data. In all reality, progress is what a coach is tracking. Coaches want to make sure that individuals are improving. So if they did 14 push-ups the first time and then 18 the next time, both times on the toes, the conclusion can be made that the athlete is getting better.

When assessing muscular endurance, there are two ways to run the protocols. One would have the athlete perform as many as possible (AMAP). By performing AMAP, a cadence of 60 bpm is required. The athlete stays on cadence until they cannot perform any more repetitions or can no longer maintain the cadence. Once either of those occurs, the test is stopped. I prefer the cadence method because everything is controlled with cadence. How many repetitions the athlete can perform would truly represent muscular endurance. The other way to run the protocol is to allow the athlete to perform AMAP in a certain amount of time. The time is typically 60 seconds. However, this has the potential to introduce another variable - a person that can perform the movements faster is going to be at an advantage. Anaerobic power should not influence a muscular endurance assessment. If a metronome is not available, then running a 60-second protocol is better than not assessing muscular endurance.

The other typical assessment to measure muscular endurance is a sit-up test or a curl-up test. There are multiple ways to run a full sit-up test. 1) The individual places their hands behind their head with elbows facing forward with their feet flat on the ground with the knees at 90-degrees. Always make sure you are standardizing how the movement happens.

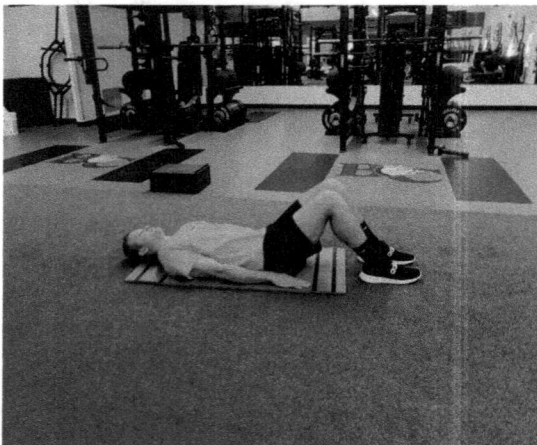

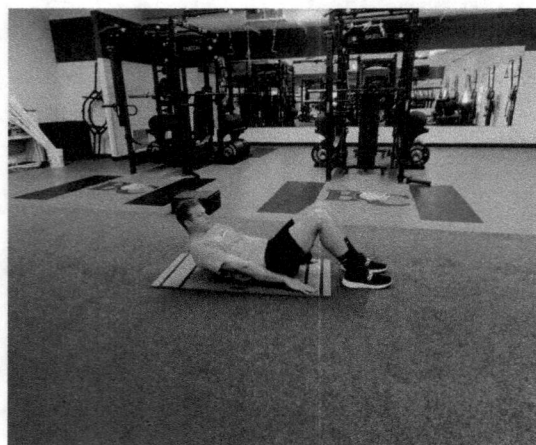

The individual comes up all the way to where the elbows touch the upper part of the thigh. A repetition is counted only if those elbows touch the upper thigh. Another standard test is typically a curl-up test. The hands are placed on the ground next to the body with their feet flat on the ground with the knees at 90 degrees.

The individual slides their hands up two inches (5.08 cm) to record a repetition. A problem with the curl-up test is that the neck is not supported; thus, some individuals may complain of neck soreness. A 60-second protocol may be used, but speed may influence the muscular education results.

Muscular Strength

One-Repetition Maximum

Muscular strength is a little different than muscular endurance. Muscular endurance looks at the force output of the muscle over numerous repetitions. With muscular strength, we are determining how much force a muscle can produce for a single repetition. This is typically measured through a one-repetition maximal effort (1RM). A coach will need resistance training equipment to be able to assess a 1RM. Large muscle groups are tested, and a coach wants to determine how much force an athlete can produce. A typical 1RM test is a flat press or a bench press. The bench press will assess the upper body pushing muscles. Every muscle that is needed to push in the upper body is utilized during that movement.

Another typical 1RM assessment is for lower body pressing muscles. These muscle groups are typically assessed through a back squat or a leg press. This would determine how much an athlete can press with the lower body muscles. There are slight differences between the squatting motion and leg press motion, but again we would use those to strengthen the lower body. There are other muscles in the body besides upper body pushing and lower body pressing. A coach can use different protocols for muscle groups involving upper body pulling muscles. A similar protocol can be utilized to assess those muscles also. It is typically done through a bent-over row or seated row exercise. When looking at overall strength, the three basic movements to assess are upper body push, an upper body pull and a lower body press.

The results obtained by these assessments are represented in load, either in pounds or kilograms. A coach can review the results a couple of different ways: absolute strength and relative strength. Absolute strength is the total number that a person can push, pull or press. An athlete's body mass doesn't matter with absolute strength. If they can bench press 300 lbs. (136 kg), their absolute strength is 300 lbs. (156 kg). Relative strength is the value when an athlete's body mass is taken into account. The number represents how much strength they have per unit of body mass. If an athlete weighs 220 lbs. (100 kg) and can bench press 300 lbs. (136 kg), their relative strength is 1.36 times their body mass.

Absolute Weight Lifted (1RM) in lbs / lifter's Body Weight in lbs = Relative Strength

A relative strength number can give a coach an indicator that allows them to look at how strong an athlete is pound per pound. Below is a table that offers approximately where an individual should be based on body mass

There is also a way to look at muscular strength without taking an athlete to maximal effort. Instead, a coach can predict muscular strength based on multiple repetitions. For example, if an athlete bench presses 220 lbs. (100 kg) for numerous repetitions, a coach can determine or predict the athlete's 1RM.

This is used if an athlete doesn't have much resistance training experience or a coach who is not comfortable taking individuals to maximal effort.

Weight room muscular strength numbers are determined through what is referred to as a dynamic motion. Dynamic, at its simplest term, refers to an object moving. In this case, an athlete is moving a resistance to determine muscular strength.

Hand Grip Dynamometer

A coach may determine muscular strength through static testing. Static is the opposite of dynamic and refers to not moving. Static muscular strength testing requires specialized equipment. First, a device to measure grip test is needed; this piece of equipment is a hand dynamometer. An athlete squeezes the hand dynamometer as hard as they can. Next, muscular strength is recorded in pounds or kilometers. Finally, the number obtained from the athlete's score is compared against normative data to see how well they did on the test.

A benefit of the grip test is that a coach can look at the right and left sides. Comparing right-hand strength versus left-hand strength, an athlete will typically be stronger in their dominant hand. Therefore, a coach would want to make sure that there is no significant difference between the left and right sides within certain sports and specific activities.

There is also a pulling dynamometer.

The pulling dynamometers are more specialized equipment, and typically they are not the easiest to utilize, but if a coach would prefer a static strength measurement versus a dynamic measurement, dynamometers are an option. Then, they would be able to perform that assessment with that equipment.

A coach must determine whether they want to perform a dynamic or static muscular strength test. A coach can look at both absolute and relative values with either dynamic or static muscular strength assessments. If dynamic muscular strength is utilized, a 1RM can be performed; otherwise, a coach can predict the 1RM values using a prediction equation.

Agility

Agility is a performance attribute that covers a variety of abilities, including the ability to react and respond, coordinate movement, balance, display quickness, orient the body and move efficiently. A key aspect of agility in many sports is the ability to change directions. Changing direction requires skilled body control as one decelerates, stops and then accelerates in a new direction. Two classic change of direction tests are the pro-agility test and the T-test.

The pro-agility test requires a stopwatch and three cones placed in a straight line with each cone placed five yards apart. The athlete starts at the middle cone and sprints to the left five yards, changes direction and sprints 10 yards to the far cone, and then changes direction again and sprints back through the middle cone.

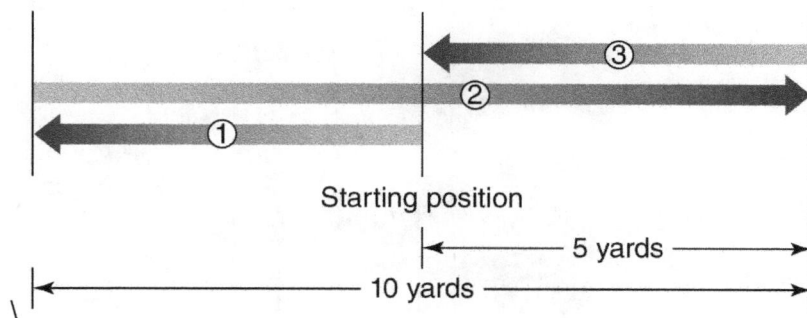

Haff, G. G., and Triplett, N. T. *Essentials of Strength Training and Conditioning-NSCA* (4th ed). Champaign, IL: Human Kinetics, 2016.

The pro-agility is considered a 180-degree change of direction test. However, sports often require the combination of changing direction and changing movement patterns (i.e. forward, backwards, lateral). The T-test provides an excellent evaluation of changing direction and movement pattern. The T-test requires the following equipment:

- Four cones
- Tape measure that is at least 10 yards long
- Stopwatch

The cones are arranged in a T shape with three cones across the top of the T that are five meters apart. The fourth cone is placed 10 yards away from the middle cone. Cone A is the base of the T, cone B is the middle cone at the top of the T, cone C is the cone on the left end of the top of the T, and cone D is the far right cone on the top of the T. The athlete sprints 10 yards from cone A to cone B, then shuffles laterally to the left to cone C, shuffles right 10 yards to cone D, and then shuffles back 5 yards left to cone B. To complete the T-test the athlete runs backwards from cone B through cone A.

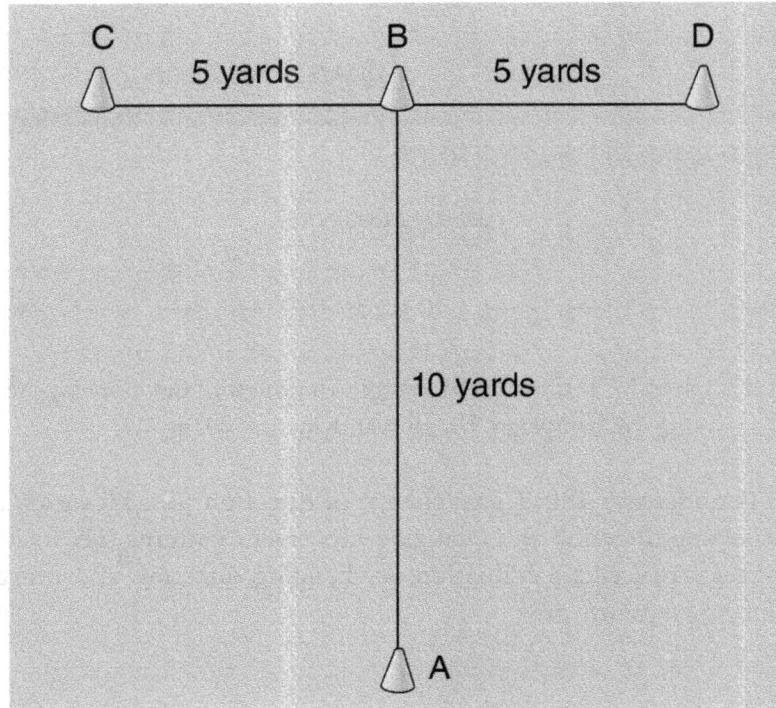

Haff, G. G., and Triplett, N. T. *Essentials of Strength Training and Conditioning-NSCA* (4th ed).
Champaign, IL: Human Kinetics, 2016.

Body Composition

The next area of assessment is body composition. When assessing body composition, the goal is to put the body into two categories: fat mass and fat-free mass. To be able to determine this, the assessment of an athlete's body density is determined. It is typically said that muscle weighs more than fat; the truth is that one kilogram of muscle weighs the same amount as a kilogram of fat. But obviously, you would notice that it takes a lot more value of fat to weigh the same as muscle. Thus the difference is in density. Muscle is a lot more dense than fat, therefore 1 kilogram of muscle takes up less space than 1 kilogram of fat. That would equate to the whole body. The more dense the body is, the higher amount of fat-free mass it contains. To determine the body's density, what is looked at by a coach is how much the body displaces a substance.

Hydrostatic Weighing

Hydrostatic weighing works under the Archimedes' Principle. An explanation of the Archimedes' Principle is beyond the chapter's scope, but it examines the displacement of an object in a fluid. In the case of hydrostatic weighing, that is, the human body in water. Thus, how dense the body is underwater can be determined by the volume of water that is displaced. Anything denser than water will sink like a stone will sink.

Anything less dense than water, like fat, will float in water–since the body is roughly 65% water, that will cancel out when in water.

If a brick is placed in a bucket of water, it does not displace a lot of water. However, if a balloon, which is a lot less dense than water, is placed in a bucket of water, it will float on top. Once that balloon is pushed underwater, it takes up a lot of space, and the water will come out of the bucket, thus having a large displacement of the water. This displacement of water in hydrostatic weighing allows a coach to measure the relative weight. So it is with this assessment the body can be divided into fat mass and fat-free mass.

Hydrostatic weighing is a learned skill for both the practitioner and the athlete. The practitioner needs to be skilled in how to run the assessment and the use of the equipment. The athlete needs to learn how to properly exhale air from the lungs to get an accurate measurement.

Air Displacement Plethysmography (ADP)

There is a different technology that eliminates some of the skills required to obtain a precise measurement. In addition, that technology allows using air displacement to measure volume instead of using water displacement.—ADP.

ADP places a person in a capsule and based on how much they displace the air within the capsule to determine body density.

The two previous assessments of hydrostatic weighing and ADP are clinical tests, and expensive equipment is needed. The purpose of presenting those two tests was to establish the importance of measuring body density. The use of displacement measurements is not the only way to determine the body's density. The following two body composition assessments are more practical ways for a coach to assess an athlete's body density, ultimately giving a coach body composition.

Bioelectrical Impedance Analysis (BIA)

BIA can be accomplished in two ways. It is either a handheld device or a scale. There are also BIA devices that incorporate both handheld and scale. What is typically used in the field is a handheld device. The athlete simply grabs the device and based on a small electrical current being sent through the body, the device will determine how much of that signal is impeded. Based on the amount of impedance, body density will be predicted. For the best results from a BIA, the device should be used after an eight-hour fast. What I typically recommend is once an athlete wakes in the morning to take the measurement.

Skinfolds

Another method of determining body density is through the use of skinfold measurements. Unlike the simplicity of the BIA device, with the skinfold measurement, the practitioner does need to be skilled in using a skinfold caliper. Skinfolds are measured throughout the body. First, the practitioner pinches the skin and adipose tissue away from the muscle tissue. Next, the skinfold calipers measure the width of the fold in millimeters that are made from the skin and adipose tissue. Finally, body density is estimated by adding the total number of measures and using one of the following equations based on the number of skinfolds used, anywhere from two to seven. It does take practice to be proficient actually to measure skinfolds.

Throughout the section, a lot was discussed about body density. In all reality, coaches want to know what an athlete's fat mass is. This is represented by percent body fat (%BF). Once body density is determined, %BF can be predicted. The coach needs to use the correct prediction equations based on several variables: age, sex, ethnicity and training. The equations are listed below.

Flexibility

The last assessment category that will be looked at in this chapter is flexibility. Flexibility is when an athlete moves their joints through a range of motion (ROM). There are several standardized assessments that a coach can utilize to assess an athlete's flexibility.

Sit and Reach

The first standardized assessment is a sit and reach test. The athlete sits on the ground with the legs fully extended. The athlete then places one hand on top of the other so that their middle fingers line up. The athlete will then reach as far as they can while still maintaining their legs fully extended. A sit-and-reach box allows an individual to push against a metal slide that measures the distance an athlete can reach. The toe line of a sit and reach box lines up at 27 cm. If an athlete can push further than their toe, it would be quantified with a number higher than 27 cm. Anything less than 27 cm would represent less than the ability to reach their toes.

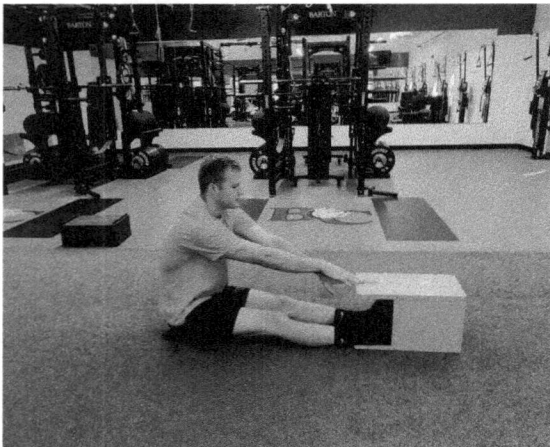

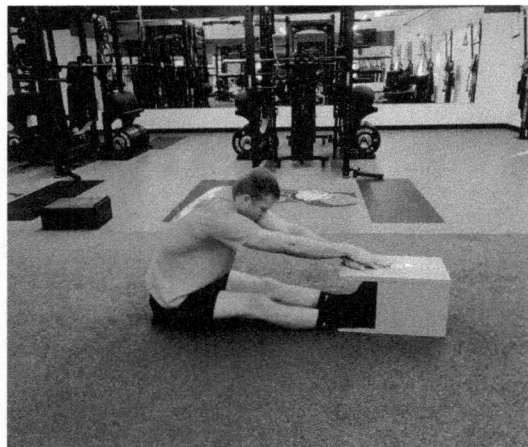

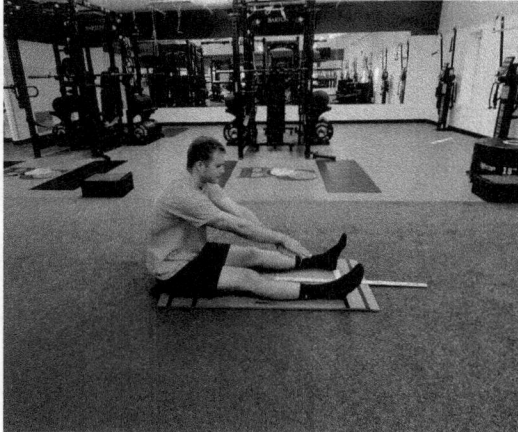

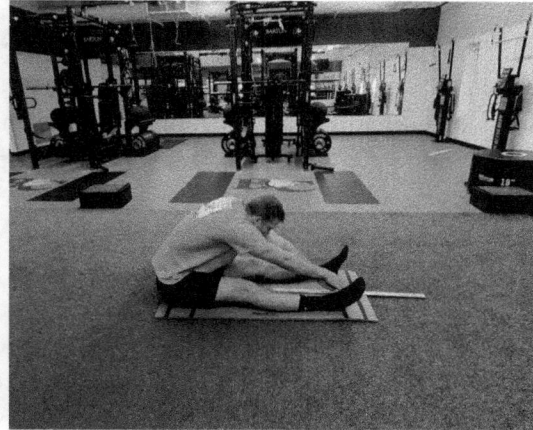

The value obtained by the athlete is compared to the normative data based on age and sex.

The sit and reach test allows a coach to compare the athlete's results to normative data. A coach would perform this assessment without a sit and reach box by placing a ruler on top of a stair and having the athlete put their feet against the base of the stair. The limitation of the sit and reach does not paint the whole picture of the ROM of the human body. It only represents the posturer side of the lower body and lumbar spine.

Goniometry

A coach can measure the ROM of each joint through the use of goniometry. Goniometry is a direct measurement of a joint angle using a goniometer.

What is the ROM of an athlete's elbow? A goniometer is used to look specifically at different joint angles throughout the body. For example, a coach can look at complete extension and flexion of the elbow to determine if the elbow joint would have a normal ROM. Goniometry is best utilized to determine if there are limitations to an individual's ROM. These (limitations) could be due to post-injury or post-surgery as an athlete is preparing themselves to return to play. A coach can use tables that show the ROM of specific joints to determine if the athlete is back to within normal limits (WNL).

A strength and conditioning coach who works strictly in performance-based work may not use much goniometry. Most athletes will have normal ROM, thus, joint angles will not indicate much for a coach.

Functional Movement Screen (FMS)

The FMS is a series of seven tests that are designed for an athlete to move their body through a specific ROM. Not much coaching is needed or wanted through these tests because a coach wants to see how an athlete moves through the particular ROM. A coach then critiques the motion. For example, one of the tests is an overhead squat. An athlete is asked to take a dowel and raise it over their head. Then the athlete will squat down as far as they can. Based on how fluid that motion is and how well it is completed, the test is scored on a scale from 3 to 0. A score of three would indicate the athlete can perform the test flawlessly. If the test can be completed with modification, it is scored as a two. For example, if

the heels are elevated on that overhead squat, the athlete can then perform the test flawlessly. If the test has been modified and the athlete cannot complete the motion, the test is scored as a one. The athlete will receive a zero score if there is pain during the test. Even if the athlete can perform the test flawlessly, but there is pain, it still is zero (0) score. Pain is an indicator that something is wrong and a coach needs to take pain seriously. The pain should be identified and dealt with.

Overall there are seven tests. Each test can be scored with a three at best. That means the best an athlete can score on the FMS is 21. Notes should be scribed on each test that indicated score, pain and asymmetries between left and right sides on some of the tests.

The FMS is a total body movement screening tool. You can see tests on the list that would allow a coach to look at the left and right sides of the body to see asymmetries. The example that was given is the overhead squat. The seven tests of the FMS are the deep squat, hurdle step, in-line lunge, shoulder mobility, active straight-leg raise, trunk stability push-up, and rotary stability.

Putting it All Together

In wrapping this up, let's look at all these assessments together. We are trying as coaches to determine all these different variables of an individual. Aerobic power is the ability for an individual to use oxygen to go to maximal effort. The three tests we looked at were the Pacer/Beep test, Cooper's test and the Queen's step test. Secondly, we want to determine anaerobic power. How much energy can a person produce without oxygen? Three tests were looked at: RAST, Margaria-Kalamen Stair Climb Test and the Sargent Jump Test. We started by looking at power output, both the use of oxygen and without.

Next, the body's ability to produce force was looked at. What was examined was a force through multiple repetitions and force produced for a single repetition. Multiple repetitions or muscular endurance can be assessed through calisthenic movements, for example, push-ups, sit-ups or curl-ups. The force produced by a muscle group for a single repetition is evaluated using a 1RM or measured through a static assessment of a hand dynamometer. In addition, a coach can predict a 1RM through a prediction equation. Once a maximal force is determined for a group of muscles, a coach can look at the value as an absolute number or relative number based on body weight.

To determine an athlete's body fat percentage, you must first determine its density. The body's density is determined through hydrostatic weighing, APD, BIA or skinfolds. Once the density is determined, the athlete's %BF can be estimated using a prediction equation.

Finally, the category of flexibility was discussed. This is the body's ability to go through a ROM. A coach can use a Sit and Reach Test, Goniomery, or the FMS. Each of these has its benefits, and a coach should review the needs of an athlete before a flexibility assessment is used.

Within these areas, numerous other tests can be utilized by coaches. What was presented in this chapter is far from an all-inclusive list. What is shared is some of the assessment tools that a coach can utilize to determine the different assessment categories. There are more tests out there, but for this chapter, what was presented are the tests that can be utilized with little equipment and are not too technical.

NSCA 1RM Testing Protocol

1. Instruct the individual to warm up with a light resistance (i.e., 50% of anticipated 1RM) that easily allows 5-10 repetitions.

2. Provide a 1-min rest period.

3. Estimate a warm-up load that will allow the individual to complete 3-5 repetitions by adding
    a. 10-20 lb or 5-10% for upper body exercise
    b. 30-40 lb or 10-20% for lower-body exercise

4. Provide a 2-min rest period.

5. Estimate a conservative, near-maximum load that will allow the individual to complete 2-3 repetitions by
    a. 10-20 lb or 5-10% for upper body exercise
    b. 30-40 lb or 10-20% for lower-body exercise

6. Provide a 2- to 4-min rest period.

7. Make a load increase
    a. 10-20 lb or 5-10% for upper body exercise
    b. 30-40 lb or 10-20% for lower body exercise

8. Instruct the individual to attempt a 1RM.

9. If the individual was successful, provide a 2- to 4- min rest period, and go back to step 7

If the individual failed, provide a 2- to 4-min rest period, decrease the load by subtracting
- 15-20 lb or 5-10% for lower-body exercise or 5-10 lb or 2.5-5% for upper-body exercise

AND then go back to step 8

Continue increasing or decreasing the load until the individual can complete on repetition with proper exercise technique. *Ideally, the individual's 1RM will be measured within five testing sets.*

Adapted from: Baechle, T. & Earle, R., eds. *Essentials of Strength Training and Conditioning.* Champaign, IL, Human Kinetics. 2000

References: Chapter 19

1. Haff, G. G., and Triplett, N. T. *Essentials of Strength Training and Conditioning-NSCA* (4th ed). Champaign, IL: Human Kinetics, 2016.

2. Topend Sports
    https://www.topendsports.com/testing/tests/index.htm

Note: Additional testing materials (procedures, skin fold equations, and norm charts are available in the appendix)

SECTION 6

AUXILIARY TRAINING METHODS

20
AUXILARY TRAINING METHODS: OVERVIEW OF ECCENTRIC/FLYWHEEL TRAINING

By: Paul Cater
Professional Strength and Conditioning Coach

In a conversation with a colleague, we discussed a common theme: the focus on general preparation exercise in strength progression. In a collective background covering youth, college and professional sports development, we came to consensus that there is a disconnect between the exercises prescribed, the culture built around those exercise outcomes, and performance in competition itself. Auxiliary Training is a broad topic of "what essentially comes first"–this hits at the heart of the greater context of this book: holistic athlete development, across all sports and spectrums of resources. How can we train sustainably and in environments with variable coaching and equipment resources?

This chapter will focus on what is efficient when coaches are operating with potentially less resources, time and/or equipment to gain the greatest transfer of power to the given sport. Efficient transfer has everything to do with the order of exercises selected by the coach for the athlete to perform and determined by the ultimate goal of the program. But how does a coach or athlete determine the needs in a training landscape where traditional linear periodization block models are challenged by continual sports practice and seasonal involvement?

INTRODUCTION

Every time an athlete trains, a decision is made of what exercises to do first, second, third, etc. In the context of a competing athlete, these decisions should be directed by what adaptation is desired for competing at a higher level in their given event or sport. What guides the decisions are the basics of physiology, biomechanics and bioenergetics upholding the immutable principles of fatigue and specific adaptation. While the freedom of exercise prescription and infinite combinations of exercise during a given training session can be the topic of much debate, the spirit of this book is to provide a simplistic view of choosing exercise order of importance based on sports performance outcomes. While not comprehensive in scope of periodization theory or design, this chapter will help you guide your program design and order exercises in variable environments.

The goal of this chapter is to help give definition and context to auxiliary exercise relative to athletic power-based outcomes, with definitions including, but expanded beyond single joint, low intensity exercises primarily seen in hypertrophy, muscle endurance or active recovery phases. It will provide a practical overview of auxiliary training exercises, from the perspective of maximizing power and training proportional deceleration for athletic development.

In assessing auxiliary exercises, we must include basic principles of periodization and ordering of general and specific exercises dependent on individual needs. Strength and subsequent power development for sport, is in essence sought after to transfer to greater sports performance. The mix of primary and auxiliary is highly dependent on what the coach deems is best for optimal transference; therefore this chapter on "auxiliary methods" must be viewed in light of movement towards peak performance in and supporting the primary exercises to allow for that greatest transfer.

Secondary in this chapter is the prioritization of Specific Development Exercises, with a backup of general compound barbell exercises; this secondary importance on the *general strength* exercises enables more of a continual transference of power through longer competitive cycles throughout the entire yearly training cycle. And since many professional, and now youth sport scenarios, demand longer competition phases, the context of this chapter will be viewed in this light of prolonged optimization of peak power production relative to sport.

Two extremes seem to exist based on who is directing the strength and conditioning program:

- On one hand there is the assumption that by gaining a certain level of strength, an athlete can progress to the next stage of sport development.
- Conversely, all an athlete has to do is perform the sport activity with regularity.

This chapter will bring balance to the two, using an auxiliary assignment method and tools relative to its implementation.

Identifying Performance Needs

Within the needs analysis for a given sport, the exercise order is established within each session that is in line with the periodized program outcomes based on an individual's unique foundational level and phase within the competitive cycle; it often ends up boiling down to pushing an individual's power curve and the ability to reproduce peak power over a course of time. Yet, as alluded to, there may be a disconnect between simply becoming more powerful and performing on the field or track or court.

It is widely accepted that there are standards for relative strength and correlating performance levels. Associated standards for optimal transference for track and field events were established in Bondarchuk's seminal "Transfer of Training in Sport." The NSCA establishes exercise strength standards relative to male and female Division 1 sports. For example, a female softball pitcher should be power cleaning 122 pounds, squatting 184 pounds and bench pressing 117 pounds. (Fundamentals of Strength and Conditioning, 3rd Edition)

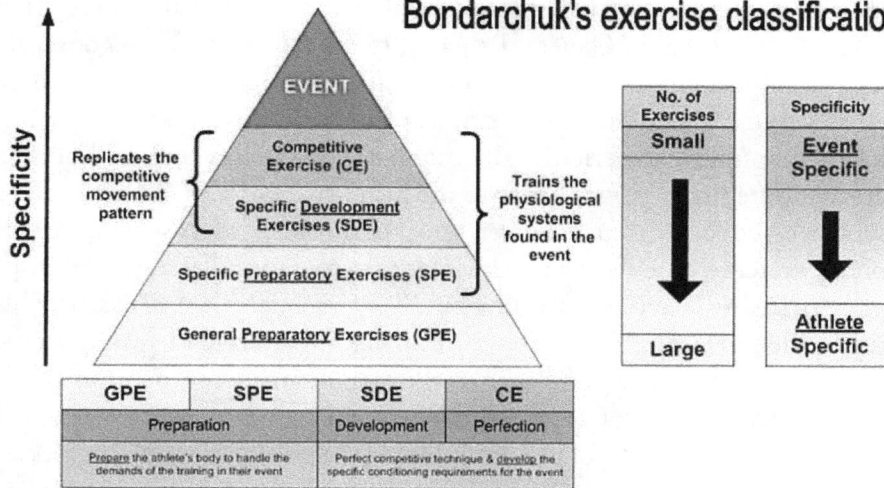

Bondarchuk's exercise classifications

These established standards can help determine the primary exercise in the given program, but how they are blended chasing greater power for greater transference has to take into account multiple variables, the biggest of which is the amount of competitive exercise that is already being performed on a daily basis. Sports like baseball, whereby the competitive cycle is long and frequency of competition high, obtaining neural adaptation (and therefore maintenance in-season) the mix of primary and auxiliary exercise will be dependent on the type of resistance a coach and athlete has at their disposal, but most importantly the volume of competitive exercise an athlete is already accomplishing during the day. For example, if a baseball player is already taking 200 max effort swings in a day, what patterns and intensities should a coach prescribe?

Velocity Based Training metrics, force plates, motion capture and other advanced analysis can help to determine the order the power stroke training and accessory exercise needs to be implemented, a trained coach's eye can often determine at which point form breakdown correlates to acceleration and top speed inefficiency. These form deficiencies can be backed up by higher tech help noting velocity and postural variations. Generally speaking, auxiliary exercise models address the deficiencies of phases of power development of any given primary exercise.

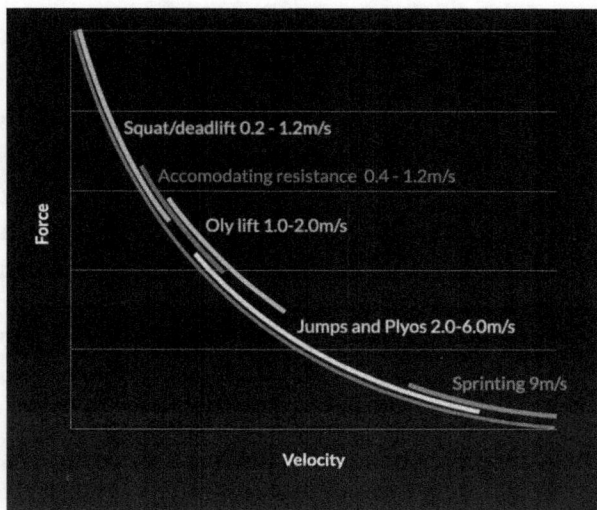

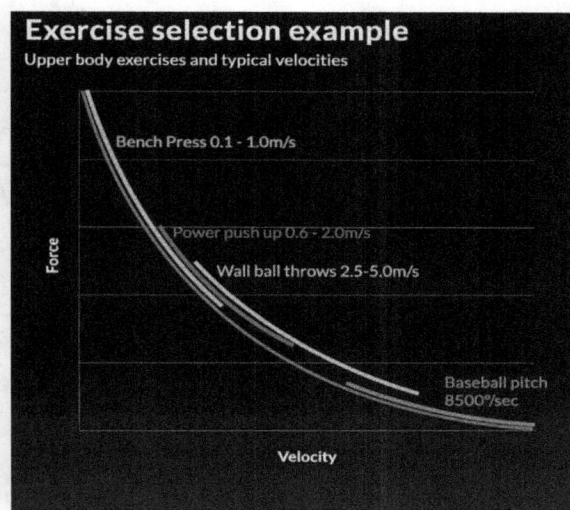

Exercise selection example
Upper body exercises and typical velocities

Because power exercises require the highest level of skill, concentration and energy (Fleck & Kramer, 1997). And if auxiliary exercises fall in General Preparatory Exercise (GPE) categories, then all types of strength exercises can be implemented to support Specific Preparatory Exercises (SPE's), including compound multi-joint barbell strength exercises that can be secondary in nature.

Different philosophies on how to periodize the core barbell exercises are based on specificity or volume/intensity to create desired adaptation; however the primary exercise is chosen in the programming, the velocity of moving a given load through a given range of motion and its specific classification should determine selection of exercises to complement primary or core exercises for a given program block. **What phase of concentric displacement does the auxiliary exercise need to assist?** This can be determined by deficiency in the different phases of power moving the given mass through time and space.

Programming and periodization for exercises to ultimately affect competition outcomes is a very complex and highly individual endeavor based on how certain foundations have already been achieved over the course of the athletes training lifetime or buildup to what Bondarchuk defines as sports "form" blocks leading into peak competition. Transition to peak form is an interdependent relationship between exercises that maintain a base of strength and power while engaging relative levels of specificity. Linear models that separate each General or Specific Exercise usually don't account for the variables of training and competition; while good in theory, they are insufficient in accounting for intra-correlatory factors of each exercise in progressing an athlete towards a desired sports form and competitive peak.

Therefore, it is important to account for where an athlete has already mastered a general or specific outcome and blend exercise programming with the highest level of desired transference; this unique blend–determined by supported testing and correlation to sport performance–will ultimately determine the primary and auxiliary exercises of a program. While it is beyond the scope of this chapter to standardize what correlations exercise, once mastered, will have on competition, or determine the election of specific training or chronological age related needs determining percentage of general, specific or competitive exercise within a program matrix, we can examine the complimentary exercises that support primary exercises selected.

DETERMINING PRIMARY SUPPORT EXERCISE

Form and Function

Traditional strength and conditioning texts have defined *auxiliary* (or *assistance*) exercises as single joint exercises that train smaller or isolated muscle areas. (Fleck and Kramer, 1997) Relative to this chapter, the definition could be broadened to not only those exercises assisting the primary compound exercises, for aesthetic or conditioning purpose, but the main barbell exercises to obtain overall power outcomes through training synergist muscle groupings and/or helping in deficient points in the compound exercises force-velocity curves. While the power exercises such as the snatch, power clean, hang clean and jerk, squat, deadlift and bench press are viewed as *primary*, what is programmed later in the given session to support that Force-Velocity outcome can be viewed as *auxiliary (NSCA, 2000)*. Auxiliary exercises are particular to what the greatest need is at the time for the sport skill defining their position or event. We can boil it down to four basic needs: starting, acceleration, top speed and deceleration.

Exercise Classification	Exercise	Need	Type of Resistance
CE	Bullpen Practice	Not maintaining load/hip hinge in windup of delivery	No load
SPE	Single Leg Squat Squat	Cueing more glute involvement in pattern particular to windup	Free Weight
GE: **Primary Support** **Auxiliary A**	Clean	General Loading Sequence	Barbell
Secondary Support **Auxiliary B**	Deadlift	Maintaining Load in hip in first pull	Flywheel
Tertiary Support **Auxiliary C**	Glute Ham Bridge	Supporting posture in first pull	Body Weight

The ability to safely increase functional intensity and magnitude of force in functional movement patterns may support the prioritization of more specific exercises in programming, as seen in program modeling that places higher priority on specific exercises in building base foundations. While beyond the scope of this chapter, the *Generalist* versus *Specialist* periodization model debate (well framed by Anatyliy Bondarchuk in terms of what to prioritize in program design for greater transference of power in sport) provides the backdrop from which to understand how to both classify and determine what is auxiliary. Energy, effort and prioritizing general power exercises, such as the power clean, may not be as efficient or effective as exercises in functional vectors with similar power ability, but more optimally placed as a secondary, and within this context, an auxiliary exercise or support exercise.

Relative to the *General* versus *Specialized Preparation and Development* and ultimately *Competitive Exercise* ordering, there are innovative technologies which have helped to evolve the definition of auxiliary exercise by safely increasing force and rate of force development in functional vectors; what is programmed as *primary* and subsequently *auxiliary* can be influenced by the *type of resistance* utilized in the exercise in achieving the desired training outcome, as higher neural adaptation can be achieved with greater loading paradigms. Higher force, rate of force development and innervation displacement both in concentric and eccentric phases can be produced in pathways once only in the realm of bi-lateral, axial and Olympic style free-weight training, potentially moving exercises up in the order of exercise selection and specific programming importance.

Moreover, those general compound exercises can be performed with alternative modes of resistance utilizing pneumatic, magnetic, motorized and rotary inertia flywheel, utilizing cables and straps, helping to re-frame how primary exercises can be delivered and ultimately programmed. Whatever general or specific priority is chosen, the mode of exercise once viewed as auxiliary (utilizing cables and straps) in conjunction with Special Preparation Exercise can change program prioritization. What is auxiliary particular to power development, may not necessarily be single-joint, isolated muscle group exercises that are limited by intensity and magnitude of force. These exercises may best compliment the desired power outcomes and sport transference philosophies based on the primary exercise or series within a program.

Yet before we discuss the expanding types of auxiliary exercises, we need to establish what they are in fact supporting. Though it has been presented that barbell exercise can in fact be a secondary and supportive in order of importance during a session, for the sake of this chapter we will look at the Olympic

Weightlifting as a correlatory competitive sport, and therefore what exercises can help with deficiency or higher performance. In a purely traditional sense, or in renditions of weightlifting competitions, as seen in CrossFit, Olympic Weightlifting exercises are the sport themselves and will make the discussion of what to program in support; fortunately, the potential deficiencies observed in an Olympic barbell exercise are metaphorical to much of sport in terms of initial drive, acceleration and top speed and bracing situations.

While exercises comprising *single joint* movement and *lesser intensity* in the training program are typically deemed auxiliary, for the specific topic of this book, the definition may include what those exercises implemented to augment, or even take the place of the core compound exercises relative to optimizing power for sport. If more corrective needs are taken care of with more compound exercise with greater intensity potential, less traditional auxiliary exercises need to be programmed. This is significant in terms of saving time and energy to maintain a balance of strength, elasticity and ultimately pushing the peak power curve in and out of season.

The expansion of the definition of auxiliary assistance exercise works well within the framework of athletic development models, putting a premium on specific exercise closely mimicking the competitive sport scenarios. Configuring programs in the classical sense of *power, core,* then auxiliary or *assistance* based on volume and intensity to move adaptation becomes based on fatigue paradigms, rather than movement specificity during phases of the training cycle. That is, what exercises are selected as *primary* or *core* should be determined by desired performance outcomes rather than bettering that specific exercise. Based on Bondarchuk's exercise classification chart (on page 373), it could be inferred that any exercise coming after the more specific classification could be deemed as accessory in nature. And what could be traditionally deemed as auxiliary, if done with adequate intensity to mimic competition, could in fact be classified as primary in importance and order of programming.

Auxiliary Exercise Modes

Once a program's primary exercises are set, a coach can determine how to best support those primary exercises based on determined deficiencies and needs analysis of the athlete in general. *Many times the limited factor is based on leverage inefficiency, not necessarily creating more strength. Strength should be viewed through the lens of maintaining leverage and optimal mechanical advantage at higher velocity.* If we view exercise selection—both primary and its auxiliary support—as a leverage issue, then we can address issues of time and energy to reserve for training the actual sport event and its given energy systems, strength training will remain in proper context rather than a means to its own end.

Ultimately the metrics of the sport itself can help determine the training pathway in real time. In the case of baseball, swing and throwing form and velocity deviations from an established previous baseline or "optimal" can help in determining what is prioritized in exercise prescription. This can also be triangulated with loss of previous relative strength or range of motion measurements. Yet in this very complex assessment; it could be generally stated that in-season athletes practicing their competitive exercise hundreds of times a day do not add more of the same exercise as priority in specific preparation or development. General adaptation and detraining principles can underpin the necessity for more priority on general preparation as needed in the primary supportive role. And whereby time and energy are factors in implementing this programming, the higher force developing compound exercises take priority. Yet, still they can be viewed as auxiliary because they support the primary competitive exercises. Furthermore, if the exercise is comprehensive in magnitude, rate of force development and in complete range of motion, finishing auxiliary exercises for the smaller stabilizer are not as necessary.

So, if in-season auxiliary exercises become the traditional primary compound exercises, which exercises do we select? A coach must prescribe the mode of compound which addresses deficiency in the competitive exercise itself. Once the limiting factor of an exercise or performance outcome is determined, auxiliary exercises can be programmed in addition to primary exercise. Often these supportive exercises can be trained on separate phases and days of the week, as well later in individual sessions.

Three different phases can be dictated by the gravity-dependent physical properties outlined by Isaac Newton hundreds of years ago and as the basis of modern-day physics. The three modes or phases of moving weight are first and foremost in resistance training–the application of force greater to that mass is exerted in its innate, unmoving state. Secondarily, is the acceleration of that mass through propulsive measures until momentum and ultimately maximum velocity or top speed is achieved. Thirdly, is the capacity to slow down that velocity. While the second and third modes have a particular relationship to propulsion of mass through longer ranges of displacement (where momentum may be both the goal and limiting factor of exercise) and proportional contending with that very momentum, the first phase of moving weight can be the easiest to demonstrate with auxiliary barbell exercises.

The power clean could be an example of an auxiliary support exercise to address the specific need of an athlete to develop a higher rate of force development during an in-season program. Yet the prescription of this primary support exercise are components of the exercise to achieve better form. Usually the needs of these exercises (the regressions and progressions) mirror the needs of the competitive exercise betterment. It is through this lens we assign what is *auxiliary*, using it as a tool rather than a means to itself. We are merely trying to gain greater context of what is supportive in nature to better sports performance and become more adept at efficient programming, especially in-season. Working with other sport coaches, athletic training, physical therapists, sport scientists and other practitioners developing the athlete can help to assess what we can call *leverage deficiency*, and ultimately what is needed.

For this chapter, we will use the power clean as an accepted tool to increase the rate of force development needs, and as alluded to previously, this exercise can reveal the deficiency itself, determining regressions reasonably applied within the time, energy and logistical constraints of the training scenario.

To determine the assistance needed to support progress in the power clean, we can break down the exercise into three parts and relative exercises to address deficiency in those parts. Though beyond the scope of this chapter is to go into depth of this exercise, we can use basic analysis principles for this exercise to guide the auxiliary assignment.

Starting/Drive Phase - Overcoming inertia, 'Sticking Points'

Force is needed to overcome gravity and the inertial load. In sprinting, it is the human body and gravity that is not in motion. In weightlifting, particularly in the first pull of a clean, a greater force is needed to overcome the weight of the barbell and gravity. One could look at increasing the propulsive phase of the power clean with another exercise: the deadlift. By increasing an athlete's deadlift 1 rep max, more weight can be moved faster potentially up through the phases of acceleration and maximal barbell velocity. Therefore, the deadlift or clean pull is an auxiliary accessory to the Olympic power clean.

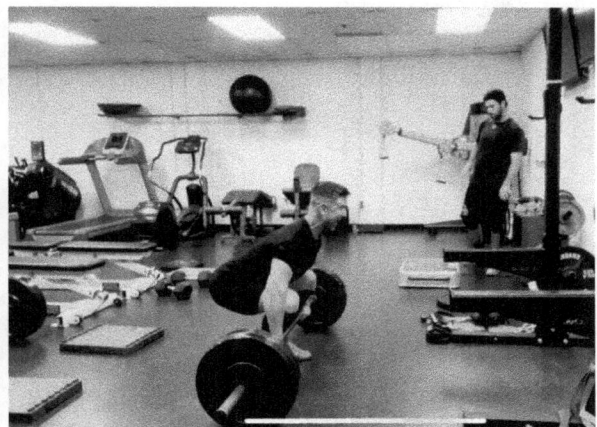

As further auxiliary exercises can help the deadlift, we look at types of exercises and resistance that can supplement. Simply adding more weight could very well be classified as auxiliary force adaptation for the first pull of the power clean to augment the power clean. If you don't have force plates and velocity measurement relative to displacement, simple observation in speed and technique can highlight what portion of the compound movement to assist and augment.

While these phases and associated exercises are specific to the power clean, they can represent a greater representation of auxiliary exercises for sprinting or any endeavor to more efficiently create momentum, just as sprinting 100 meters can also be looked at in terms of these stages and what exercises (other than the practice of sprinting) can support higher levels of performance. In the case of the power clean, if the athlete is pulling too slow from the floor, and/or not able to maintain position during the first pull, affecting loading sequence up the chain of events, more practice at variable loads and velocity or positions need to be implemented.

Transition Phase : Acceleration Phases, "Creating Momentum"

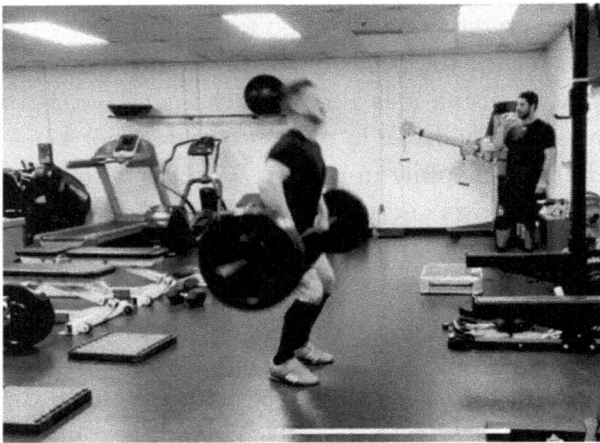

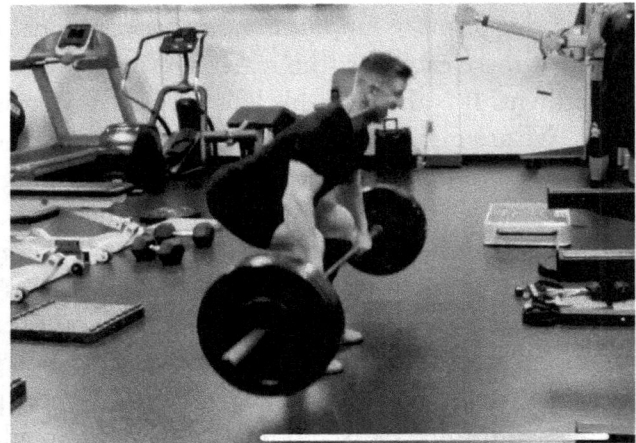

Need: Quickly producing force in the right direction.
Target: Acceleration in Second Pull
Example: RDL to Hang Clean

Peak Velocity: Mechanics of Maintaining Velocity, Maintaining Momentum and Position

The first exercise that comes to mind is the high pull exercise. Using a relatively lighter weight than power clean 1RM, the athlete practices the third pull phase of the lift in effort to train bar path and contraction through longer displacement. This will have an effect when performing the Olympic power clean of pulling longer before receiving, or catching the barbell. Prescribing this exercise may be an effort to address mechanical issues the coach or athlete has identified.

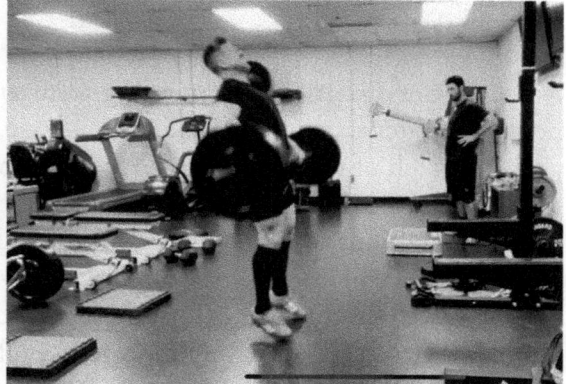

Need: Velocity
Target: Second Pull Velocity and Trajectory
Auxiliary Prescription: Upright rows, High Pulls

Deceleration: The capacity to handle proportional deceleration force

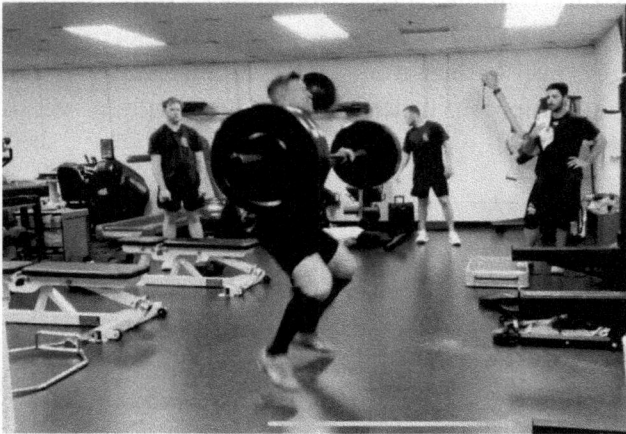

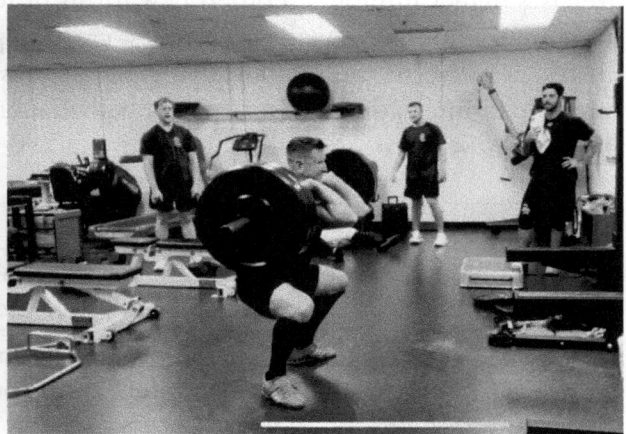

Auxiliary exercise augmenting eccentric phases and therefore deceleration ability, may be of **equal importance** to achieve and maintain optimal performance in sport, as many sport-specific demands and associated injury risk factors are particular to the proportional deceleration of force that is produced. If equal force and rate of force development is not programmed for, programming is not complete and may increase the potential for injury. Addressing both the difficulty and potential solutions through auxiliary eccentric at variable velocities and overloading paradigms is essential for mimicking sport-like movements. Aside from sport specificity to better change direction and achieve higher movement velocities, eccentric training has great adaptation advantages.

DETERMINING SECONDARY SUPPORT METHODS:

Form and Velocity

Much of the discussion surrounding form and mechanics in achieving and maintaining top speed is postural awareness and mechanical advantage. We can see this in later stages of the 100m dash and final pull and catch of the power clean. The training for these outcomes are accommodative resistance methods whereby greater innervation and subsequent adaptation of muscle to stabilize and hold form outside of normal bounds of momentum and inertial shift. In other words, an athlete is able to train through longer displacement at velocities (and relative loads) not limited by normal gravitational limitations. The ability to do this allows for training effect to allow for the athlete to achieve mechanical form and advantage necessary to maintain posture, pull and continued mechanical advantage during the specific or competitive exercise.

Particular to achieving the continued mechanical advantage and leverage at high rates of movement velocity, is implementing methods of accommodating resistance. Innovation in this area has allowed for more training stimulus and adaptation in longer lines of pull to practice leverage and postural capacity at places 'before' and 'after' traditional sticking points, and in different force vectors particular to sport.

Depending on variables pertaining to athlete training age, phase of program periodization, available equipment, specific needs and injury history, certain programs can prioritize auxiliary or assistance exercises higher in program order; new forms of resistance training can provide higher load-velocity in what are traditionally auxiliary exercises, creating priority for those exercises especially in sport-specific phases. Relative to these innovative types of resistance, non-barbell modes of resistance training can mimic load-intensities and velocities of barbell exercises; equipment usually relegated to 'auxiliary' status only, can now mimic the barbell in compound exercises.

Primary Support Mode				
Mode	Force Development	Rate of Force Development	Peak Velocity	Deceleration
Primary Support & Competitive Lift Exercises	Core Compound: Squat Deadlift Bench	Dynamic Compound: Clean & Jerk Snatch Throws	Ballistic Resistance: Jumps Throws	Reciprocal: Landing/Receiving Flywheel Motorized
Associated Velocities	0.18-1.2m/s	1.0-2.0 m/s m/s	>2.0 m/s	Proportional to concentric velocity
Movement Signature	Push First Pull	Hinge Second Pull	Postural Third Pull	Timing
Muscle Grouping	Anterior	Posterior lat/glute pennate muscle	shoulder/spine stabilizer biceps	

Application of innovative types of resistance, which can not only accessorize beyond exercise classification (multi-joint, compound, isolated), but in some cases supplant the compound exercises traditionally trained with barbell resistance training, will be included in this chapter as auxiliary, even though they may be able to stand on their own. Innovative technology in administering force and velocity through greater ranges of motion not limited by traditional sticking points and momentum shifts, may not be available or realistic for many in program design, they can highlight the limitations—and solutions—for programming with primary barbell, giving context for auxiliary or accessory exercises in general.

Contending with Momentum

Effective strength and conditioning programming requires logical sequences of exercises during a given training session. While there are seemingly unlimited combinations of exercise groupings based on the multiple variables for each individual athlete, as well as varying philosophies and bias of preferred exercises to increase an athlete's power profile, uniformity exists ordering primary, secondary and tertiary exercises in a session: *multi-joint, high force movements requiring greater coordination and focus are of primary importance* while exercises augmenting or complimenting the those movements are secondary. This effort to move heavier loads at greater rates of velocity in certain vectors to create momentum; ironically, achieving this goal necessitates programming auxiliary lifts to manage these momentum shifts, or lack thereof in concentric only training.

While developing the prime movers through compound exercises higher in relative power production should be prioritized to meet the desired performance outcomes, auxiliary exercises are important in reinforcing the movement pattern, training synergists within the compound exercise and address potential 'inertial gaps' particularly in the acceleration and maximum velocity phases of the resistance exercise. With inertia being a tendency of an object to stay at rest or continue in its state of movement, during sport the body is challenged to overcome inertia as one stops, starts, accelerates, decelerates, jumps and changes direction. To perform optimally, the body has to be trained under all these varying conditions.

Accommodative Resistance Types

Accommodative Resistance methods utilizing chains are within the same scope of cam configurations in isolated machine weights. Methods of negating momentum shifts, and providing more stimulus at various desired points through displacement can play a lead role in power development. While accommodative resistance techniques using bands, chains or pneumatics are valid in achieving higher maximum voluntary contraction and rate of force development in larger ranges, they are devoid of coupled eccentric overloading paradigms important in developing the ability to decelerate. Improportional deceleration capacity may lead to subsisting rates of injury within athlete populations even as training methods and venues continue to advance. Gravity-independent auxiliary training methods are enabling maximum voluntary contraction through greater concentric displacement through the principles of accommodative resistance.

The ability to innervate more muscle fibers at higher rates and duration of force development through range is important. When limited to an inertial mass equal to "sticking point," more speed and different leveraging strategies must be taken to lift the appropriate weight. For example, to aid in this in the power clean, accessory exercises pulling dumbbells, working back extensions, and using chains for developing more power through the first pull of the exercise can be used. Placing more tension at various points of extension where usually momentum takes over (at the top end range), or where there is typically less engagement of the muscle and lower rates of force development, can be beneficial is developing greater power through concentric phases of muscle action.

Adding additional loading stimuli like rubber bands and chains account for momentum shift and sticking points to add resistance through greater range of motion; rubber bands allow for more resistance at the top end of the range of a squat for example, where the inertial load gains momentum and becomes easier as the natural levers gain more advantage. Other apparatus like chains, allow for more load at the bottom of the range of the exercise by proportionally loading as the lifter ascends out of the bottom of the squat.

Advances in accommodation methods using pneumatic, hydraulic and motorized resistance has allowed for greater variable control of consistent resistance through range of motion while negating momentum shift. The "sticking point" can be consistent throughout the entire range and at higher movement velocity. This is significant in both physiological adaptation and logistical set ups. While these types of resistance demand elaborate set ups of air compressors, motors and external power sources, they can determine the extent to which gravitational inertia (e.g.; barbells and medballs) need to be thrown, dropped or constrained with additional apparatus like bands or chains, to gain more strength and ultimately power through range of motion. The ability to efficiently apply external load through functional ranges is important for specific power development and ultimately efficient programming for sport.

Isoinertial Training

Because there is no free-flight of momentum in isoinertial resistance, voluntary contraction can occur through longer ranges of displacement. *Isoinertial* resistance, whereby the resistance stays constant through space, may prove to be an important tool to not only increase concentric power through extension, but proportional deceleration. Safer training practices to induce eccentric overload may be superseded by safer performance as proportional braking capacity is developed within the athlete's strength and power skill sets.

Yet, more accurately matching strength curves and the dynamic collection of forces to move an object (or your own body) is Fluid Resistance. A classic example is the hydrostatic pressure in water. Air resistance is a factor in biking as a steady force to overcome along with gravity and weight of the object. While an athlete's ability to extend powerfully in the concentric phase of movement is key, the ability to decelerate with high rates of force and velocity in the eccentric phase of movement is equally important to athletic performance. Eccentric training can be specifically programmed and augmented in the entire spectrum of athletic development, especially for specific rehab, injury prevention or overloading principles.

Advances in novel resistance training technologies have enabled coaches and athletes to circumnavigate logistical and injury risk factors typically associated with high rates of momentum shift and supramaximal overloading schemes in the attempt to obtain *eccentric overload*. Isoinertial Flywheel and Mechanized resistance devices are proving efficient in achieving eccentric loading stimuli without unnecessary chronic or accumulative stresses in the joint and tendon.

Attempts to gain higher force capacity in ranges not traditionally trained due to the momentum of inertia load once overcome and the typically inadequate load in coupled eccentric phase to gain sufficient deceleration adaptations are key. To produce greater power through greater range in extension, variable and accommodative loading schemes may be utilized. For example, using chains or bands during a back squat may increase the neural activation due to augmenting load at bottom or top ends of the range of motion. Relative to sprinting, towing or pushing sleds enhance the ability to load through functional ranges.

Because while these foundational movement patterns and exercises can be the basis of any program, methods addressing limitations in safety, logistics and efficiency–as well as the inherent gravitational inertia shift seen in momentum and disproportionate eccentric loading paradigms– observe with gravity-dependent "free-weight" are becoming more mainstream in the quest for greater power and function.

Flywheel Variations

In Flywheel devices, the concentric force output is matched with immediate and proportional eccentric force as the released energy is immediately recaptured around the cone or cylinder. This coupling of contraction phases can potentially mimic the loading and velocity of sport more efficiently than eccentric overloads working on the opposite ends of the force-velocity curve and often absent of specific movement patterns and proportional concentric force development parameters.

A main benefit derived from flywheel resistance, is the proportional nature of coupled concentric-eccentric force production. The magnitude to which eccentric overload is gained, and at which point in the eccentric phase depends on the directive the coach gives the athlete to redirect the rotary inertia.

The many benefits of eccentric training are employed in rehab and performance training. The *mode* of eccentric training varies on the specific needs and resources of the athlete-coach partnership. Some xamples of eccentric modes are augmented body-weight plyometrics, motorized resistance, and eccentric hooks for the squat and bench. In resistance training programming, *overload* can simply refer to intensity prescription greater than what the athlete is accustomed to. The overload principle can refer to manipulating exercises, rest periods and increasing assigned loads. (Haff & Triplett, 2016)

While *eccentric overload* is important for muscle health and performance, it comes with inherent logistical and injury risk factors. To achieve overload during the eccentric phase of the back squat for example, there must be a proportional higher load during the downward eccentric phase than what can be performed in the upward concentric phase at the "sticking point"–or point of least mechanical advantage. Therefore, loads have to be augmented during the downward phase which can be labor-intensive or logistically complex. Supramaximal loading in the eccentric phase has to be performed at slower velocities and becomes less specific to the higher rates of force production observed in sport.

To train high rates of eccentric force development, progressively loaded plyometrics can be prescribed, yet can be associated with higher injury risks. While the strength and conditioning practitioner has to be comfortable and competent with prescribing progressive overload, avoiding injury during training is paramount. The height of depth jumps, for example, can be increased, but it is often a guessing game at which point either tendon or joint may become overloaded, and injury occurs.

Instances of eccentric overload during overloaded barbell movements, in conjunction with progressive plyometrics, can work at opposite ends of the force-velocity curve, yet are associated with inherent injury risks, but also may not be as efficient in developing proportional eccentric force development relative to concentric force ability. These capacities, often trained separately, may become dissociated with performance that demands coupled concentric-eccentric phases at various points along the force-velocity curve and for variable durations.

Metabolic Considerations in Auxiliary Programming

Auxiliary exercise is often prescribed to enhance metabolic work capacity at the end of a training session. When integrating fatigue resistance protocols, it may be advantageous to utilize differing forms of accommodative resistance to safely contend with momentum shifts and deceleration. Performing complex movement patterns under fatigue with gravity biased inertia (such as free weights) demands a very high level of skill, strength base and ultimately training age. Furthermore, repeated weightlifting exercises like the power clean demand a training environment and equipment to drop weight consistently. The necessity to drop, throw or perform isometric holds in fatigue protocols can be specific in nature, but often lack the ability to incorporate deceleration patterns. This lack of eccentric phase of exercise is not specific to sport and injury prevention due to demands of sport and where injury often occurs.

Incorporating accommodative resistance types can lead to more efficient programming because of the incorporated deceleration phases of the exercises. Time under tension, greater muscle activation and the relative hormonal responses to eccentric overload make it optimal to incorporate into fatigue resistance, auxiliary programmed "finishers." A study comparing the barbell and flywheel high-pull exercise demonstrated higher blood lactate production when using the Versapulley rotary inertia device. (Nunez et al., 2017) The ability to produce similar concentric and eccentric force paradigms for longer because of less mechanical demand is significant when considering metabolic training protocols for auxiliary exercises specific to transfer to sport.

Corrective Considerations in Auxiliary Programming

Also relative to efficient auxiliary programming for sports transfer needs are the single-joint exercises focusing on one muscle/muscle grouping and its function for maintaining posture, alignment and synergy in the compound general, specific and ultimately competitive exercises. Eccentric overload can be beneficial for producing a strength and hypertrophic effect through incorporating high rates of eccentric overload specific to sport demands. Increased functional lean muscle mass that can be used both for greater acceleration and brake force should be the outcome of programmed auxiliary exercises that are acutely and chronically corrective in nature for greater power outcomes. Accommodative resistance whereby proportional eccentric overload can be incorporated with each rep can reduce training time, the number of necessary auxiliary exercises and provide functional benefit of increased deceleration capacity at variable velocities.

Efficient Exercise Prescription: Function of time and energy

For athletes contending with longer competitive cycles and/or needing to maintain higher performance levels over time, adjusting primarily the order of exercise, rather than load intensities of the same exercises–as seen in Bondarchuk's periodization methodology–may prove effective in sustained high-performance levels and efficiently guide auxiliary support exercise assignment. Adjusting exercise selection to drive adaptation can potentially limit the need for high numbers of single joint exercises observed more in traditional hypertrophy preparatory phases, and assistance exercise "finishers" to account for lack of adaptation from the primary exercise pallet.

For example, a professional baseball player contends with a 7-month competitive cycle. During the season, his program prioritizes exercises particular to his throwing motion. This may be sufficient to maintain performance until his relative lower body strength diminishes to a point where his specific strength exercises are not sufficient to maintain form, and general lower body strength exercises need to be prioritized. This may demand that the primary exercise of order is general in movement like the back squat, because of their mastery of specific movement patterns, and, as alluded to previously, the relative light loading paradigms of the specific exercises mimicking the throwing or hitting motion. Yet, if there is an adequate strength base, more SPE's will take precedence during the season, especially if those exercises can be adequately and safely loaded.

But as specific development or competitive exercise modes are increasingly over or unloaded, these specific preparation exercises can also be looked at as supportive in nature to what is more specific and translational to sport performance. *Many times, auxiliary exercise is relegated as time fillers, metabolic finishers or means for hypertrophy aesthetics.*

Because strength training is captured in the sport of Olympic Weightlifting competition itself, we must seek to constantly provide the right amount of strength in the context of tension balance. Some exercises compress, while others expand; while limb length, relative strength, speed and a multitude of other variables both genetically determined and trained determine success, sport performance is about maintaining and progressing elastic harmony and tension balance.

Manipulation of load, leverage, mechanical, vector, velocity and range to invoke greater length-tension relationship through greater displacement, contend with the limiting factors posed by gravitational inertia in the aid of greater power. These principles of auxiliary exercise are in fact demonstrated within the microcosm of Olympic Weightlifting as multiple pull points; torso angles and muscle groups lift the weight off of the ground. As the backdrop and "purpose statement" of what can be defined as "auxiliary," the question of inertia must be addressed.

Whether adhering to traditional barbell-based resistance training or endeavoring to progressively load in vectors more specific to sport, similar issues persist in gaining strength and speed in those vectors. Newton's first and second laws of motion pertain to force applied to accelerate mass: "the inertial resistance is equal to the accelerative force applied to the object from the opposite direction. Overcoming the inertial and gravitational force demands muscle to produce force above the load. Once the initial force is applied to the object, the amount of force applied does not have to be as great through the range or through multiple repetitions."

EXAMPLE:

Auxiliary exercises are corrective in nature and work primarily towards supporting technical efficiency for mechanical advantage. Ultimately better leverage is what drives selection; the ability to do more or longer resides in the primary strength move and in practice conditioning. If needs of training are indicated by form breakdown at any stage of power, and backed up by available analytics, then appropriate exercise selection for phase or individual workout can be programmed.

A baseball pitcher is struggling to maintain balance through the loading of his drive leg during wind up. This is affecting efficient storage of potential energy and timing of mechanics. The tempo of his sequence is rushed, affecting a multitude of issues pertaining to velocity, pitch location and health. In the weight room, his power testing is in the higher percentile. While box jumps are prescribed in conjunction with trap bar deadlift, there is a lack of hinge sequencing at lower depths and longer sequence of load displacement. While the pitcher has a history of hang clean and is able to front rack a bar into a front squat, it is not prescribed due to potential risk of injury.

Without getting into the intricacies of intensity, volume and recovery, and simply looking at exercise selection order, below is an example of the order of the day, week and ultimately the month phase itself in terms of desired form adaptation for the specific problem. In this example, the days have different General or Specific biases in the effort to expand and compress in an effort to retain tension balance through the week. Various types of resistance have been added to train the desired sequence issue.

IN SEASON BASEBALL PITCHER						
	Day 1: General A	Day 2: Specific Development	Day 3: General B	Day 4: Specific Preparation	Day 5: Specific Development	Day 6: Competition Exercise
SPE Primary Need	Single Leg Squat	**Alternate Skater Drive** -Cylinder Flywheel (Kbox)	**Banded Skaters (Elastic)**	**Standing Hip Rotations** -Conical Flywhele (Versapulley)	**Unloaded Skater Jumps**	
COMPETITION	Bullpen	**Catch**	**Bullpen**	**Throw**	**Throw**	**PITCH**
GPE (A) Primary Support (Auxiliary A)	Power Clean	**Back Squat**	**FFE Split Squat (Iso Inertial Flywheel)**	**Cable Press**	**MB Ballistic Throw**	
GPE (B) Secondary Support Strength (Auxiliary B)	RDL	**DB Bench Press**	**SL RDL**			
C) **Correctives, Astethics, Muscular Endurance**	Glute Ham Raise					

As previously mentioned, accommodative resistance methods, such as iso inertial flywheel, provides higher loading paradigms in functional vectors and acts as an intermediary between the *compressive* Competitive Exercise and *expansive* General Exercise spectrum. The idea of GPEs being corrective in nature fits into the theory that exercises limited by velocity and sticking points due to gravitational interia constraints actually have greater end range capacity and even under heavier inertial loads can act ironically as decompressors.

When discussing auxiliary training, much of the conversation should be around the topic of recruitment patterns, fatigue and ultimately the order of importance in prescribing exercises in a macro or micro cycle. Generally, for coaches and athletes with a potentially young training age—yet specific to power development for athletic development—the order of importance in light of neural fatigue is important to determine. While exercises comprising single joint movement and lesser intensity in the training program are typically deemed auxiliary, for the specific topic of this book, the definition may include what those exercises implemented to augment, or even take the place of the core compound exercises relative to optimizing power for sport.

In my own training and coaching experience over the last 20 years, I have often become enamored with and biased towards what I am good at, what is easily progressed and measured, and what was the norm in my high school and collegiate experience. For example, I excel at back squatting. Much of my priority in programming, and subsequent auxiliary exercises support the outcome of me squatting more. Yet, I have to reflect and analyze what is best for the player to perform on the field. In the great mix of variables that goes into the pathway for individual programming like training age, injury history, position, time of the year, travel schedule, etc., there is the basic question of what is first and what is second in order. On a given day I may have 15 minutes with a player, and I get two to three exercises with them as they go from skills practice to the game. That exercise may be the back squat, but may be something more specific and farther away from general strength. It is in this light of training, often in season or in conjunction with sports practice, and of course, with the proportional amount of time practicing strength that did not in fact lead to better performance on the field or court.

If for healthy populations the compound exercises, ultimately the Olympic lifts (or their equivalent derivatives), can be done to support specific and competitive power development there, does not need to be an extensive prescription of traditional auxiliary exercise to fill time, scratch a training feeling or satisfy a coach or athlete's ego. Injured populations or those trying to achieve aesthetic looks will ultimately have different needs than that of an athlete achieving greater power transference for their particular sport.

While traditional strength and conditioning programming demands multi-joint exercises working larger muscle groups via barbell exercises progressively overloaded based on the percentage of 1RM, this can vary depending on how specific the exercise is in preparation or development in enabling the competitive exercise itself. The barbell exercises can be scaled up or down depending on variable skill, equipment, or injury limitations, and attempt to represent the natural human movement patterns of hinge, squat, push and pull that form the foundation of athletic development. The extent to which program design progresses, regresses or replaces these core exercises is a function of available equipment and individual training philosophies to overcome problems presented to gaining strength and subsequent power for an athlete.

Limited or Austere Training Scenarios

Program design is especially relevant for populations in austere environments with limited equipment and structural resources, and/or a diverse spectrum of training ages who don't have the time to master complex barbell power exercises or the resources to maintain long term adaptations. To get around these potentially limiting variables, there are innovative technologies that have the potential to consolidate weight room and programming for those in austere or remote locations. You can still deliver important elements of power and proportional deceleration capacity. For example, the simple non-motorized and highly portable coupled concentric/eccentric phases of flywheel training have particular interest in advancing peak, average and repeated power ability for those without access to complex training sites and systems and who need to apply sport specific power adaptations.

Whether in austere training environments where equipment and resources are limited, or in highly complex performance training setups, the intensity within those exercises programmed first (the primary exercises) affect the type and volume of auxiliary exercise–those exercises supporting those primary exercises and their objectives. Too often the complimentary exercises have to be employed in high volume because the intensity of the primary exercise was not present. This is more evident as more functional movement exercises constitute more priority in programming for sport.

Key Takeaways:

- Primary exercises are determined by competition needs.
- Core Compound "Big Lifts" act as primary support to Specific Exercises during In Season.
- Primary exercises supported by four phases of auxiliary needs:
  - Drive
  - Acceleration
  - Top Speed
  - Deceleration
- Flywheel allows for proportional eccentric overload and rhythmic properties particular to sport.
- More comprehensive, higher intensity auxiliary support exercises reduce time training.
- Less secondary support auxiliary exercises are needed with higher intensities of primary support exercises.
- Portable accommodative resistance methods are ideal for primary and auxiliary exercise programming remote, austere or limited resourced training scenarios. Accommodative Resistance Innovations may aid in the training of the four modes of power development.
- Traditional Specific Exercises are deemed auxiliary and lack adequate intensity for sport transfer.
- The effort to mimic specificity can lead to high volume of exercise and inadequate intensities.
- General Preparation barbell exercises can be "auxiliary" tools in transfer of power.
- Deficiency in power development assessed in Drive, Acceleration, Top Speed and Deceleration phases.
- Innovative methods efficient link between General Preparation and Competitive Exercises.

REFERENCES: Chapter 20

1. Bondarchuk, Anatoliy. *Transfer of Training in Sports, vols. 1 & 2*. Ultimate Athlete Concepts: Muskegon, MI, 2007 and 2010.

2. Caruso, J.F., Coday, M.A., Monda, J.K., Ramey, E.S., Hastings, L.P., Vingren, J.L., Potter, W.T., Kraemer, W.J., Wickel, E.E. "Blood lactate and hormonal responses to prototype flywheel ergometer workouts." *J Strength Cond Res* 24 (2010): 749-756.

3. Fernandez-Valdes, B., Sampaio, J., Exel, J., Gonzalez, J., Tous-Fajardo, J., Jones, B., Moras, G. "The Influence of Functional Flywheel Resistance Training on Movement Variability and Movement Velocity in Elite Rugby Players." *Frontiers in psychology* 11 (30 June 2020): 1205. https://doi.org/10.3389/fpsyg.2020.01205

4. Fleck and Kramer. *Designing Resistance Training Programs*. Champaign IL: Human Kinetics, 1997.

5. Gonzalo-Skok, O., Tous-Fajardo, J., Valero-Campo, C., Berzosa, C., Bataller, A. V., Arjol-Serrano, J. L., Moras, G., Mendez-Villanueva, A. "Eccentric-Overload Training in Team-Sport Functional Performance: Constant Bilateral Vertical Versus Variable Unilateral Multidirectional Movements." *International journal of sports physiology and performance* 12, no. 7 (August, 2017): 951–958. https://doi.org/10.1123/ijspp.2016-0251

6. Hamill, J., Knuten, K. M., Derrick, T. R. *Biomechanical basis of human movement*. Lippincott, Williams & Wilkins: Philadelphia, PA, 2015.

7. Hedayatpour & Falla 2016

8. Nunez, F. J., de Hoyo, M., Lopez, A. M., Sanudo, B., Otero-Esquina, C., Sanchez, H. and Gonzalo- Skok, O. "Eccentric-concentric Ratio: A Key Factor for Defining Strength Training in Soccer." *International Journal of Sports Medicine* 40, no. 12 (November, 2019): 796-802.

9. Nunez, F. J., Suarez-Arrones, L. J., Cater, P., Mendez-Villanueva, A. "The high-pull exercise: A comparison between a versapulley flywheel device and the free weight." *International Journal of Sports Physiology and Performance* 12, no. 4 (April, 2017): 527–532.

10. Ratamess, N. *ACSM's foundations of strength and conditioning.* Wolters Kluwer: Philadelphia, PA, 2022.

11. Smith, Joel @justflysports

12. Suarez-Arrones, L., Lara-Lopez, P., Torreno, N., Saez de Villarreal, E., Di Salvo, V., and Mendez-

13. Villanueva, A. "Effects of Strength Training on Body Composition in Young Male Professional Soccer Players." *Sports* 7, no. 5 (May, 2019): 104.

14. Tobers, Jacob, Instagram account @vbtcoach

15. Włodarczyk, M., Adamus, P., Zieliński, J., Kantanista, A. "Effects of Velocity-Based Training on Strength and Power in Elite Athletes-A Systematic Review." *International Journal of Environmental Research and Public Health* 18, no. 10 (May, 2021): 5257. https://doi.org/10.3390/ijerph18105257

GLOSSARY

Acceleration: The rate of change of velocity with respect to time is called acceleration.

Agonist: Muscles creating the same joint movement are termed agonists.

Antagonist: Muscles opposing or producing the opposite joint movement are called antagonists. The antagonists must relax to allow a movement to occur or contract concurrently with the agonists to control or slow a joint movement.

Auxiliary Support: Those exercises which support the primary support exercise. These tend to be relative to fatigue resistance and or better function of the preceding exercise.

Cardiac Output: Total amount of blood pumped per minute by the heart.

Cluster Set: Cluster training is a method used successfully in the training of Olympic weightlifters and other athletes. It involves inserting intraset rest intervals in between reps, inserting intra set rest intervals in between smaller groups of reps, or reducing rest intervals in between sets and including a rest interval in the middle of a set (rest redistribution).

Competitive Exercise: The sport event within which an athlete participates. These exercises are repeatable within both competition or practice.

Compound Exercise: Exercise featuring a combination of movements, like a squat to press.

Concentric: If a muscle visibly shortens while generating tension actively, the muscle action is termed concentric.

Core Lift or Core Exercise: Exercise generally utilizing multiple muscles and multiple joint actions.

Deceleration: The term decelerate is used to describe a decrease in velocity.

Displacement: Displacement is the difference between the initial and final positions of the object.

Dorsi Flexed: foot flat, toes not pointed, top of foot pulled towards the leg

Dynamic stretching: Stretching while simultaneously moving

Eccentric: When a muscle is subjected to an external torque that is greater than the torque generated by the muscle, the muscle lengthens, and the action is known as eccentric.

Eccentric Overload: Eccentric overloading strategies are to help develop greater forces in the deceleration. Bigger engine will necessitate bigger brakes.

Ejection Fraction: The percentage of blood ejected from the left heart when it contracts. Not all the blood is emptied from the left heart when it contracts.

Flywheel Training: Utilizes kinetic energy transferred to a flywheel. This allows for eccentric overload and variable resistance throughout the movement.

Force *(F)* **:** The push or pull impacted on an object and is the product of mass multiplied by acceleration. In the weight room, body weight and external resistance (barbells, resistance bands, medicine balls, etc.) are often used as resistance forces in order to bring about positive adaptations of the musculature, skeletal and connective tissues. Force is typically measured in Newtons (N). $N = 1kg . 1\ m/s2$

Force-Velocity Curve *(FV)***:** The force-velocity curve is a physical representation of the inverse relationship between force and velocity.

General Prepartaion Exercise (GPE): Exercises used for strength and conditioning but not directly correlated to improvement of the sport event. Low-level athletes will have transfer from basic progression of general exercise.

Glucagon: (pronounced: GLOO-kuh-gon) A hormone that raises blood sugar (glucose). It is made in the pancreas. When blood sugars are low, glucagon tells the liver to send sugar into the blood, which goes to the cells for energy. When someone with diabetes has a very low blood sugar level, a dose of glucagon can help raise their blood glucose quickly.

Glucose: The main type of sugar in the blood and is the major source of energy for the body's cells. Glucose comes from the foods we eat or the body can make it from other substances. Glucose is carried to the cells through the bloodstream. Several hormones, including insulin, control glucose levels in the blood.

Homeostasis: A self-regulating process achieving a relatively stable equilibrium between interdependent elements within the body.

Hypohydration: taking in less water than is lost from the body

Inertia: The inertia of an object is used to describe its resistance to motion.

Insulin: A hormone that lowers the level of glucose (a type of sugar) in the blood. It's made by the beta cells of the pancreas and released into the blood when the glucose level goes up, such as after eating. Insulin helps glucose enter the body's cells, where it can be used for energy or stored for future use. In diabetes, the pancreas doesn't make enough insulin or the body can't respond normally to the insulin that is made. This causes the glucose level in the blood to rise.

Iso Inertial: A type of resistance used in exercise training which maintains a constant inertia throughout the range of motion, facilitating a constant resistance and maximal muscle force in every angle.

Momentum: Momentum is the quantity of motion of an object.

Olympic Lift: A sport that involves lifting a loaded barbell from the ground to up overhead using explosive power.

Placebo: A control treatment that is known to have no effects.

Plantar flexed: toes pointed, top of foot points away from leg

Power: Force over the time that it takes to produce that force.

Primary Exercise: The prescribed exercise that most directly influences the power training transfer goal of the phase. This is most relative to the specific Preparatory and/or Developmental Exercises in Bondarchuk's periodization. More closely mirrors the muscle function of competitive sport exercises (i.e., eccentric utilization ratios and concentric contraction phase velocity).

Primary Support: Exercises which support the primary exercise and main focus of the training session, as determined by the established need of the training phase. This is primarily determined by the competitive cycle (in-season, out of season) and training age of the athlete. If the athlete's training base has been established, primary exercises and their supportive auxiliary exercises may consist of general preparation exercises such as the back squat, placed lower in the order of importance in the training session.

Rate of Force Development (RFD): A measure of explosive strength, or simply how fast an athlete can develop force.

Rotary Inertia: Rotational inertia is a property of any object which can be rotated. It is a scalar value which tells us how difficult it is to change the rotational velocity of the object around a given rotational axis.

Specialized (or Specific) Preparatory Exercise (SPE): Exercises that reproduce the Competitive Exercise in its separate parts. Exercises using similar muscle groups and work demand to advance main movements specific to a particular sport, but in the form of a different movement.

Specific Developmental Exercise (SDE): Exercises that reproduce the Competitive Exercise in its separate parts, it combines the same muscles and systems as the competitive movements. Often referred to as "specific strength" or "special strength."

Static stretching: When you hold a stretching position for 30 to 60 seconds without moving.

Strength: The work or force that can be produced. Also is the ability to produce force at a given velocity.

Stroke Volume: The amount of blood pumped in each heartbeat (or stroke)

Superset: Supersets involve consecutive performance of two different exercises (either for the same muscle group or different muscle groups, i.e., agonist-antagonist, unrelated). Many times the term compound set is used to describe supersets of different exercises involving the same muscle groups.

Synergist: Muscles act as a synergist, or neutralizer when a muscle contracts to eliminate an undesired joint action of another muscle.

Velocity (V): The change in position of an object in reference to time.

Velocity Based Training: Training strategy in which the velocity or speed of the movement is matched with the desired strength characteristic.

APPENDIX

Embracing the "D"

Dynamics of Discipleship Coaching

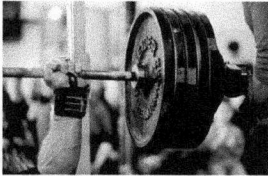

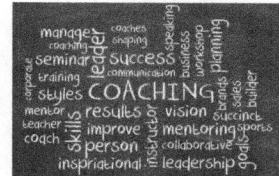

D²⁶

Desire

Dedication   **D**evotion

Designated

Direction	**D**efinition	**D**ialogue
Discipline	**D**etermination	**D**evelopment
Demonstration	**D**iscipleship	**D**ynamics
Duration	**D**iscernment	**D**elivery
Dependability	**D**isposition	**D**uty

Defense   **D**ecisive

Delighted   **D**eployed

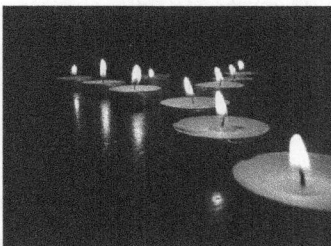

Dignity

Destiny

Divinity

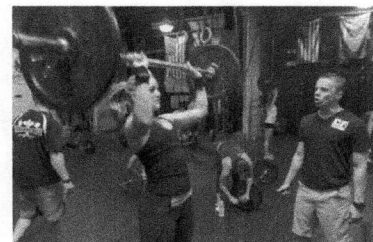

APPENDIX B

Sport _____

Annual Plan (Macrocycle)

Month	January	February	March	April	May	June	July	August	September	October	November	December
Season (Mesocycle)												
Training Phase (Microcycle)												
					Auxillary Training Priority							
Agility												
Speed												
Plyometrics												
Energy System Develoment												

Labeling

Mesocycle		**Training Phases**		**Agility, Speed & Power**		**Energy System Development**	
Pre-season		E - endurance		Priority:	H- High		O - Oxidative
In-season		H - Hypertrophy			M - Medium		G - Glycolytic
Post-season		BS - Basic Strength			L - Low		A - ATP / CP
Off-season		S & P - Strength and Power					

Periodization Scheme

Phase Specifics	% 1 RM	Rettition Range	Sets	Rest Periods	Duration
Endurance					
Hypertrophy					
Basic Strength					
Strength & Power					

APPENDIX C

TABLE 13.10 Percentiles by Age Groups and Sex for Partial Curl-Up

Percentile*	Age and sex									
	20-29		30-39		40-49		50-59		60-69	
	M	F	M	F	M	F	M	F	M	F
90	75	70	75	55	75	55	74	48	53	50
80	56	45	69	43	75	42	60	30	33	30
70	41	37	46	34	67	33	45	23	26	24
60	31	32	36	28	51	28	35	16	19	19
50	27	27	31	21	39	25	27	9	16	13
40	24	21	26	15	31	20	23	2	9	9
30	20	17	19	12	26	14	19	0	6	3
20	13	12	13	0	21	5	13	0	0	0
10	4	5	0	0	13	0	0	0	0	0

*Descriptors for percentile rankings: 90 = well above average; 70 = above average; 50 = average; 30 = below average; 10 = well below average.

Reprinted, by permission, from American College of Sports Medicine, 2014, *ACSM's guidelines for exercise testing and prescription*, 9th ed. (Baltimore, MD: Lippincott, Williams, and Wilkins), 101.

TABLE 13.11 Fitness Categories by Age Groups and Sex for Push-Ups

Category	Age and sex									
	20-29		30-39		40-49		50-59		60-69	
	M	F	M	F	M	F	M	F	M	F
Excellent	36	30	30	27	25	24	21	21	18	17
Very good	35	29	29	26	24	23	20	20	17	16
	29	21	22	20	17	15	13	11	11	12
Good	28	20	21	19	16	14	12	10	10	11
	22	15	17	13	13	11	10	7	8	5
Fair	21	14	16	12	12	10	9	6	7	4
	17	10	12	8	10	5	7	2	5	2
Needs improvement	16	9	11	7	9	4	6	1	4	1

Source: Canadian Physical Activity, *Fitness & Lifestyle Approach: CSEP-Health & Fitness Program's Appraisal & Counselling Strategy*, Third Edition, © 2003. Reprinted with permission from the Canadian Society for Exercise Physiology.

TABLE 13.19 Percentile Ranks for the 12-Minute Run

Percentile	Age (years) and distance					
	20-29		30-39		40-49	
	km	miles	km	miles	km	miles
MEN						
90	2.90	1.81	2.82	1.75	2.72	1.69
80	2.78	1.73	2.67	1.66	2.57	1.60
70	2.62	1.63	2.56	1.59	2.46	1.53
60	2.54	1.58	2.48	1.54	2.40	1.49
50	2.46	1.53	2.40	1.49	2.30	1.43
40	2.37	1.47	2.32	1.44	2.22	1.38
30	2.29	1.42	2.24	1.39	2.14	1.33
20	2.20	1.37	2.14	1.33	2.06	1.28
10	2.06	1.28	2.01	1.25	1.95	1.21
WOMEN						
90	2.59	1.61	2.53	1.57	2.43	1.51
80	2.46	1.53	2.40	1.49	2.27	1.41
70	2.35	1.46	2.27	1.41	2.20	1.37
60	2.27	1.41	2.19	1.36	2.11	1.31
50	2.20	1.37	2.14	1.33	2.04	1.27
40	2.12	1.32	2.04	1.27	1.96	1.22
30	2.03	1.26	1.95	1.21	1.90	1.18
20	1.95	1.21	1.88	1.17	1.82	1.13
10	1.82	1.13	1.75	1.09	1.70	1.05

Adapted, by permission, from ACSM, 2014, *ACSM's guidelines for exercise testing and prescription*, 9th ed. (Philadelphia: Wolters Kluwer Health/Lippincott Williams & Wilkins), 88.

TABLE 13.14   Maximal Rate of Oxygen Consumption, 1.5-Mile (2.4 km) Run Time, Sit-and-Reach Test, and Body Composition: Percentile Rankings for 20- to 29-Year-Old Males

Percentile rank	$\dot{V}O_2$max (ml·kg⁻¹·min⁻¹)	1.5-mile (2.4 km) run time, min:s	Sit-and-reach test*		Body fat (%)
			in.	cm	
99	60.5	8:29			4.2
90	54.0	9:34	22	55.9	7.9
80	51.1	10:09	20	50.8	10.5
70	47.5	10:59	19	48.3	12.6
60	45.6	11:29	18	45.7	14.8
50	43.9	11:58	17	43.2	16.6
40	41.7	12:38	15	38.1	18.6
30	39.9	13:15	14	35.6	20.7
20	38.0	14:00	13	33.0	23.3
10	34.7	15:30	11	27.9	26.6
01	26.5	20:58			33.4

*Sit and reach for 18- to 25-year-old men.

Adapted from American College of Sports Medicine, 2014, *ACSM's guidelines for exercise testing and prescription*, 9th ed. (Baltimore, MD: Lippincott, Williams, and Wilkins).

TABLE 13.15   Maximal Rate of Oxygen Consumption, 1.5-Mile (2.4 km) Run Time, Sit-and-Reach Test, and Body Composition: Percentile Rankings for 20- to 29-Year-Old Females

Percentile rank	$\dot{V}O_2$max (ml·kg⁻¹·min⁻¹)	1.5-mile (2.4 km) run time, min:s	Sit-and-reach test*		Body fat (%)
			in.	cm	
99	54.5	9:30			11.4
90	46.8	11:10	24	61.0	15.1
80	43.9	11:58	22	55.9	16.8
70	41.1	12:51	21	53.3	18.4
60	39.5	13:24	20	50.8	19.8
50	37.8	14:04	19	48.3	21.5
40	36.1	14:50	18	45.7	23.4
30	34.1	15:46	17	43.2	25.5
20	32.3	16:46	16	40.6	28.2
10	29.5	18:33	14	35.6	33.5
01	23.7	23:58			38.6

*Sit and reach for 18- to 25-year-old women.

Adapted from American College of Sports Medicine, 2014, *ACSM's guidelines for exercise testing and prescription*, 9th ed. (Baltimore, MD; Williams &Wilkins).

TABLE 13.16 Maximal Rate of Oxygen Consumption, 1.5-Mile (2.4 km) Run Time, Sit-and-Reach Test, and Body Composition: Percentile Rankings for 30- to 39-Year-Old Males

Percentile rank	$\dot{V}O_2$ max (ml·kg^{-1}·min^{-1})	1.5-mile (2.4 km) run time, min:s	Sit-and-reach test*		Body fat (%)
			in.	cm	
99	58.3	8:49			7.3
90	51.7	10:01	21	53.3	12.4
80	48.3	10:46	19	48.3	14.9
70	46.0	11:22	18	45.7	16.8
60	44.1	11:54	17	43.2	18.4
50	42.4	12:24	15	38.1	20.0
40	40.7	12:58	14	35.6	21.6
30	38.7	13:44	13	33.0	23.2
20	36.7	14:34	11	27.9	25.1
10	33.8	15:57	9	22.9	27.8
01	26.5	20:58			34.4

*Sit and reach for 26- to 35-year-old men.

Adapted from American College of Sports Medicine, 2014, *ACSM's guidelines for exercise testing and prescription*, 9th ed. (Baltimore, MD; Williams & Wilkins).

TABLE 13.17 Maximal Rate of Oxygen Consumption, 1.5-Mile (2.4 km) Run Time, Sit-and-Reach Test, and Body Composition: Percentile Rankings for 30- to 39-Year-Old Females

Percentile rank	$\dot{V}O_2$ max (ml·kg^{-1}·min^{-1})	1.5-mile (2.4 km) run time, min:s	Sit-and-reach test*		Body fat (%)
			in.	cm	
99	52.0	9:58			11.2
90	45.3	11:33	23	58.4	15.5
80	42.4	12:24	22	55.9	17.5
70	39.6	13:24	21	53.3	19.2
60	37.7	14:08	20	50.8	21.0
50	36.7	14:34	19	48.3	22.8
40	34.2	15:43	17	43.2	24.8
30	32.4	16:42	16	40.6	26.9
20	30.9	17:38	15	38.1	29.6
10	28.0	19:43	13	33.0	33.6
01	22.9	24:56			39.0

*Sit and reach for 26- to 35-year-old women.

Adapted from American College of Sports Medicine, 2014, *ACSM's guidelines for exercise testing and prescription*, 9th ed. (Baltimore, MD; Williams & Wilkins).

TABLE 13.25   Equations for Calculating Estimated Body Density From Skinfold Measurements Among Various Populations

SKF sites[a]	Population subgroups	Sex	Age	Equation	Reference
S7SKF (chest + abdomen + triceps + subscapular + suprailiac + midaxilla + thigh)	Black or Hispanic	Women	18-55 years	Db (g/cc)[b] = 1.0970 − 0.00046971 (S7SKF) + 0.00000056 (S7SKF)^2 − 0.00012828 (age)	Jackson et al. (57)
S7SKF (chest + abdomen + triceps + subscapular + suprailiac + midaxilla + thigh)	Black or athletes	Men	18-61 years	Db (g/cc)[b] = 1.1120 − 0.00043499 (S7SKF) + 0.00000055 (S7SKF)^2 − 0.00028826 (age)	Jackson and Pollock (55)
S4SKF (triceps + anterior suprailiac + abdomen + thigh)	Athletes	Women	18-29 years	Db (g/cc)[b] = 1.096095 − 0.0006952 (S4SKF) − 0.0000011 (S4SKF)^2 − 0.0000714 (age)	Jackson et al. (57)
S3SKF (triceps + suprailiac + thigh)	White or anorexic	Women	18-55 years	Db (g/cc)[b] = 1.0994921 − 0.0009929 (S3SKF) + 0.0000023 (S3SKF)^2 − 0.0001392 (age)	Jackson et al. (57)
S3SKF (chest + abdomen + thigh)	White	Men	18-61 years	Db (g/cc)[b] = 1.109380 − 0.0008267 (S3SKF) + 0.0000016 (S3SKF)^2 − 0.0002574 (age)	Jackson and Pollock (55)
S2SKF (triceps + calf)	Black or white	Boys	6-17 years	% BF = 0.735 (S2SKF) + 1.0	Slaughter et al. (103)
S2SKF (triceps + calf)	Black or white	Girls	6-17 years	% BF = 0.610 (S2SKF) + 5.1	Slaughter et al. (103)
Suprailiac, triceps	Athletes	Women	High school and college age	Db (g/cc)[b] = 1.0764 − (0.00081 3 suprailiac) − (0.00088 3 triceps)	Sloan and Weir (104)
Thigh, subscapular	Athletes	Men	High school and college age	Db (g/cc)[b] = 1.1043 − (0.00133 3 thigh) − (0.00131 3 subscapular)	Sloan and Weir (104)
S3SKF (triceps + abdomen + thigh)	Athletes	Men or Women	18-34 years	%BF = 8.997 + (S3SKF) − 6.343 (gender[c]) − 1.998 (race[d])	Evans et al. (28)

[a]SSKF = sum of skinfolds (mm); Db = body density.

[b]Use population-specific conversion formulas (see table 13.26) to calculate %BF from Db.

[c]Male athletes = 1; female athletes = 0.

[d]Black athletes = 1; white athletes = 0.

Adapted, by permission, from V. H. Heyward, 1998, *Advanced fitness assessment and exercise prescription*, 3rd ed. (Champaign, IL: Human Kinetics), 155.

www.ingramcontent.com/pod-product-compliance
Lightning Source LLC
Chambersburg PA
CBHW080415030426

42335CB00020B/2458